Neonatal Emergencies

Neonatal Emergencies

Richard M. Cantor, MD, FAAP, FACEP
Associate Professor of Emergency Medicine
Pediatric Emergency Department
State University of New York—Upstate Medical University
Syracuse, New York

P. David Sadowitz, MD
Associate Professor of Emergency Medicine
Pediatric Emergency Department
State University of New York—Upstate Medical University
Syracuse, New York

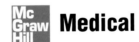

New York Chicago San Francisco Lisbon London
Madrid Mexico City Milan New Delhi San Juan
Seoul Singapore Sydney Toronto

ISBN 0-07-147020-4
MHID 978-0-07-147020-9

CIP application is on file with the publisher.

This book was set in Garamond Light by Newgen.
The editors were Anne Sydor and Karen G. Edmonson.
The production manager was Philip Galea.
Project management was provided by Newgen North America.
The cover designer was Kiley Fusco.
China Translation & Printing, Ltd. was printer and binder.

This book is printed on acid-free paper.

McGraw-Hill books are available at special quantity discounts to use as premiums and sales promotions, or for use in corporate training programs. To contact a representative please e-mail us at bulksales@mcgraw-hill.com.

CONTENTS

CONTRIBUTORS

Jahn Avarello, MD
Director, Pediatric Emergency Medicine
Huntington Hospital
Attending, Pediatric Emergency Medicine
North Shore University Hospital
Manhasset, New York

Richard M. Cantor, MD, FAAP, FACEP
Associate Professor of Emergency Medicine
Pediatric Emergency Department
State University of New York-Upstate
    Medical University
Syracuse, New York

Derek Cooney, MD
Assistant Professor
Department of Emergency Medicine
State University of New York-Upstate
    Medical University
Syracuse, New York

Norma Cooney, MD
Assistant Professor
Department of Emergence Medicine
State University of New York-Upstate
    Medical University
Syracuse, New York

James D'Agostino, MD
Assistant Professor of Emergency Medicine
    and Pediatrics State University of
    New York-Upstate Medical University
Syracuse, New York

Lisa Keough, MD
Assistant Professor
Department of Emergency
    Medicine
State University of New York-Upstate
    Medical University
Syracuse, New York

Jeff Lapoint, DO
Resident Physician
Department of Emergency
    Medicine
State University of New York-Upstate
    Medical University
Syracuse, New York

Jennifer Mackey, MD, FAAP
Assistant Professor
Department of Emergency Medicine and
    Pediatrics
State University of New York-Upstate
    Medical University
Syracuse, New York

Deborah J. Mann, MD
Assistant Professor
Department of Emergency
    Medicine
State University of New York-Upstate
    Medical University
Syracuse, New York

Jeanna Marraffa, PharmD
Assistant Professor
Departments of Emergency Medicine and
  Medicine
Section of Clinical Pharmacology
State University of New York Upstate
  Medical University
Syracuse, New York

Jamie L. Nelsen, PharmD, DABAT
Assistant Professor
Department of Emergency Medicine
State University of New York-Upstate
  Medical University
Syracuse, New York

P. David Sadowitz, MD
Associate Professor of Emergency
  Medicine
Pediatric Emergency Department
State University of New York-Upstate
  Medical University
Syracuse, New York

LaLainia Secreti, MD
Assistant Professor
Department of Emergency Medicine
State University of New York-Upstate
  Medical University
Syracuse, New York

Brian Stout, MD
Assistant Professor
Department of Emergency Medicine
State University of New York-Upstate
  Medical University
Syracuse, New York

Trisha Tavares, MD
Assistant Professor
Department of Pediatrics
State University of New York-Upstate
  Medical University
Syracuse, New York

Linnea Wittick, MD
Fellow in Pediatric Emergency Medicine
Department of Emergency Medicine
State University of New York-Upstate
  Medical University
Syracuse, New York

PREFACE

The delivery of emergency care to infants and children remains both a challenge and a privilege. It can be one of the most humbling yet rewarding experiences for the emergency health care provider. This text was developed to assist our colleagues in the evaluation and treatment of children of a young age. The genesis of this text arose from both clinical experience and an obvious need within the practice of emergency medicine for a greater emphasis to be placed on these high risk infants. At such young developmental and chronological ages, these patients present with a miriad of undifferentiated complaints. Their histories may be short but the complexity of their problems may indeed be quite complex. The goal of this text is to guide the provider in a systematic approach to any and all problems within this fragile population.

The text is divided into sections based on organ systems. There will be much crossover within each section, only highlighting the commonalty of complaint that can result from a multitude of disparate medical problems. We are hopeful that our readers find it to be a useful tool in addressing the needs of the very young infant.

Richard M. Cantor, MD, FAAP/FACEP
P. David Sadowitz, MD

ACKNOWLEDGMENTS

To my valued friend and colleague Dr. Sadowitz, who has always served as a wonderful role model for excellence in the delivery of pediatric care.

To my mentors Drs. Oski, Tunnessen, and Stockman, who have empowered me with the work ethic I practice today.

To my patients who have provided me with the blessed coverage of caring for them.

To my wife Nina, and my children Gillian and Liza, who energize, love, and support me every moment of everyday.

Richard M. Cantor

To my friend and colleague Dr. Cantor, whose wisdom, knowledge and wit have made this project a great learning experience.

To those who have taught me by their example and experience, my gratitude for their wisdom and patience.

To students and practitioner of emergency medicine; it is my hope that the material in this book will be a valuable tool in the quest to provide excellent care to children in a busy ER setting.

To my wife Cheryl and my children Amy, Ben, Jared, Emily, Elizabeth, Ryan, Jordan, Mitchell, and Madeline for their constant love and support that have encouraged me in this endeavor.

To my God whose unfailing love and grace is the foundation of my life.

P. David Sadowitz

CHAPTER 1

HEENT Emergencies of the Infant

Deborah J. Mann, MD

▶ INJURIES ASSOCIATED WITH THE BIRTHING PROCESS

The head of the newborn should be inspected for the presence of scalp protuberances, lacerations, abrasions, and abnormal hair patterns. The fontanelles are normally soft and flat, and should be palpated with the infant in the sitting position. Cranial sutures should also be palpated and should be open with up to several millimeters of distance between them. Passage through the birth canal may cause cranial sutures to overlap resulting in a temporary skull deformity called molding. Molding typically resolves in 2-3 days after delivery. Failure to resolve may indicate craniosynostosis, whereas widely split sutures may indicate

increased intracranial pressure and hydrocephalus. The trauma of vaginal or assisted delivery may cause scalp swelling such as caput succedaneum or bleeding, which causes cephalohematomas and subgaleal hemorrhages. Child abuse must be suspected in all cases of head or facial trauma in infants.

CAPUT SUCCEDANEUM

Caput succedaneum is an area of edema over the presenting part of the head. It is common after vaginal delivery and may give the newborn's head a cone-shaped appearance. The edema is due to pressure exerted by the cervix and vaginal walls upon the presenting part of the infant's head during the birthing process.

This swelling may or may not cross suture lines and resolves in the first few days of life. No treatment is necessary.

CEPHALOHEMATOMA

Cephalohematoma is a collection of blood under the periosteum (Figure 1–1). It is a common complication of childbirth and is present in 1-2% of newborns.[1] On palpation, cephalohematomas are fluctuant but do not cross suture lines. The edges of a cephalohematoma become more distinct over the first few days of life as opposed to caput succedaneum, which resolves in the first few days of life. As the hematoma resolves and the breakdown of red blood cells occurs, the risk of hyperbilirubinemia increases. Cephalohematomas resolve over a period of weeks to months and require no treatment.

The risk of cephalohematomas increases with the use of forceps and in vacuum-assisted deliveries. If a cephalohematoma crosses a suture line then suspect an underlying skull fracture and rule out child abuse. If a skull fracture is suspected or there are neurologic symptoms, a CT of the head is indicated.

SUBGALEAL HEMATOMA

Subgaleal hematoma results from trauma to the scalp with subsequent bleeding into the potential space between the skull periosteum and the scalp galea aponeurosis (Figure 1–1).

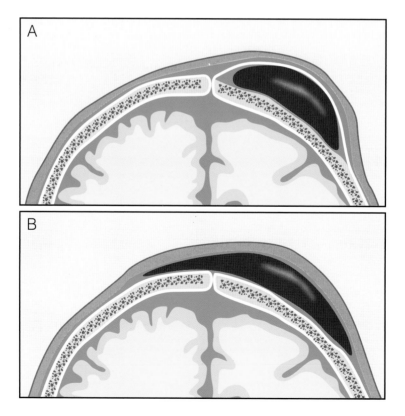

Figure 1–1. Cephalohematoma versus subgaleal hematoma.

Because this space has no containing membranes or boundaries, the subgaleal hematoma may extend from the orbital ridges to the nape of the neck. This vast space can easily accommodate up to half of a neonate's blood volume and allow life-threatening hemorrhage. Once bleeding begins, it can be difficult to control because of potential coagulopathy. Because of this, physicians must maintain a high index of suspicion and treat aggressively to prevent mortality.

Early signs of subgaleal hemorrhage include pallor, hypotonia, tachycardia, tachypnea, and increasing head circumference.[2] Late signs include anemia, a fluctuant and boggy scalp, and hyperbilirubinemia.[3]

The diagnosis is generally a clinical one and should be suspected in any infant or child with a boggy fluctuant scalp. The swelling may obscure the fontanelle and cross suture lines, which distinguishes subgaleal hemorrhage from cephalohematoma. Periorbital or periauricular ecchymosis may be present. In the newborn, the swelling often develops insidiously over 8-72 hours of age. Subgaleal hematomas occur in up to 45 per 10,000 vacuum-assisted deliveries.[4] After 72 hours, the presence of a subgaleal hematoma in an infant or child is indicative of trauma and again, child abuse must be excluded.

Treatment is aimed at controlling hemorrhage and coagulopathy if present with transfusion of packed red blood cells and fresh frozen plasma. Pressure-wrapping of the head should be considered in consultation with neurosurgery because it may cause increased intracranial pressure, decreased cerebral perfusion, and even herniation.

▶ BRUISING OF THE INFANT HEAD & FACE; CHILD ABUSE

Child abuse is a problem that cannot be ignored. An estimated 1 million suspected

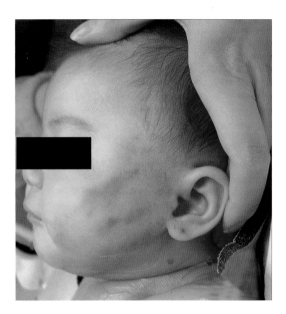

Figure 1–2. Facial bruising suggestive of nonaccidental trauma. *Source:* From Strange GR, Schafermeyer RW, Ahrens WR, et al. *Pediatric Emergency Medicine*, 3rd ed. New York, NY: McGraw-Hill, 2009.

abuse cases are reported in the United States each year.[5] Head injuries are the primary cause of child abuse-related fatalities, which means that all physicians must consider child abuse when evaluating any infant with head or facial trauma (Figure 1–2). This is particularly true in nonambulatory children, as less than 1% of nonambulatory children sustain accidental cutaneous injuries.

The head is the most common site for nonaccidental bruising.[6] Other patterns of bruising that are consistent with abuse include bruises to the face and ears, bruises that are not over bony prominences, multiple and clustered bruises, bruises of uniform shape, or patterned bruises (bruises that mirror the form of the striking object).[7-15] However, fatal nonaccidental head injury and nonaccidental fractures may occur in the absence of bruising.

Bruises must never be interpreted in isolation, but must always be assessed in the

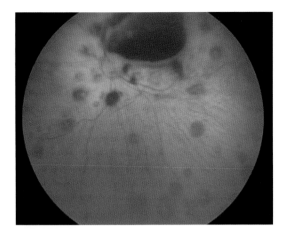

Figure 1–3. Retinal hemorrhages in nonaccidental trauma. *Source:* From Knoop KJ, Stack LB, Storrow AB. *Atlas of Emergency Medicine,* 2ⁿᵈ ed. New York, NY: McGraw-Hill, 2005.

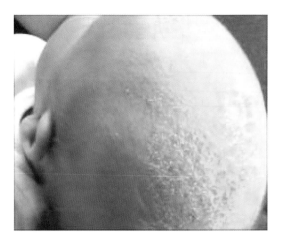

Figure 1–4. Cradle cap (seborrheic dermatitis).

context of the patient's medical and social history, developmental stage, the explanation given for the bruises, and a full clinical examination. It is the primary responsibility of the physician to report any suspected abuse.

In all cases of unexplained or suspicious bruising, a full skin examination and head-to-toe assessment for other injuries must be performed. The examination should include inspection of the fundi for retinal hemorrhages (Figure 1–3), inspection of the mouth for injuries, and an age-appropriate genital examination. Diagnostic tests should include a head computed tomography (CT) scan in all infants with suspected head trauma, even in the absence of bruising or hematomas. Fatal nonaccidental head injury may occur without bruising.[16]

▶ RASHES OF THE NEWBORN SCALP & FACE

CRADLE CAP (SEBORRHEA)

Cradle cap is seborrheic dermatitis that occurs in up to 50% of all infants. It is generally seen in infants less than 3 months of age and is rare after 12 months. It is characterized by a nonpruritic, yellowish, patchy, greasy, scaly, crusty, skin rash of the scalp (Figure 1–4). When the flexural folds and intertriginous areas are involved, erythema is predominant rather than scale. It occurs where the concentrations of sebaceous oil glands are heaviest, and is therefore frequently prominent around the ears, eyebrows, eyes, and nose. When the face and body are involved it is known as seborrheic dermatitis.

The condition is benign, self-limiting, and does not cause discomfort in the infant. Treatment includes washing with mild baby shampoo and gently combing away the scale. If seborrheic dermatitis is persistent, a 2% ketoconazole shampoo is generally an effective treatment. In resistant cases, 1% hydrocortisone lotion may be used topically up to 3 times a day. This should be distinguished from atopic dermatitis, which is typically pruritic, occurs after 3 months of age, and relapses after treatment.

ACNE NEONATORUM

Acne neonatorum occurs in up to 20% of newborns and presents as closed comedomes on

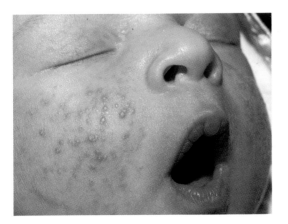

Figure 1–5. Acne neonatorum. *Source:* From Wolff K, Goldsmith LA, Katz SI, et al. *Dermatology in General Medicine,* 7th ed. New York, NY: McGraw-Hill, 2008.

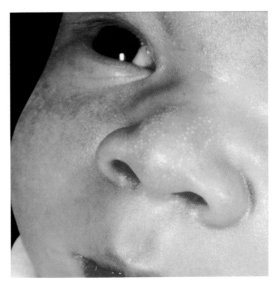

Figure 1–6. Milia. *Source:* From Wolff K, Goldsmith LA, Katz SI, et al. *Dermatology in General Medicine,* 7th ed. New York, NY: McGraw-Hill, 2008.

the forehead, nose, and cheeks (Figure 1–5). Neonatal acne is thought to be the result of maternal or infant androgens that stimulate sebaceous glands. The acne is self-limiting, usually resolves within 4 months, and does not require treatment. However, if the acne is extensive or persistent for more than 4 months, then treatment with topical 2.5% benzoic peroxide lotion may be considered.[17] When neonatal acne is severe and unrelenting, look for signs of hyperandrogenism. Investigate for adrenal cortical hyperplasia, virilizing tumors, and endocrinopathies.[18]

MILIA

Milia, commonly known as milk spots, are very common and occur in up to 50% of newborn infants.[19] These small 1- to 2-mm, pearly white papules occur on the face and are caused by the retention of keratin within the dermis (Figure 1–6). While most milia are seen on the nose and cheeks, they may be present on the upper trunk, limbs, penis, and mucous membranes. No treatment is necessary because

they typically resolve spontaneously within the first month of life.

[crystallina .
[rubra .

MILIARIA

Miliaria is caused by the partial closure of eccrine sweat glands. It may affect up to 40% of infants and is usually seen in the first month of life.[20] Several clinical subtypes exist, but miliaria crystallina and miliaria rubra are most common.

Miliaria crystallina is due to superficial eccrine duct closure with the subsequent development of 1- to 2-mm vesicles that have no surrounding erythema. They occur in greatest concentration on the head, neck, and trunk. Vesicle ruptures are followed by desquamation over hours to days.

Miliaria rubra, commonly known as heat rash, is due to deeper obstruction of eccrine sweat glands.[21] Small erythematous papules and vesicles develop over covered areas of skin. Treatment includes avoidance of overheating, removal of excess clothing, and cool baths.

▶ MALFORMATIONS OF THE SKULL

CRANIOSYNOSTOSIS

Skull deformities in the newborn are not uncommon, but they still pose a diagnostic and therapeutic challenge. The challenge is distinguishing benign conditions, such as positional skull flattening, from the more serious condition of craniosynostosis.

The newborn skull is composed of seven bones separated by connective tissue, sutures, and fontanelles (Figure 1–7). This arrangement allows the transient distortion of the

skull during the birthing process and permits the rapid growth of the brain. Fontanelle and suture closure occur in a predictable pattern (Tables 1–1 & 1–2). Craniosynostosis is the premature fusion of one or more cranial sutures and may result in an abnormal head shape.

In primary craniosynostosis, the skull compensates for the expanding brain with growth at nonossified sutures. Premature fusion of a cranial suture prevents growth of the skull perpendicular to the affected suture. As the brain increases in size, it forces compensatory growth parallel to the fused suture. The resultant skull deformity is thus dependent upon the particular suture or sutures affected. Multiple sutures that fuse while the brain is still growing pose an increased risk of elevated intracranial pressure.

In secondary craniosynostosis, the brain fails to grow and the sutures fuse in a manner that causes microcephaly. Intracranial pressure is usually normal and surgical intervention is rarely needed.

The underlying cause of craniosynostosis is unclear. However, craniosynostosis involving a single suture is often sporadic and occurs as an isolated defect. In contrast, craniosynostosis

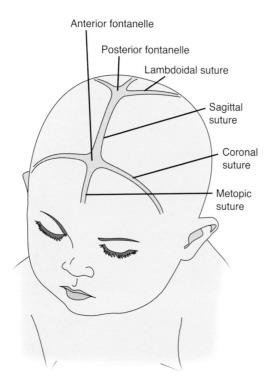

Figure 1-7. Infantile fontanelles.

▶ TABLE 1–1. **AGE OF FONTANELLE CLOSURE**

Fontanelle	Closure
Posterior	2 months
Anterior lateral	3 months
Posterior lateral	1 year
Anterior	2 years

▶ TABLE 1–2. **AGE OF SUTURE CLOSURE**

Suture	Age Closure Begins
Metopic	2 months
Sagittal	22 months
Coronal	24 months
Lambdoid	26 months

involving multiple sutures is often part of a larger syndrome with additional abnormalities. Common syndromes are Crouzon and Apert syndromes.

Craniosynostosis is often present at birth, but the skull deformity may not be apparent until after the first few months of life. Diagnosis is dependent primarily upon physical examination. Radiographic studies including plain radiography of the skull and CT of the head are used to characterize the structural abnormalities. CT is better at identifying sutures than plain films and can be used to evaluate the extent of fusion. Despite the advantages of CT, a specific diagnosis may be difficult when abnormalities overlap with multiple syndromes. Molecular diagnosis is available for Apert and Crouzon syndromes.

Diagnosis is important because complications of craniosynostosis include increased intracranial pressure and inhibition of brain growth with associated impairment in cognitive and neurodevelopment function.

Lambdoid synostosis must be differentiated from positional skull flattening (also called deformational plagiocephaly, occipital plagiocephaly, posterior plagiocephaly, and plagiocephaly without synostosis). The incidence of positional skull flattening has increased, in part because of campaigns that promote supine sleeping positions to prevent sudden infant death syndrome.[22,23] The incidence of the more common positional skull flattening is 1 in 300 live births versus the rarer lambdoid synostosis, which affects 3 in 100,000 live births.[24,25] Risk factors for positional skull flattening include limited head rotation, supine sleeping position, and decreased activity levels.

Infants with a typical rounded head at birth may be deformed at a few weeks or months of age. Positional skull flattening is best diagnosed by examining the infant's head from the top vertex view. The position of the ear is the most reliable indicator in distinguishing positional skull flattening from lambdoid synostosis. In positional skull flattening, the ipsilateral ear is displaced away or anteriorly from the flattened area.[26] In contrast, in lambdoid synostosis, the ipsilateral ear is displaced posteriorly toward the fused suture or flattened area of the skull.[27]

If positional skull flattening is recognized, the parents should be instructed to alternate the infant's sleep positions on the right and left occiput and to limit seating (eg, baby carriers, strollers) that maintains the head in a supine position. Parents should also be encouraged to give the infant supervised "tummy time" each day. All infants should follow up with their primary care doctor.

If craniosynostosis or hydrocephalus is suspected, a careful history and examination should be done to exclude signs and symptoms of an elevated intracranial pressure. Signs and symptoms of increased intracranial pressure specific to the neonate and young infants include bulging fontanelle, widened cranial sutures, prominent scalp veins, poor head control, and upward gaze palsy ("setting sun" eyes). General symptoms of increased intracranial pressure are papilledema, vomiting, and lethargy. In all cases of suspected increased intracranial pressure, a head CT should be ordered to evaluate for suture fusion and hydrocephalus. All infants with suspected elevated intracranial pressure should be seen emergently by neurosurgery.

HYDROCEPHALUS

Hydrocephalus is a disorder in which the cerebral ventricular system contains an excessive amount of cerebral spinal fluid (CSF) and is dilated by the increased intracranial pressure. The prevalence of congenital and infantile hydrocephalus is estimated at 0.48-0.81 per 1000 live births.[28] The excess of CSF is attributed to an imbalance in its production and absorption. CSF is produced by the choroid plexus of the lateral and 4th ventricles. It circulates through the ventricular system and is reabsorbed into the systemic venous circulation. There are a multitude of causes of hydrocephalus, but preterm infants with intraventricular hemorrhage (IVH) are at particular risk. Thirty-five percent of preterm infants with IVH develop hydrocephalus.[29] Regardless of the cause, symptoms are similar and are caused by increases in intracranial pressure. The acuity of symptoms is related to the rapidity of increases in the intracranial pressure.

Anatomic or functional obstruction of the CSF flow is the most common cause of hydrocephalus. Dilation of the ventricular system ensues proximal to the obstruction and eventually the subarachnoid space over the hemispheres is obliterated (Figure 1–8). The vascular system is then compressed causing venous pressures within the dural sinus to rise. Eventually, the ependymal lining of the ventricles is disrupted and CSF moves directly

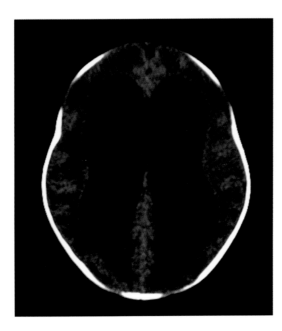

Figure 1-8. Hydrocephalus. *Source:* From Strange GR, Schafermeyer RW, Ahrens WE, et al. *Pediatric Emergency Medicine,* 3rd ed. New York, NY: McGraw-Hill, 2009.

into brain tissue, causing interstitial edema of the periventricular white matter.

In infants, as CSF accumulates, the cranial sutures spread and the skull expands. Skull expansion allows the intracranial pressure to be spread over a greater surface area, which prevents acute increases in intracranial pressure. This chronic hydrocephalus typically results in a substantial enlargement of the head. Marked enlargement of the head does not occur with acute increases in CSF or after fusion of cranial sutures, which result in significantly increased intracranial pressure.

The signs and symptoms of hydrocephalus derive from increased intracranial pressure. Neonates and infants may present with bulging fontanelles, widened cranial sutures, frontal bossing (an abnormal skull contour in which the forehead becomes prominent), prominent scalp veins, poor head control, and upward gaze palsy. Examination may also reveal spasticity in the extremities, especially in the legs. Excessive head growth may be noted on serial measurements of head circumference noted on growth charts.

In cases of rapid increases in intracranial pressure or delayed diagnosis of hydrocephalus, the infant may present in extremis as the brain stem is affected. These infants will appear ill and are often unresponsive with dilated pupils, papilledema, respiratory failure, posturing, hypertension, and bradycardia. Emergent neurosurgical consultation and intervention is needed.

Diagnosis of hydrocephalus may be made by antenatal ultrasonography, CT of the head, or erial head measurements plotted on growth charts and confirmed with ultrasound.

Survival in untreated hydrocephalus is very poor. Approximately 50% of affected children die before the age of 3 years and few survive until adulthood.[28] The prevalence of children with hydrocephalus is rising because of the advent of intracranial shunting leading to improved survival. Intracranial shunts were developed to divert excess accumulation of CSF and avert the development of hydrocephalus. Treatment with a surgical shunt does not cure hydrocephalus, but treats the symptoms and stops progression of neurologic deterioration. These shunts are composed of proximal tubing with a one-way valve that is placed in the ventricle, plus a distal tube that drains fluid to an extracranial site, most often the peritoneal cavity. This configuration is commonly known as a ventriclulperitoneal (VP) shunt (Figure 1–9). Other common extracranial drainage sites include the right atrium, pleural cavity, gallbladder, urinary bladder, ureter, stomach, fallopian tube, bone marrow, mastoid, and thoracic duct.

Intracranial shunts are life saving but are prone to malfunction and failure, accounting for many pediatric visits to the emergency department. Mechanical failure of intracranial shunts including infection is 40% in the first year after placement.[28] The majority of mechanical malfunctions in the first year are due to obstruction of the ventricular catheter,[28] which

Ventriculoperitoneal Shunt Placement

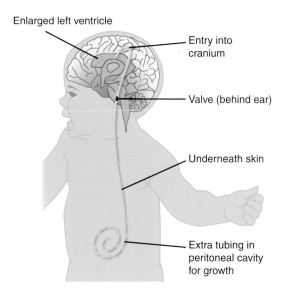

Enlarged left ventricle

Entry into cranium

Valve (behind ear)

Underneath skin

Extra tubing in peritoneal cavity for growth

Figure 1–9. Diagram of a ventriculo-peritoneal shunt.

is believed to occur because the shunt over drains and substantially reduces the size of the ventricles. This decrease in ventricular size causes the ends of the catheter to lie against the ependyma and choroid plexus, blocking the holes at the end of the catheter. Fracture of the tubing, overdrainage, and migration are less common causes of mechanical failure.

The clinical presentation of mechanical intracranial shunt failure is varied and is dependent on the rate of rise of the intracranial pressure, the child's age, the location of the catheter's distal tip, as well as timing of the shunt placement and other comorbid conditions. The progression of shunt malfunction may be insidious and the symptoms are often vague and nonspecific. Parents or caregivers of children with shunts that have had a previous malfunction are often adept at identifying subsequent episodes of shunt malfunction. This experience makes them useful resources for the treating physicians when the symptoms are vague. As always, the physician needs to screen for signs and symptoms of increased intracranial pressure.

Shunt infection is a common complication and occurs in up to 10% of shunts and at a slightly higher rate in newborns. Most shunt infections occur within 6 months of shunt placement.[30] Infecting organisms are usually part of the patient's own skin flora and include, most commonly, *Staphylococcus epidermidis*.[28] Less frequently seen pathogens include *S aureus*, enteric bacteria, diphtheroids, and *Streptococcus* species.[31]

Shunt infections should be suspected in any child with persistent fever. However, the clinical presentation for shunt infection is highly variable and often occurs in the absence of fever. Irritability and meningeal signs may be present. Check the surgical site for signs of infection such as erythema, edema, and purulent drainage. If shunt infection is suspected then neurosurgery should be consulted. Definitive diagnosis requires analysis of the CSF. Tapping of the shunt should be done by or with consultation of a neurosurgeon. In the presence of shunt infection, operative removal of the shunt and the placement of a temporary external ventricular drain are required. Appropriate antibiotic therapy should be started in consultation with a neurosurgeon.

If shunt malfunction with infection are suspected, then a CT scan of the head and a shunt series (a series of radiographs covering the entire course of the shunt tubing) is recommended. Neurosurgery should be consulted in all cases of intracranial shunt malfunction with infection.

▶ OPHTHALMIC PROBLEMS

A good eye examination in the infant is dependent on patient cooperation. Infants and younger children are best examined in the upright position, in the comfort of their parent's arms. Examination of the newborn infant's eyes may be particularly difficult because the eyelids are often edematous after delivery. Most infants will open their eyes spontaneously if held upright in a room with low ambient lighting.

The eye examination should note the positioning and spacing of the eyes as well as the appearance of the sclera and conjunctiva and the condition of the eyelids. The presence of eye discharge or excessive tearing may indicate a pathologic condition. Pupillary size and reactivity should be evaluated. The presence of the red reflex must be documented. Extraocular movements should be symmetrical and can be elicited by holding the child in a vertical position and gently rocking them from side to side. The tracking of objects or a penlight is age dependent and should be expected at 3 to 4 months of age.

The scleras are normally white, but subconjunctival hemorrhages are common with trauma to the head and face that can occur during delivery. The sclera may have a light blue coloration in premature infants, but a deep blue sclera should prompt consideration of osteogenesis imperfecta.

The conjunctiva should be inspected for hemorrhage, inflammation, or purulent discharge. Silver nitrate administration for prevention of ophthalmia neonatorum due to gonococcal infection frequently causes chemical conjunctivitis. In all cases of conjunctivitis, a bacterial cause should be excluded.

The cornea in most newborns is approximately 10 mm in diameter.[32] An enlarged cornea greater than 12 mm may suggest glaucoma. The cornea should be clear and transparent. All patients that present with a "red eye" need a fluoroscein examination to exclude corneal abrasion, corneal ulcer, or herpes keratitis.

Pupils should be round and reactive to light. Pupillary reaction is seen consistently after 32 weeks of gestational age. A red reflex should be present when eyes are examined using an ophthalmoscope (Figure 1–10). Ophthalmoscopic examination should begin at a distance of a few feet with the beam of light projected on the upper face, and then the distance is reduced to focus the beam onto to each fundus. The lens setting of the ophthalmoscope should be zero. If visualization of the red reflex is difficult, the otoscope may be used. First remove the magnifying glass from the examiner's line of vision,

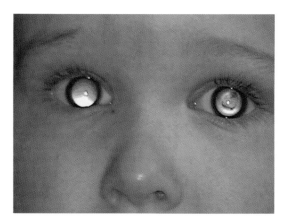

Figure 1–10. The red reflex.

then look through the otoscopic aperture and aim the beam of light at the fundus. Evaluate for the red reflex. Absence of the red reflex indicates abnormalities of the lens (congenital cataract), retina (retinoblastoma), or vitreous.

RED EYE

Ophthalmia Neonatorum

Conjunctivitis in infants less than 4 weeks old is called ophthalmia neonatorum and might be aseptic or septic. Aseptic conjunctivitis is becoming less common and is often due to silver nitrate solution administered for the prophylaxis of bacterial conjunctivitis. The most common cause of septic conjunctivitis is *Chlamydia trachomatis*. Other causes of septic conjunctivitis are *Neisseria gonorrhea*, *Staphylococcus aureus*, *Streptococcus pneumoniae*, *S viridans*, *Staph epidermidis*, and herpes simplex virus (HSV). The incidence of septic neonatal conjunctivitis in the United States ranges from 1-2%. Common features of septic conjunctivitis include erythema of the conjunctiva and eyelids with purulent discharge. Although the clinical presentations of neonatal conjunctivitis vary with etiology, there is significant overlap making physical examination alone an unreliable diagnostic tool. A Gram stain and culture of the conjunctival exudate and a culture of the conjunctival epithelium should be done in all cases.

Chemical Conjunctivitis

At one time, aseptic neonatal conjunctivitis was most often chemical conjunctivitis caused by the administration of silver nitrate solution for prophylaxis of infectious conjunctivitis. This is becoming less common as the use of erythromycin ointment has replaced silver nitrate solution in the prophylaxis of bacterial conjunctivitis. Silver nitrate is typically administered on the first day of life. The presentation of chemical conjunctivitis is one of mild, transient conjunctival erythema and tearing that spontaneously resolve in 2 to 4 days. No treatment is needed.

Chlamydial Conjunctivitis

Chlamydia trachomatis is the most common infectious cause of ophthalmia neonatorum in the United States with an incidence of 6.2 per 1000 live births. *C trachomatis* is transmitted to newborns via exposure to an infected mother's genital flora during vaginal delivery. There are case reports of transmission of *Chlamydia* infection after cesarean section with and without ruptured membranes. The risk of acquired neonatal chlamydial conjunctivitis in infants born to infected mothers is between 20% and 50%.[33-35] None of the current prophylactic regimens to prevent ophthalmia neonatorum are effective in preventing chlamydial conjunctivitis or extraocular infection such as pneumonia.[36]

The typical incubation period for chlamydial conjunctivitis is 5 to 14 days after delivery. Presentation prior to 5 days is rare.[37] Clinically, the infant may have a range of symptoms from mild scleral hyperemia with a watery eye discharge that becomes mucopurulent, to eyelid swelling with chemosis and pseudomembrane formation (Figure 1–11).

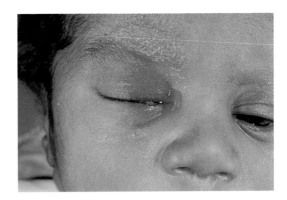

Figure 1–11. Chlamydial conjuctivitis.
Source: From Shah BR, Lucchesi M. *Atlas of Pediatric Emergency Medicine.* New York, NY: McGraw-Hill, 2006.

Blindness is much rarer than in gonococcal conjunctivitis and much slower to develop. Blindness is not caused by corneal damage as in gonococcal disease, but as a result of eyelid scarring and pannus formation. The pannus is a membrane of granulation tissue that develops if a patient is left untreated for more than 2 weeks.[38] With prompt treatment healing occurs without complications.

Chlamydia should be suspected in any infant less than 1 month old with conjunctivitis. The "gold standard" for the diagnosis of *C trachomatis* is culture of a sample taken from the everted eyelid.[39] Samples for culture must include conjunctival epithelial cells because *C trachomatis* is an obligate intracellular organism. Exudates are not adequate for the testing of *C trachomatis*. Additional testing should include Gram stain and culture to exclude *Neisseria gonorrhea*. Also consider nucleic acid amplification tests (NAAT); however, although NAATs have high sensitivity and specificity in the diagnosis of genital infections in women, there is insufficient data in neonatal *C trachomatis* infections to replace isolation cultures as the "gold standard."[33]

Erythromycin (50 mg/kg per day PO in 4 divided doses) for 14 days is the treatment of choice for *C trachomatis* conjunctivitis and pneumonia, as recommended by the American Academy of Pediatrics Committee on Infectious Disease and the Centers for Disease Control.[39,40] Treatment failure after a course of erythromycin occurs in up to 20% of cases of chlamydial conjunctivitis. Infants should receive close follow up, and may require a second course of erythromycin (50 mg/kg per day PO in 4 divided doses for 14 days) should the infection fail to resolve with the first course of therapy.

Treatment for chlamydial conjunctivitis should not be started without a positive diagnostic test. The administration of oral erythromycin and azithromycin has been associated with infantile hypertrophic pyloric stenosis. This risk appears greatest when the medications are given within the first 2 weeks of life.

Alternative therapies are not well studied and the American Academy of Pediatrics and the Centers for Disease Control continue to recommend oral erythromycin as first-line therapy for chlamydial infections. When starting oral erythromycin therapy in the newborn, the parents should be counseled regarding the potential risk of infantile hypertrophic pyloric stenosis (IHPS) and the infant should be closely monitored for signs of obstruction.

Gonococcal Conjunctivitis

Gonococcal conjunctivitis tends to be more severe than the other forms of ophthalmia neonatorum and has the greatest potential for harm to the newborn. Before the advent of routine newborn prophylaxis of ophthalmia neonatorum with silver nitrate ophthalmic solution, gonococcal conjunctivitis was the leading cause of blindness in the United States. Gonococcal infections in pregnant women in developing countries are estimated at less than 1% and the risk of perinatal transmission occurs in 30% to 50% of cases.[41,42]

The eye is the most frequent site of gonococcal infection in the newborn and symptoms typically arise at 2 to 5 days after birth. The infection is typically bilateral and severe (Figure 1–12). Clinical features include profound lid edema, chemosis, and copious and purulent discharge. Corneal ulcers may occur and rapidly progress to corneal perforation if treatment is delayed.

The diagnosis of gonococcal conjunctivitis is suspected in the newborn who develops conjunctivitis after the first day of life or who seems to have chemical conjunctivitis that is severe and persistent. In these cases a Gram stain of the exudate should be done and examined for Gram-negative intracellular diplococci. In addition, cultures of the exudate on a modified Thayer-Martin medium should be done. If Gram-negative diplococci are noted on the Gram stains, additional cultures of the anus and oropharynx should be done.

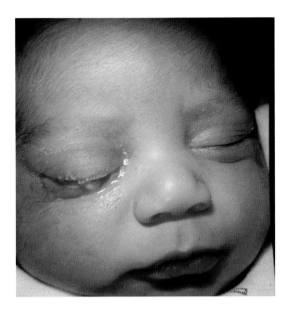

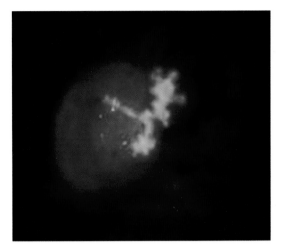

Figure 1–13. Dendritic filling defect seen in herpetic keratitis.

Figure 1–12. Gonococcal conjuctivitis. *Source:* From Shah Br, Lucchesi M. *Atlas of Pediatric Emergency Medicine.* New York, NY: McGraw-Hill, 2006.

Treatment of gonococcal conjunctivitis is a single dose of ceftriaxone (25-50 mg/kg, not to exceed 125 mg IV or IM). Infants with gonococcal conjunctivitis should be hospitalized. Infants should be observed for response to antibiotic therapy and monitored for signs and symptoms of disseminated disease. All cases of suspected gonococcal conjunctivitis should be tested for coinfection with *Chlamydia trachomatis.*

Herpetic Conjunctivitis

Herpes simplex virus (HSV) can cause neonatal keratoconjunctivitis, but this is rare and usually associated with a generalized herpes simplex infection. It presents in the first 2 weeks of life with nonspecific lid edema, moderate conjunctival hyperemia, and nonpurulent, often serosanguineous, drainage that may be unilateral or bilateral. A culture for HSV is indicated if a corneal epithelial defect is noted. Microdendrites or geographic ulcers are more

common in neonates on inspection of the cornea with fluoroscein staining than the typical dendrites seen in adult patients (Figure 1–13). Treatment is intravenous acyclovir. Consult an ophthalmologist immediately for evaluation and treatment recommendations if HSV keratitis is suspected.

CORNEAL ABRASION

Corneal abrasions in the newborn are not uncommon and often present with an inconsolable infant. In addition to crying, the infant may present with a red eye with persistent tearing, blepharospasm, and photophobia (Figure 1–14). One to two drops of tetracaine 0.5% ophthalmic solution, a topical anesthetic, are placed in the eye. This often calms the infant and facilitates the examination. Fluoroscein is instilled and the cornea inspected under a Wood's lamp (blue cobalt light). The fluoroscein adheres to epithelial defects in the cornea and makes the abrasion appear to glow under the Wood's lamp.

Most corneal abrasions are believed caused when infants inadvertently scratch

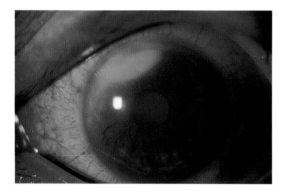

Figure 1–14. Corneal abrasion in a neonate.
Source: From Knoop KJ, Stack LB, Storrow AB. *Atlas of Emergency Medicine*, 2nd ed. New York, NY: McGraw-Hill, 2005.

their own eyes, but the presence of a foreign body should be excluded. The eye should be copiously irrigated with normal saline. Topical antibiotics are recommended for all corneal abrasions as prophylaxis against the development of a bacterial corneal ulcer. Consider prescribing erythromycin ophthalmologic ointment. Most abrasions heal in 24 hours and should be followed up by an ophthalmologist. Parents should be instructed to give appropriate oral analgesics and to keep fingernails short or covered.

► ABSENT RED REFLEX: LEUKOCORIA

Leukocoria means "white pupil" and is the term used for the clinical finding of a white pupillary reflex (Figure 1–15). Leukocoria is caused by abnormalities with the retina, lens, or vitreous. It is often the initial manifestation of a number of intraocular and systemic diseases.

Evaluation for leukocoria is part of the routine eye examination. In the first year of life, asymmetry of the red reflex during examination using a direct ophthalmoscope or penlight is the most common presentation

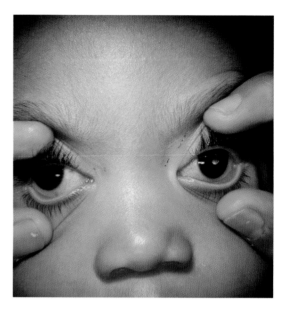

Figure 1–15. Leukocoria. *Source:* From Shah BR, Lucchesi M. *Atlas of Pediatric Emergency Medicine.* New York, NY: McGraw-Hill, 2006.

of leukocoria. The presence of leukocoria should impart a sense of urgency on the part of the practitioner. First, the presence of nonaccidental head injury must be excluded. Vitreous hemorrhage is most often the result of trauma, including nonaccidental head trauma, in the infant.[43] All infants with suspected nonaccidental head trauma should have an emergent eye examination performed by an ophthalmologist. Otherwise, all children with newly recognized leukocoria in whom trauma is not suspected need urgent ophthalmologist and pediatric referral within 1week to exclude retinoblastoma and other life- or sight-threatening conditions. Other conditions that cause leukocoria include persistent fetal vasculature, retinopathy of prematurity, cataract, toxocariasis, and vitreous hemorrhage. Other conditions not discussed here that may present with leukocoria include uveitis, Coat disease, optic disc abnormalities, and retinal dysplasia.

RETINOBLASTOMA

Retinoblastoma is the most common intraocular tumor of childhood and exists in sporadic and heritable forms. Approximately 1 in 15,000 live births are affected with retinoblastoma and the annual incidence is 11 per 10^6 children under the age of 4 years.[44,45] This means an estimated 200-500 new cases of retinoblastoma occur in the United States every year. The majority of cases are diagnosed in children less than 2 years of age.[46]

Approximately 25% of retinoblastoma cases are bilateral, which is always inherited and typically presents in the first year of life. However, 95% of these patients will have no previous family history of retinoblastoma. Unilateral disease is usually sporadic and diagnosed after the first year of life.[47,48]

If left untreated retinoblastoma will grow to fill the eye and destroy the globe. Metastasis usually begins after 6 months, and death occurs within a few years. The most common route of metastasis is direct extension to the central nervous system (CNS) via the optic nerve or the choroid to the orbit. However, tumor cells may disperse through the subarachnoid space to the contralateral optic nerve or through the CSF to the CNS. Hematogenous spread to the lung, bone, and brain occurs. Lymphatic dissemination of tumor cells into the conjunctivae, eyelids, and extraocular tissues occurs as well.

The most common clinical presentation of retinoblastoma is leukocoria (Figure 1–16). Strabismus is the second most common clinical finding associated with retinoblastoma.[49] All children with either leukocoria or strabismus, or both, should be evaluated by an ophthalmologist. However, other clinical signs may herald the disease and include: decreased vision, ocular inflammation, vitreous hemorrhage, hyphema, orbital cellulitis, proptosis, glaucoma, eye pain, and fever. A family history of retinoblastoma should include questions about the possible occurrence of other

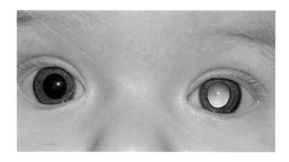

Figure 1–16. White pupil in a neonate with retinoblastoma.

eye tumors, eye loss, and cancers, especially osteogenic sarcoma, which has a strong association with retinoblastoma.

The diagnosis of retinoblastoma is made based upon the clinical examination, and the presence of intratumoral calcification on CT of the orbit or ocular ultrasonograhy.

CATARACT

A cataract is an opacification of the lens. Congenital cataracts are present at birth or in early infancy.[50] The incidence of congenital cataracts in the United States is 1.2 to 6.0 cases per 10,000 live births. If undetected and untreated, a cataract may cause partial or total blindness in an infant. Most congenital cataracts are associated with intrauterine infections, rubella being the most common cause. Other intrauterine infections associated with cataracts include rubeola, chicken pox, toxoplasmosis, herpes simplex virus, herpes zoster, poliomyelitis, influenza A, Epstein-Barr virus, syphilis, and cytomegalovirus. Unilateral cataracts are usually sporadic events; they account for approximately one-third of congenital cataracts and are associated with ocular abnormalities, intrauterine infection, and trauma. Bilateral cataracts are often inherited; they are indicators of a number of systemic, genetic, and metabolic disorders and require a full work-up. Metabolic and systemic diseases are found in as many as 60% of bilateral cataracts patients. Cataracts may also occur as a result of high-dose, long-term corticosteroid therapy.[50]

An irregular or asymmetric red reflex is the most common clinical finding indicative of a congenital cataract. This finding should prompt urgent ophthalmologic and pediatric follow-up, the goal being to prevent visual loss due to deprivation amblyopia. Cataract surgery is the treatment of choice and is most effective in preventing visual loss if preformed prior to 17 weeks of age.

PERSISTENT FETAL VASCULATURE

Persistent fetal vasculature (PFV) is caused by the failure of the embryonic primary vitreous and hyaloid vasculature to involute during gestation. In addition to leukocoria, the involved eye is often mildly micro-ophthalmic with a shallow anterior chamber and prominent vessels on the iris. Infants with PFV may develop glaucoma, cataracts, intraocular hemorrhage, or retinal detachment.[51,52] Refer all patients with leukocoria or suspected PFV to an ophthalmologist.

RETINOPATHY OF PREMATURITY

Retinopathy of prematurity (ROP) is a disease that affects the immature vasculature of the retina in premature infants. The neovascularization of the retina may be aggressive and progress to retinal detachment and blindness. All babies that weigh less than 1500 g at birth or are younger than 32 weeks gestational age at birth are at risk of developing ROP. The incidence of ROP has increased as smaller and younger infants have survived. The factors that play a role in the pathogenesis of ROP are still not well understood, but risk factors have been identified. They include assisted

ventilation for more than 1 week, surfactant therapy, intraventricular hemorrhage, bronchopulmonary dysplasia, sepsis, elevated arterial oxygen tension, and large volumes of blood transfusions.[53,54] ROP presents with leukocoria when retinal detachment has occurred and an emergent ophthalmologic consult is recommended. Patients with ROP are at increased risk for strabismus, glaucoma, and cataracts.

TOXOCARIASIS

Toxocariasis, also known as visceral larval migrans, is most commonly found in children 1 to 5 years of age. Common complaints are poor vision and strabismus. Ocular changes may be the only manifestation of the disease caused by the dog ascarid (*Toxocara canis*) or cat ascarid (*T catis*). Frequently there is no antecedent history of symptomatic visceral larval migrans. The infection often causes uveitis, which is the presence of inflammatory cells and debris in the vitreous and may result in the development of a secondary cataract. Both these changes produce leukocoria. Additionally, a whitish subretinal granuloma or large inflammatory mass (nematode endophthalmitis) may develop and be seen on funduscopic examination. These findings may be confused with retinoblastoma. All patients with leukocoria should be referred urgently to an ophthalmologist.

VITREOUS HEMORRHAGE

Vitreous hemorrhage causes leukocoria when there is extensive organization of the blood to form a clot prior to its degradation. The most common cause of vitreous hemorrhage in children is trauma, including nonaccidental head trauma. Vitreous hemorrhage should prompt a careful history, physical examination, and work-up to exclude shaken baby syndrome. Vitreous hemorrhage is also associated with a number of other conditions: retinopathy of prematurity, persistent hyperplastic primary vitreous, leukemia, and other blood dyscrasias.

▶ PERSISTENT TEARING: EPIPHORA

Tears keep the eyes moist and clear of debris. The tear film contributes to corneal clarity and the transmission of a focused image to the retina. Tears are produced by the lacrimal glands and drain through the lacrimal drainage system (Figure 1–17). The punctum is the opening on the medial surface of each eyelid and serves as the entrance to the canaliculus, which drains tears into the lacrimal sac. Tears collect in the lacrimal sac and drain into the nasolacrimal duct, which empties into the nose via the inferior meatus.

The valve of Hasner located at the distal end of the nasolacrimal duct is a mucosal flap that prevents air from tracking into the lacrimal duct system when the nose is blown.

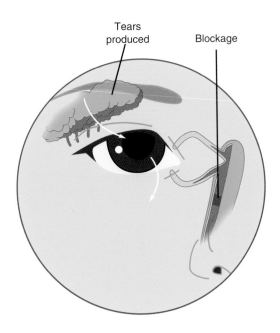

Figure 1–17. The lacrimal duct apparatus.

Nasolacrimal duct obstruction is the most common cause of persistent tearing, infection, and eye discharge in children. The differential for epiphora includes dacryostenosis, dacrocystitis, and glaucoma, all of which are discussed here. Additional causes of persistent tearing include corneal abrasion, conjunctivitis, and eyelid abnormalities such as trichiasis (ingrown eyelashes) and entropion (inversion of the eyelid).

DACRYOSTENOSIS: NASOLACRIMAL DUCT OBSTRUCTION

Dacryostenosis is the most common cause of persistent tearing in children and occurs in up to 20% of newborn infants.[55] Six percent of children will have epiphora due to nasolacrimal duct obstruction in the first year of life.[56] Blockage can occur at any point along the lacrimal drainage system, but most frequently occurs at the membrane of Hasner.

Infants with nasolacrimal duct obstruction present with a history of persistent or intermittent tearing without blepharospasm or photophobia. On examination no nasal drainage is noted, despite excessive tearing. There may be crusting or matting of the eyelashes in the absence of conjunctivitis.

First line treatment of nasolacrimal duct obstruction is lacrimal duct massage. To perform lacrimal duct massage, moderate pressure is applied over the lacrimal sac in a downward direction. This massaging motion forces tears from the lacrimal sac into the nasolacrimal duct and increases the hydrostatic pressure enough to open the valve of Hasner, which relieves the obstruction. Parents should practice on themselves and then perform this on the child at least 3 times a day. Parents should be instructed to keep their fingernails short and to wash their hands before massaging the infant's nasolacrimal sac.

Nasolacrimal duct obstruction resolves spontaneously in 90% of infants by 6 months.[56]

If nasolacrimal duct obstruction fails to resolve spontaneously by 12 months of age, then probing of the lacrimal duct by an ophthalmologist is recommended.

DACRYOCYSTITIS

Acute dacryocystitis is an ophthalmologic emergency and a complication of nasolacrimal duct obstruction. Mucopurulent drainage from the puncta occurs when bacteria grows in tears retained in the lacrimal sac. This infection is most frequently caused by alpha-hemolytic streptococci, *Staphylococcus epidermidis*, and *S aureus*. On examination the lacrimal sac may be erythematous and swollen with increased warmth and tenderness on palpation.

Acute dacryocystitis requires admission for intravenous antibiotics and consultation with an ophthalmologist. Complications of acute dacryocystitis include preseptal cellulitis, orbital cellulitis, sepsis, and meningitis.

GLAUCOMA

Congenital glaucoma is present at birth, but may not be recognized until infancy or early childhood. It is a rare condition that occurs in 1 in 10,000 live births.[57] It is characterized by improper development of the eye's aqueous outflow system. Impaired drainage of aqueous fluid from the anterior chamber leads to increased intraocular pressures, which causes damage to the optic nerve and blindness. As the intraocular pressure increases, peripheral vision is lost, followed by the progressive loss of central visual, and, eventually, complete blindness. Surgical intervention is required for definitive treatment.

The typical triad of symptoms for infantile glaucoma includes epiphora (chronic or intermittent tearing), photophobia, and blepharospasm. All symptoms are results of increased intraocular pressure, which causes globe distension

and ocular enlargement known as an "ox eye" or buphthalmos. Distension of the cornea secondary to elevated intraocular pressure causes corneal edema, which is seen as a cloudiness or haziness of the cornea on inspection. The corneal edema causes tremendous glare, which leads to photophobia. The photophobia causes tearing and blepharospasm. Increases in corneal size secondary to increases in intraocular pressure are not seen in other conditions with epiphora. The normal corneal diameter in infants is 10 mm, increasing to 12 mm by 2 years of age. A horizontal corneal diameter greater than 12 mm, or asymmetry in corneal diameters, suggests glaucoma.[58,59] All infants and children with suspected glaucoma need an urgent ophthalmologic consultation.

The goal of therapy in glaucoma is to preserve sight. Treatment of infantile glaucoma is surgical because of the rapidity of ocular damage and loss of sight. Medications are most often used postoperatively.

▶ NASAL PROBLEMS

The external nose is a pyramid-shaped structure composed of bony and cartilaginous structures. The nasal septum divides the two nostrils. The superior, middle, and inferior turbinates make up the lateral nasal walls. The turbinates are erectile structures made of mucosa and spongy bone covered by mucous membrane. The nasal turbinates swell and contract in response to changes in temperature, crying, allergen exposure, and illness.

These structures are best examined with the child in the sitting position. The child's head is tilted back while the examiner sits directly opposite the patient. The examiner holds the otoscope, with an ear speculum attached, in their dominant hand. Simultaneously the examiner uses their nondominant hand to stabilize the patient's head by resting the ulnar aspect of the hand against the forehead and using the thumb to elevate the tip of the nose.

The normal nasal mucosa is pink and moist. The vestibules should be patent and visible to the levels of the middle turbinates. The septum should be in the midline.

The nasopharynx is located posterior to the nasal cavity and is superior to the soft palate and oropharynx. The paired choanae form the anterior border of the nasopharynx and are divided by the nasal septum. Airflow through the nose begins at the nostrils as the negative pressure of inspiration draws air back through the nasal passages to the choanae and then to the larynx, trachea, and into the bronchi.

Infants are obligatory nasal breathers from birth to 6 weeks and thereafter prefer to breathe through their noses until 6 months of age.[60-63] The characteristic upturned nose of infancy and their relatively large tongue allow the infant to breathe and swallow simultaneously while breastfeeding. The posterior portion of the tongue exerts upward pressure on the soft palate during feeding that forms a seal that temporarily blocks the oral airway. This blockage of the oral airway combined with nasal breathing during feeding ensures swallowing without aspiration. This dynamic process has been described as the "veloglossal sphincter."[64] This process makes mouth breathing more cumbersome than nasal breathing for infants. For these reasons occlusion of the infant's nose is serious and can prove fatal.

CHOANAL ATRESIA

Choanal atresia is the most common congenital anomaly of the nose. Choanal atresia is caused by the persistence of the bucconasal membrane or bony septum in the posterior nares and occurs in approximately 1 in 7000 births. Girls are affected more frequently. Most cases are unilateral.[65]

Bilateral choanal atresia is a life-threatening emergency that typically presents shortly after birth. These infants typically have symptoms of severe upper airway obstruction and cyclical cyanosis. As the infant struggles ineffectively to breathe through the nose, the infant becomes cyanotic and then begins to cry, which allows the child to breathe through the mouth and resolves the cyanosis. When the infant stops crying or attempts to feed, the cyanosis recurs. Bilateral choanal atresia requires the insertion of an oral airway to keep the infant's mouth open and the oral airway patent, allowing the infant to breath. If the oral airway fails to alleviate respiratory distress and prevent recurrent cyanosis, then endotracheal intubation is necessary. Surgical correction of the obstruction is required.

Unilateral choanal atresia may go undetected in the newborn nursery and not become apparent until the infant develops an upper respiratory infection (URI). The swelling of the nasal mucosa and associated secretions of the URI block the normally patent nare and symptoms mimicking those of bilateral choanal atresia occur. These infants have stridor, labored breath sounds, and cyanosis that worsens during feeding and improves during crying. Unilateral choanal atresia may also present with chronic unilateral rhinitis.[66]

In infants with suspected choanal atresia, a size 5-8 French catheter should be passed from the nose into the oropharynx.[64,65] The catheter should be passed a distance of at least 3 to 3.5 cm from the alar rim. If the catheter cannot be passed, then choanal atresia is suspected. An obstruction due to mucosal swelling and turbinate hypertrophy will allow the catheter to pass into the pharynx, and the obstruction is determined to be functional, not mechanical.

The diagnosis of choanal atresia is confirmed by CT scan with intranasal contrast that shows narrowing of the posterior nasal cavity at the level of the pterygoid plate. For best results it is recommended that nasal secretions be suctioned and a topical vasoconstrictor be applied to nasal mucosa prior to the CT scan.

Infants that have respiratory distress or difficulty feeding should be admitted to the hospital. An oral airway must be established and gavage feeding may be needed. Definitive treatment is surgical and requires otolaryngology consult. Up to 60% of infants with choanal atresia have other associated anomalies, including anomalies of heart and eyes that warrant cardiology and ophthalmology consults.[66]

▶ ORAL PROBLEMS

The exam of the newborn infant's mouth should include inspection and palpation. Examination of the mouth begins with visual inspection of the lips for their overall shape, color, and for anatomic defects.

Sucking pads are areas of thickened epithelium on the lip mucosa. These may be present at birth and cause is unknown. They resolve spontaneously and require no treatment. The oral mucosa should be moist. The lips and oral cavity should be free of ulcerations. Ulcerations are associated with herpetic stomatitis, aphthous ulcers, metabolic disorders, and drug reactions. Small white shiny masses called epithelial pearls are common on the gingiva. Epithelial pearls often occur in clusters. White bumps seen in the midline at the junction of the hard and soft palate are Epstein pearls. Both epithelial pearls and Epstein pearls are normal findings in the infant. The palatine tonsils are generally not visible until the infant is 6 to 9 months of age. Palpation is important as some cleft palate abnormalities may not be seen, but are palpable. A cleft uvula should raise the suspicion of a palate defect. With palpation of the mouth, the normal and awake newborn will usually suck the examiner's finger. The examiner's finger will be drawn into the infant's mouth as the tongue moves back and forth against the palate. A small, cyst-like mass, called a ranula, may be felt on the floor of the mouth. These masses are benign and are caused by the obstruction of salivary glands. Natal teeth, if present, should be checked for looseness. Loose natal teeth pose a potential aspiration risk and should be extracted.

THRUSH: OROPHARYNGEAL CANDIDIASIS

Thrush is the most common infection of the oral cavity in healthy newborns. It is caused by an overgrowth of the fungus *Candida albicans*, which is part of the normal flora of the gastrointestinal and genitourinary tracts in humans. *Candida albicans* typically causes disease when the balance of normal flora is disrupted by the use of antibiotics, or there is a compromised immune system due to disease or the use of steroids. The former instance includes antibiotics administered directly to the infant, to the mother during delivery, or to a breastfeeding mother.

Symptoms typically develop in the first few weeks of life. Initially the parent may notice a white film in the mouth that looks like milk or formula that will not go away. The infant may be fussy or have difficulty feeding because of pain. The infant may pass the infection to the mother's nipples during breastfeeding. The mother may notice reddened tender nipples and unusual pain while nursing or between feedings.

On examination white plaques may be noted on the buccal mucosa, palate, tongue, or the oropharynx (Figure 1–18). These plaques do not scrape off with a tongue blade. In addition, pinpoint areas of bleeding are seen underneath the plaques when they are scraped.

The diagnosis is usually a clinical one and is confirmed when plaque scrapings viewed with a KOH preparation reveal budding yeasts, with or without pseudohyphae. Treatment consists of topical antifungals such as miconazole gel, which has a superior cure rate and lower rate of recurrence than nystatin suspension.[67] The breastfeeding mother with symptoms of candidiasis of the nipples should apply the same topical antifungals to the nipples and

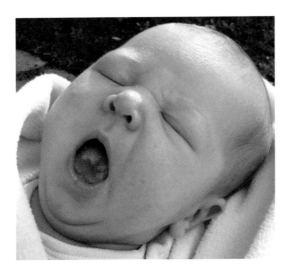

Figure 1–18. Oral candida.

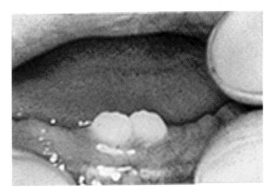

Figure 1–19. Natal teeth.

areolas after nursing. Breastfeeding should not be interrupted. If symptoms in the breastfeeding woman or infant are persistent, consider oral fluconazole.

NATAL TEETH

Natal teeth are relatively rare and occur in approximately 1 in 3,000 births. The majority of natal teeth occur as isolated events, but may run in families or be associated with some syndromes. Natal teeth are typically seen on the lower gum located where the future lower central incisors will be (Figure 1–19). These teeth are usually poorly formed with a weak root structure, which frequently makes the teeth wobbly and therefore an aspiration risk. To prevent aspiration, loose natal teeth should be extracted.[68]

ORAL INJURIES

Orofacial injuries in the nonambulatory infant are often the hallmark of abuse.[69] A careful and thorough oral examination is necessary in any infant with orofacial injuries in whom child abuse is suspected. Some experts believe the mouth and oral cavity may be a focus for physical abuse because of its significance in communication and eating.[70] Oral injuries most commonly feature bruising or laceration of the lips.[14] Oral injuries may be inflicted with instruments, such as eating utensils and pacifiers that are forced into the mouth, or perhaps with bottles during forced feeding. This mechanism can cause bruising or laceration of the lips; it may also tear the frenulum; bruise the gingiva or alveolar mucosa; lacerate, bruise or contuse the tongue; bruise the soft palate and uvula; and puncture the posterior oropharynx. The infant with perforation of the posterior pharynx may present with subcutaneous emphysema, fever, drooling, and respiratory distress. Gagging the infant may cause bruising at the corners of the mouth. Smothering the infant may tear the frenulum of the upper lip and be associated with facial petechiae.

All injuries to the head, face, and mouth in nonambulatory infants must be distinguished from abuse. The reported mechanism of injury must be consistent with physical findings, and it must fit with the developmental capabilities of the injured infant. The infant must have a full head-to-toe examination to exclude other unexplained injuries. Multiple injuries, injuries in different stages of healing, or inconsistent history all make abuse more likely. All cases of suspected child abuse must be reported to local or state child protective services, which is mandatory in all 50 U.S. states. Consider admission to the hospital for any infant with suspected physical abuse.

REFERENCES

1. Southgate WM, Pittard WB. Classification and physical examination of the newborn infant. In: Klaus MH, Fanaroff AA, eds. *Care of the High-Risk Neonate.* 5th ed. Philadelphia, PA: WB Saunders; 2001:100.

2. Plauche WC. Subgaleal hematoma. A complication of instrumental delivery. *JAMA.* 1980;244:1597-1598.

3. Benaron DA. Subgaleal hematoma causing hypovolemic shock during delivery after failed vacuum extraction: a case report. *J Perinatol.* 1993;13:228-231.

4. American College of Obstetricians and Gynecologists, Operative vaginal delivery. *ACOG Practice Bulletin no 17.* Washington, DC: American College of Obstetricians and Gynecologists; 2000.

5. U.S. Department of Health and Human Services National Center on Child Abuse and Neglect. *The Third National Incidence Study of Child Abuse and Neglect (NIS-3).* Washington, DC: U.S. Government Printing Office; 1996.

6. Atwal GS, Rutty GN, Carter N, Green MA. Bruising in non-accidental head injured children; a retrospective study of the prevalence, and distribution and pathological associations in 24 cases. *Forensic Sci Int.* 1998;96(2):215-230.

7. Feldman KW. Patterned abusive bruises of buttocks and the pinnae. *Paediatrics.* 1992;90(4):633-636.

8. Brinkman B, Püschel K, Mätzsch T. Forensic dermatological aspects of the battered child syndrome. *Akteuelle Dermatologie.* 1979;5(6):-217-232.

9. De Silva S, Oates RK. Child homicide the extreme of child abuse. *Med J Aust.* 1993;158(5)300-301.

10. Dunstan FD, Guildea ZE, Kontos K, Kemp AM, Sibert JR. A scoring system for bruise patterns: a tool for identifying abuse. *Arch Dis Child.* 2002;86(5):330-333.

11. Ellerstein NS. The cutaneous manifestations of child abuse and neglect. *Am J Dis Child.* 1979;133:906-909.

12. Johnson CF, Showers J. Injury variables in child abuse. *Child Abuse Negl.* 1985;9:207-215.

13. Leavitt EB, Pincus RL, Bukachevsky R. Otolaryngologic manifestations of child abuse. *Arch Otolaryngol Head Neck Surg.* 1992;118(6):629-631.

14. Naidoo S. A profile of the oro-facial injuries in child physical abuse at a children's hospital. *Child Abuse Negl.* 2000;24(4):521-534.

15. Sussman SJ. Skin manifestations of the battered-child syndrome. *J Pediatr.* 1968;72(1)99-101.

16. Saternus KS, Kernbach-Wighton G, Oehmichen M. The shaking trauma in infants—kinetic chains. *Forensic Sci Int.* 2000;109:203.

17. Van Praag MC, Van Rooij RW, Folkers E, et al. Diagnosis and treatment of pustular disorders in the neonate. *Pediatr Dermatol.* 1997;14(2):131-143.

18. Katsambas AD, Katoulis AC, Stavropoulos P. Acne neonatorum: a study of 22 cases. *Int J Dermatol.* 1999;38(2):128-130.

19. Paller A, Mancini AJ, Hurwitz S. *Clinical Pediatric Dermatology: A Textbook of Skin Disorders of Childhood and Adolescence.* 3rd ed. Philadelphia, PA: Elsevier–Saunders; 2006:737.

20. Feng E, Janniger CK. Miliaria. *Cutis.* 1995; 55(4):213-216.

21. Schachner L, Press S. Vesicular, bullous, and pustular disorders in infancy and childhood. *Pediatr Clin North Am.* 1983;30(4):609-629.

22. Turk AE, McCarthy JG, Thorne CH, Wisoff JH. The "back to sleep campaign" and deformational plagiocephaly: is there a cause for concern?. *J Craniofac Surg.* 1996;7:12.

23. Hutchison BL, Hutchison LA, Thompson JM, Mitchell EA. Plagiocephaly and brachycephaly in the first two years of life: a prospective cohort study. *Pediatrics.* 2004;114:970.

24. Benson ML, Oliverio PJ, Yue NC, Zinreich SJ. Primary craniosynostosis: imaging features. *AJR Am J Roentgenol.* 1996;166:697-703.

25. Ghali GE, Sinn DP, Tantipasawasin S. Management of nonsyndromic craniosynostosis. *Atlas Oral Maxillofac Surg Clin North Am.* 2002;10:1-41.

26. Kelly KM, Littlefield TR, Pomatto JK, Ripley CE, Beals SP, Joganic EF. Importance of early

recognition and treatment of deformational plagiocephaly with orthotic cranioplasty. *Cleft Palate Craniofac J.* 1999;36:127.

27. Mulliken JB, Vander Woude DL, Hansen M, LaBrie RA, Scott RM. Analysis of posterior plagiocephaly: deformational versus synostotic. *Plast Reconstr Surg.* 1999;103:371-380.

28. Chumas P, Tyagi A, Livingston J. Hydrocephalus—what's new?. *Arch Dis Child Fetal Neonatal Ed.* 2001;85:F149.

29. Volpe JJ. Intracranial hemorrhage: Germinal matrix-intraventricular hemorrhage. In: Volpe JJ, ed. *Neurology of the Newborn.* 4th ed. Philadelphia, PA: WB Saunders; 2001:428.

30. Forward KR, Fewer D, Stiver HG. Cerebralspinal fluid shunt infections. *J Neurosurg.* 1983;59:389.

31. Shapiro S, Boaz J, Kleiman M, Kalsbeck J. Origin of organisms infecting ventricular shunts. *Neurosurgery.* 1988;22:868.

32. Gupta BK, Hamming NA, Miller MT. The eye. In: Fanaroff AA, Martin RJ, eds. *Neonatal–Perinatal Medicine: Diseases of the Fetus and Infant.* 7th ed. St. Louis, MO: Mosby; 2002:1568.

33. American Academy of Pediatrics. Chlamydial trachomatis. In: Pickering LK, ed. *Red Book: 2006 Report of the Committee on Infectious Diseases.* 27th ed. Elk Grove Village, IL, Author; 2006:252.

34. Schachter J, Grossman M, Sweet RL, Holt J, Jordan C, Bishop E. Prospective study of perinatal transmission of Chlamydia trachomatis. *JAMA.* 1986;255:3374-3377.

35. Frommell GT, Rothenberg R, Wang S, McIntosh K. Chlamydial infection of mothers and their infants. *J Pediatr.* 1979;95:28.

36. Chen JY. Prophylaxis of ophthalmia neonatorum: comparison of silver nitrate, tetracycline, erythromycin and no prophylaxis. *Pediatr Infect Dis J.* 1992;11:1026.

37. Darville T. Chlamydia. In: Remington JS, Klein JO, Wilson CB, Baker CJ, eds. *Infectious Diseases of the Fetus and the Newborn.* 6th ed. Philadelphia, PA: Elsevier Saunders; 2006:384.

38. Mordhorst CH, Dawson C. Sequelae of neonatal inclusion conjunctivitis and associated disease in parents. *Am J Ophthalmol.* 1971;71:861.

39. Johnson RE, Newhall WJ, Papp JR, et al. Screening tests to detect Chlamydia trachomatis and Neisseria gonorrhoeae infections, 2002. *MMWR Recomm Rep.* 2002;51:1.

40. Workowski KA, Berman SM. Sexually transmitted diseases treatment guidelines, 2006. *MMWR Recomm Rep.* 2006;55:1.

41. Laga M, Meheus A, Piot P. Epidemiology and control of gonococcal ophthalmia neonatorum. *Bull World Health Organ.* 1989;67:471.

42. Alexander ER. Gonorrhea in the newborn. *Ann NY Acad Sci.* 1988;549:180.

43. Schloff S, Mullaney PB, Armstrong DC, Simantirakis E. Retinal findings in children with intracranial hemorrhage. *Ophthalmology.* 2002;109:1472.

44. Devesa SS. The incidence of retinoblastoma. *Am J Ophthalmol.* 1975;80:263.

45. Tamboli A, Podgor MJ, Horm JW. The incidence of retinoblastoma in the United States: 1974 through 1985. *Arch Ophthalmol.* 1990;108:128.

46. Rubenfeld M, Abamson DH, Ellsworth RM, Kitchin FD. Unilateral vs bilateral retinoblastoma. Correlations between age at diagnosis and stage of ocular disease. *Ophthalmology.* 1986;93:1016.

47. Young JL, Smith MA, Roffers SD, et al. Retinoblastoma. In: Ries LA, Smith MA, Gurney JG, et al., eds. *Cancer Incidence and Survival Among Young Children and Adolescents: United States SEER Program, 1975-1995.* Bethesda, MD: National Cancer Institute; 1999:73.

48. Montegi T. Lymphocyte chromosome survey in 42 patients with retinoblastoma: effort to detect 13q14 deletion mosaicism. *Hum Genet.* 1981;58:168.

49. Abramson DH, Frank CM, Susman M, et al. Presenting signs of retinoblastoma. *J Pediatr.* 1998;132:505.

50. Green M. The eyes. *Pediatric Diagnosis: Interpretation of Symptoms and Signs in Children and Adolescents.* 6th ed. Philadelphia, PA: W.B. Saunders Company; 1998:15-36.

51. Hadad R, Font RL, Reeser F. Persistent hyperplastic primary vitreous. A clinicopathologic study of 62 cases and review of the literature. *Surv Ophthamol.* 1978;23:123.

52. Cheng KP, Hiles DA, Biglan AW. The differential diagnosis of leukocoria. *Pediatr Ann.* 1990;19:376.

53. Seiberth V, Linderkamp O. Risk factors in retinopathy of prematurity. A multivariate statistical analysis. *Ophthalmologica.* 2000;214:131.

54. Flynn JT, Bancalari E, Snyder ES, et al. A cohort study of transcutaneous oxygen tension and the incidence and severity of retinopathy of prematurity. *N Engl J Med.* 1992;326:1050.

55. Peterson RA, Robb RM. The natural course of congenital obstruction of the nasolacrimal duct. *J Pediatr Ophthalmol Strabismus.* 1978;15:246.

56. MacEwen CJ, Young JD. Epiphora during the first year of life. *Eye.* 1991;5 (Pt 5):596.

57. deLuise VP, Anderson DR. Primary infantile glaucoma (congenital glaucoma). *Surv Ophthalmol.* 1983;28:1.

58. Chew E, Morin JD. Glaucoma in children. *Pediatr Clin North Am.* 1983;30:1043.

59. Seidman DJ, Nelson LB, Calhoun JH, et al. Signs and symptoms in the presentation of primary infantile glaucoma. *Pediatrics.* 1986;77:399.

60. Moss ML. The veloepoglotttic sphincter and obligate nose breathing in the neonate. *J Pediatric.* 1970;67:330-331.

61. Swift PGF, Emory JL. Clinical observations on response to nasal occlusion in infancy. *Arch Dis Child.* 1973;48:947-951.

62. Nathan CA, Seid AB. Neonatal rhinitis. *Int J Pediatr Otorhinolaryngol.* 1997;39:59-65.

63. Moss ML. The veloepoglotttic sphincter and obligate nose breathing in the neonate. *J Pediatric.* 1970;67:330-331.

64. Myer CM III, Cotton RT. Nasal obstruction in the pediatric patient. *Pediatrics.* 1983;72:766.

65. Szeremeta W, Parikh TD, Widelitz JS. Congenital nasal malformtaions. *Otolaryngolo Clin North Am.* 2007;40:97.

66. Ferdman RM, Linzer JF, Sr. The Runny Nose in the Emergency Department: Rhinitis and Sinusitis. *Clin Pediatr Emerg Med.* 2007;8(2):123-130.

67. Hoppe JE. Treatment of oropharyngeal candidiasis and candidal diaper dermatitis in neonates and infants: review and reappraisal. *Pediatr Infect Dis J.* 1997;16:885-894.

68. Diley DC, Siegal MA, Budnick S. Diagnosing and treating common oral pathologies. *Pediatr Clin North Am.* 1991;38:1227-1264.

69. Kellogg N. Oral and dental aspects of child abuse and neglect. *Pediatrics.* 2005;116:1565.

70. Vadiakas G, Roberts MW, Dilley DC. Child abuse and neglect: ethical issues for dentistry. *J Mass Dent Soc.* 1991;40:13-15.

CHAPTER 2

Neurologic Emergencies

Linnea Wittick, MD

▶ NORMAL NEONATAL BEHAVIOR

To many observers, a neonate may appear to just sleep all day with occasional breaks for eating, but in actuality the normal neonate spends the day learning to make sense of a set of novel stimuli. At birth, the newborn is thrust into a new environment and must learn to survive in this new world. It must learn to respond appropriately to a bombardment of new stimuli, develop a sleep-wake cycle, regulate temperature control, determine who these new strange people are, and manage to grab a bite to eat every once in a while.

Neonates exist in several behavioral states—sleep, drowsy, alert, active, fussy, and crying—which largely dictate their posture and behavior. During their alert state, they lie in a flexed position with little motor control and with purposeless hand opening and closing.[1] They can turn their head from side to side without being able to lift it against gravity. They progress over their first month to assume a slightly more relaxed posture with the ability to hold their head in a tonic neck position. By 4 to 6 weeks of age, they can hold their chin up when in the prone position. As they age, they gain slightly better control of their sucking mechanisms as well.

Neonates must constantly learn to process new stimuli as they explore their new world. They learn to habituate to the familiar and only respond to a new stimulus, as seen when they will turn their head to a novel sound such as their mother entering a room. They recognize and prefer patterns in colors, consonants, contour, and intensity.[2] By 4 to 6 weeks of age, they consistently fixate on objects and follow objects both horizontally and vertically with their gaze. When neonates become overstimulated, they often yawn, look away, or begin to suck on their hands or lips. This response to stimuli will often affect their overall muscle tone and spontaneous movement.

Neonates also become more social over the first month of life. They are born with a visual preference for faces and show recognition memory by preferentially turning to their own mother's face. A newborn's focal length is about 8 to 12 inches, the perfect distance to gaze at their mother while being held for feedings. They move from simply having an involuntary smile to occasional social smiles by the end of the neonatal period.

The sleep-wake cycle also changes, to the relief of every parent, throughout the neonatal period. Initially, the newborn sleeps for equal amounts of time throughout the day and night. In the first week, the infant sleeps for approximately 16.5 hours each day. It will wake approximately every 2 to 3 hours for feedings. As the infant's neurologic system matures, it learns to consolidate periods of sleep so that by the end of the first month, the infant sleeps for 15.5 hours, still with an equal distribution between day and night. By two months of age, most babies will wake 2 to 3 times during the night to feed, with some infants sleeping 6 hours at a stretch. By 3 months of age, the infant sleeps approximately 15 hours a day with most of the sleeping during the nighttime hours.

▶ A WORD ABOUT THE FORMER NICU PATIENT

With the increasing number of premature deliveries, a rudimentary understanding of the basic developmental and neurologic consequences NICU infants face becomes important. Approximately 9% of all newborns require intensive care. Because some of these newborns require a prolonged NICU stay, they will likely not be seen in the emergency department (ED) during the neonatal period. However, given their complicated history and increased likelihood of having long-term medical complications, an understanding of common outcomes will be helpful to the ED physician.

Most premature infants are discharged near what should have been their term delivery date. In order to be discharged home, a premature infant must nipple all of its feeds, demonstrate steady growth, have no recurrent apneas or bradycardias, and maintain its temperature. Many may have some slight hypotonia. In general, premature infants, barring any underlying neurologic pathology, will function at the developmental level of their gestational age and not their chronologic age. They generally catch up to other children their own chronologic age by the time they reach 2 years of age. Parents may need reassurance that it is normal for their infant to lag behind for a time. However, very premature infants with a complicated NICU course are more likely to suffer significant brain injury and progress to developmental delay, cerebral palsy, and metal retardation. Five to 10% of all premature infants <1500 g develop a major motor deficiency, whereas 25% to 50% have developmental or visual difficulties.[3]

One common complication of prematurity causing neurological sequelae that should be understood when evaluating an infant is intraventricular hemorrhage (IVH). With improved care the relative number of infants sustaining these insults is decreasing, and the very fact that more infants survive extreme prematurity means that more infants with IVH survive as well. Eighty percent of infants born between 23 and 34 weeks of gestation will sustain an IVH with the incidence increasing as the birth weight decreases.[4] The fragile subepenydmal germinal matrix bleeds easily until about 36 weeks of gestation when it becomes fully developed. Eighty to 90% of these bleeds occur by day 3 of life, especially after events that quickly change cerebral blood flow such as asphyxia, RDS, pneumothorax, and rapid volume expansion. Symptoms of an acute bleed range from the completely asymptomatic infant to an abrupt onset of apnea, cyanosis, lethargy, changes in the neurologic examination, abnormal gaze, seizure, and acidosis. Diagnosis is usually made by ultrasound of the head through the anterior fontanelle at days 4 to 7 of life. Findings are usually graded to aid in diagnosis and prognosis. Grade I bleeds occur in 35% of IVH and involve only the germinal matrix or fill less than 10% of the ventricle. Only 20% of these infants develop a complication such as cerebral palsy or significant mental retardation. Grade II hemorrhages bleed through the ependyma and fill 10% to 50% of the ventricle, affecting approximately 40% of infants with IVH. Grade III hemorrhages fill over 50% of the ventricle and display a transient hydrocephalus. Of infants with grade II or grade III hemorrhages, 41% will suffer significant morbidity. Grade IV hemorrhage extends beyond the ventricle and affects the periventricular white matter. These infants face a poorer prognosis, with 86% developing CNS delay.[4] The ultrasound is repeated again in 6 weeks to follow the development of hydrocephalus and extent of bleeding and infarct. If these infants progress to having hydrocephalus, neurosurgical intervention will be needed. These infants will also need close developmental care.[4,5]

▶ THE NEUROLOGIC HISTORY

The neonatal neurologic examination may seem intimidating. Unlike an older child or adult, the physician cannot ask the patient to perform certain tasks, and the patient cannot respond to direct questioning. However, with a systematic approach and just a few tricks and modifications, the physician can still perform a successful neonatal neurologic examination.

As with any physician encounter, a neonatal examination should begin with a thorough history. In addition to questions concerning presenting signs and symptoms, several aspects of the history can influence the neurologic diagnosis. Historical features of the pregnancy and delivery are vital (Table 2–1). Did the mother notice normal fetal movements or was there a

▶ TABLE 2–1. **SUGGESTED COMPONENTS OF THE NEONATAL HISTORY**

Historical Issues	Predictive Possibilities
Was there a decrease in fetal movement during gestation?	Neuromuscular disorder
Were there paroxysmal, rhythmic movements noted during gestation?	Seizure disorder
What medications were taken prenatally?	Adverse fetal development
If breastfeeding, what medications are being taken presently?	Adverse neurologic effects
Were there low APGAR scores?	Perinatal asphyxia
Is there a family history of mental retardation, seizures, early strokes, or consanguinity?	Neurologic problems

decrease in fetal movements that could signify a neuromuscular disorder? Did she notice paroxysmal, rhythmic movements possibly indicating fetal seizures? What medications did the mother take during her pregnancy that may have affected fetal development? What medications is she taking now that could affect the infant if she is breastfeeding? Was the baby full term and were there any complications at the delivery? APGAR scores of less than 6 at 1 and 5 minutes may be indicative of perinatal asphyxia, which could now affect the baby's neurologic status. Birth weight is an important feature. A small for gestational age (SGA) infant (ie, weight less than the 10th percentile at birth), can signify a problem with fetal development. Large for gestational age (LGA) infants also present with their own set of complications from risks of hypoglycemia (infant of a diabetic mother) to complications arising from birth trauma. Both SGA and LGA infants have increased risk of morbidity and mortality compared to infants born at normal weight. Any problems the baby encountered in the nursery or NICU should be reviewed because the first days of life provide clues to the present neurologic status. The baby's normal behavior—feeding, sleep, crying, and alertness patterns—should be discussed to uncover any changes at time of presentation. A family history of mental retardation, learning disabilities, seizures, early strokes, or consanguinity should be obtained.

▶ THE NEUROLOGIC EXAMINATION

The physical examination should begin with a general assessment of the baby. Perform the examination in a calm manner with the baby feeling safe and comfortable. Keeping the baby in the mother's lap for much of the examination helps keep the baby quiet and responsive. Offering a bottle or a gloved finger to suck on can provide valuable information as well as facilitate the examination. At this point, note the general sense of the baby's overall neurologic status. The baby should be alert or arouse easily, depending on the normal feeding and sleeping pattern.[2] A lethargic or irritable baby should raise suspicions of a pathologic process. The alert baby displays spontaneous eye movements and moves in response to stimulus. When crying, a neonate should easily console. The physician should note if the infant cries appropriately to noxious stimuli and whether the cry is vigorous or weak and high pitched. The patient's vital signs should also be noted as these can have a relationship to the patient's neurologic findings.

EXAMINATION OF THE HEAD AND CRANIAL NERVES

Head Size

The head examination should begin with a measurement of the head circumference. The occipital-frontal head circumference is measured just above the ears and eyebrows, around the widest part of the head. The normal neonate's head measures about 35 cm at birth and increases about 1 cm per week.[6] The head circumference reflects the intracranial volume and, therefore, brain development.[2] [1] Microcephaly, where head circumference is less than 2 SD below the 3rd percentile for age and gender, reflects abnormal brain growth and developmental delay. This may be due to many causes such as Down syndrome, TORCH infections, and fetal alcohol syndrome (Table 2–2). Macrocephaly, a head circumference greater than 2 SD above the 97th percentile, may reflect an intracranial process such as hydrocephalus, hemorrhage, or storage diseases. The rate of growth often is more useful than a single measurement taken in time. Previous measurements from the primary physician may help determine whether an abnormal head size is indeed a pathologic process. If previous measurements are unobtainable and the physician finds an abnormal head size in the context of

▶ TABLE 2–2. **CAUSES OF DEVIATION IN HEAD CIRCUMFERENCE**

Microcephaly	Macrocephaly
Genetic	Hydrocephalus
Trisomy 21, 13,18	Dandy-Walker
Cru du Chat	malformation
Cornelia de Lange	Chiari malformation
Congenital infection	CNS infection
CMV	Meningitis
Rubella	Tumor
Toxoplasmosis	Familial
CNS infection	Syndromes
Meningitis	Glutaric academia
Encephalitis	type I
Drug Exposure	NF type I
Fetal alcohol	
syndrome	
Radiation	
HIE	
Craniosynostosis	

an otherwise normal neurologic examination, the infant should be referred to the primary physician for growth monitoring and further testing.

Fontanelles

There are several features of the infant skull that differ from an older child's examination. One of the most obvious is the presence of fontanelles (see Figure 1–7). Often, parents will report that their baby's "soft spot" has sunken during an illness, so familiarity with a normal fontanelle is important. Although 6 fontanelles actually exist, most physicians generally note only 2. The anterior fontanelle lies at the junction of the coronal and the sagittal sutures and measures 0.6-3.6 cm at birth. It normally closes by about 9-18 months of age. A large anterior fontanelle can be associated with Down syndrome, hypothyroidism, achondroplasia, and increased intracranial pressure (ICP). A small fontanelle can be secondary to abnormal brain development, congenital infections, fetal alcohol syndrome, and some genetic syndromes. The posterior fontanelle lies at the meeting of the lambdoidal and sagittal sutures and measures 0.5-1 cm. It closes anywhere between birth and 4 months of age. Fontanelles should feel flat and soft and be assessed with the infant quiet and upright. Lying supine may cause the fontanelles to falsely protrude. A depressed fontanelle can signify states of dehydration. A bulging and tense fontanelle may be a sign of increased intracranial pressure. Also, auscultate over the anterior fontanelle; the presence of a bruit may indicate an underlying arterial-venous malformation.

Head Shape

Many normal variations of the shape of the neonate's head exist. Positional plagiocephaly, caused by preferential positioning over time, can cause a misshapen head with the ear of the affected side pushed forward and the cranium appearing flat on the preferred side. Usually, mild plagiocephaly can be treated by advising the parents to alternate sides the infant lies on. More severe cases will need referral to a neurosurgeon for treatment as the neonate grows older. Molding occurs during a vaginal delivery when the bones of the cranium overlap to facilitate passage through the birth canal. The bones can be felt through the skin as they overlap at the suture lines. Parents may need reassurance that this will resolve in 1 to 2 days.

Caput secundum is generalized subcutaneous edema of the scalp that arises during a vaginal delivery. It is often an asymmetric bogginess that will cross over the suture lines. It normally resolves in 7 to 10 days. Cephalohematomas, subperiosteal hemorrhages caused by birth trauma, appear similar to caput secundum. As these are contained within the periosteum, they will not cross over the suture lines and are often unilateral. This makes it easy to differentiate cephalohematomas from caput secundum on examination. Due to the breakdown of the hemoglobin within, extensive or bilateral cephalohematomas may facilitate the development of jaundice.

Cephalohematomas (see Figure 1–1) normally resolve within 4 to 6 weeks. Calcifications felt as hard ridges along the skull may remain behind. These should not be confused with craniosynostosis, a pathologic condition of premature fusing of the sutures. This occurs most commonly along the sagittal suture followed by the coronal suture. A heaped up ridging along the suture line may be palpated along with an asymmetry of the infant's head. Normally, the sutures expand to allow for rapid brain growth. In craniosynostosis, the brain cannot grow against the closed suture, so growth increases in a direction parallel to the fused suture.[2] On examination, normal, open sutures are absent and the head displays asymmetry. Cranial radiographs or computed tomograohy (CT) scans and neurosurgic consult are indicated; surgical correction at a later date may be indicated to allow for proper brain development.

Cranial Nerves

Examination of the cranial nerves may be accomplished with simple maneuvers and observations (Table 2–3).[2] The neonate's ability to fix on and follow an object provides a gross assessment of visual patency. At 1 month, a neonate's eyesight is 20/150, causes a focal length of 8 to 12 inches, the perfect visual acuity to focus on the mother's face while feeding.

Eye movements and pupillary response should be assessed with the newborn bundled, comfortable, and in a darkened room or held vertically to facilitate eye opening.

The pupil should be examined for a red reflex. The appearance of a gray or asymmetrically colored pupil can signify congenital cataracts or retinoblastoma (see Figure 1–16) and necessitates an immediate referral to an ophthalmologist. Subconjunctival hemorrhages do not always indicate nonaccidental trauma, and may arise from birth trauma, coughing, or sneezing. These should resolve in 1 to 2 weeks.[1] A funduscopic examination may demonstrate retinal hemorrhages, which may be seen in 38% of normal vaginal deliveries.[2] However, if present after 2 weeks of age or encountered in another setting, they may be considered signs of nonaccidental head trauma.

▶ **TABLE 2–3. CRANIAL NERVE EXAMINATION**

Maneuver Performed	Cranial Nerve
Pupillary reaction to light	II, III
EOM while fixing on object	III, IV, VI
Corneal reflex	V
Withdrawal to pinprick	V
Facial expression/asymmetry	VII
Blinking to loud noise	VIII
Suck	V, VII, XII
Swallow	IX, X, XII
SCM strength, contractures	XI
Tongue fasciculations	XII

Source: From Refs. 1, 2, 6.

Eye movements can be observed while the infant fixes on and follows either a bright object or its mother's face. Jerky eye movements are a normal finding during the first few months of life as well as disconjugate gaze at rest or with eye movements.[2] Facial asymmetry, especially while crying, may show a defect in CN VII. A rough assessment of hearing may be performed by clapping near the infant and observing for reflex blinking.

MOTOR & SENSORY EXAMINATION

The motor and sensory examination occurs mostly through observation of the infant during the entire examination. The neonate usually rests with its limbs in flexed positions.[1] It will move all of its extremities symmetrically. Tone can be assessed by passively moving the limbs and feeling opposing flexion.[2] A neonate will demonstrate some amount of head control. When pulled to a sitting position by its arms, its head should not lag far behind. Tone can also be noted by holding the infant over the examination table by its trunk. The infant should be able to bear most of its weight with its feet on the table, and should not slide through the examiner's hands. Muscle bulk offers another tool to assess the baby's tone. A hypotonic baby will show less muscle bulk and possibly a single palmar crease, seen most commonly in Down syndrome but also in other syndromes with decreased tone in utero. The baby should withdraw to touch or pinprick. Normal reactions to touch should reassure the physician. Response to noxious stimuli, such as an IV insertion or a cold room or touch can also give clues to the neonate's sensory status.

REFLEXES

The neonate displays unique reflexes not seen during other stages of life[1,6] (Table 2–4). These

▶ TABLE 2-4. **PRIMITIVE REFLEXES**

Reflex	Stimulus	Response
Crawl	Place infant on abdomen	Flexes legs under and makes crawling motions
Morro	Pull arms away from supine infant and suddenly release	Arms abduct and extend, hands open, then arms flex in and hands close
Rooting	Stroke cheek or corner of mouth	Head turns to stimulus, mouth opens
Palmer/plantar grasp	Place finger along palm or sole of foot	Grasps finger or curls toes around finger
Tonic neck (fencing)	Turn head to one side while lying supine	Facial arm extension, occipital arm flexion
Stepping	Hold upright with sole of feet resting on flat surface	Makes alternating stepping movements
Swimmer's	Hold infant prone while supporting under the chest, stroke adjacent to the spine	Flexion of pelvis toward the stimulus
Protective	Place cloth over face	Arches and turns head side to side, brings hands to face

Source: From Refs. 1, 2, 6.

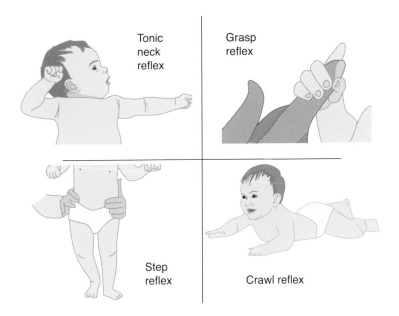

Tonic neck reflex

Grasp reflex

Step reflex

Crawl reflex

Figure 2-1. Common neonatal reflexes.

develop at approximately 28 to 32 weeks of gestation and provide a convenient way to assess the patient's tone and strength (Figure 2–1). For example, an asymmetric Morro reflex may indicate a brachial plexus injury or fractured clavicle. The inability to perform the step reflex may indicate decreased tone. Deep tendon reflexes, while often overlooked in the neonatal examination, can easily be elicited.[2] The pectoralis, bicep, brachioradialis, and knee reflex are all obtainable at this age. The overall flexor tone of the infant usually suppresses the triceps reflex and may possibly make the bicep reflex difficult to elicit. Attempt the reflex with the joint in various angles of flexion to provide the optimal tendon stretch to produce a response. Often, a knee reflex will elicit a cross adductor response, whereas a knee reflex causes the hip adductor on both the ipsilateral and contralateral sides to contract. This occurs normally in the first month of life in contrast to older children and adults. The Babinski reflex also differs from that of an adult. During the first few weeks of life, an up-going great toe is common.[6] Eliciting ankle clonus should also not cause alarm as 5 to 10 beats of clonus in a neonate is acceptable in the context of a normal neurologic examination. A grading system usually is difficult to assign to a neonate; therefore, as long as the reflexes are symmetrical throughout all extremities, the examination should be considered normal.

▶ THE CRYING INFANT

Few things become more frustrating to both parents and physicians than a crying baby. Often, parents present with an apparently otherwise healthy baby with no other complaints than "he won't stop crying!" Anxiety, stress, and depression can lead the caregiver to bring the child for an evaluation.[7] Poole et al. found that in one ED, unexplained crying in an otherwise well infant compromised 1 in 400 infant visits.[8] In the UK alone, $108 million per year is spent to evaluate crying in the first 12 weeks of life.[7]

Babies cry with the purpose of communicating their needs for attention, thirst, and hunger, or because of discomfort and pain.[7,8] The internet offers books, classes, and informational videos promising parents the ability to interpret their baby's every cry. Studies show that parents often successfully interpret their baby's needs according to their cry. Yet there exists some amount of "paroxysmal fussing" in the majority of normal babies not used to communicating with caretakers. All babies display a regular cyclic crying period without environmental factors or stimuli. One of the most well-known studies of infant crying was done by Braselton in 1962 and described a crying pattern in 80 healthy infants.[9] He states that at 2 weeks, most babies cry for an average of 1-3/4 hours per day. This increases to a peak of 2-3/4hours at 6 weeks of age and then decreases to an average of 1 hour per day by 3 months as infants became more developmentally advanced and find other ways to communicate and soothe themselves. He also notes a time dependency to the infants' crying, with the majority of time spent crying focused in the afternoon and evening. Often, the parents just need reassurance that their baby displays normal infant behavior. When parents appear especially stressed by their crying infant, techniques for dealing with their crying baby should be discussed.[10]

However, infants presenting to the ED with a complaint of excessive crying that falls outside of the range of normal crying need a complete evaluation to rule out pathologic causes of crying.[8] Five to 60% of crying infants possess a diagnosable illness as a reason for their crying. Confounding the picture, studies show that parental perceptions of crying do not correlate with the seriousness of the illness and vary widely among mothers. Therefore, the physician should seriously investigate the cause behind a complaint of excessive crying to rule out a potentially serious illness in this vulnerable population.

DIFFERENTIAL DIAGNOSIS

The differential diagnosis of the crying infant is extensive[7] (Table 2–5). A broad history and

▶ **TABLE 2-5. PATHOLOGIC CAUSES OF CRYING**

Infection	**Dermatologic**
Meningitis	Eczema
Encephalitis	Diaper dermatitis
Sepsis	Cellulitis
UTI	Abscess
Osteomyelitis	Hair tourniquet
Septic arthritis	Immunizations
Pneumonia	Insect bites
Acute otitis media	**Trauma**
Ginivostomatitis	Nonaccidental trauma
Retropharyngeal Cellulitis	Fracture
Omphalitis	Corneal abrasion
Fever	**GU**
CV- SVT	Incarcerated inguinal hernia
Myocarditis	Testicular torsion
Congenital heart defect	Hair tourniquet
Congestive heart failure	Hydrocele
GI	Balantitis
Malrotation with midgut volvulus	Complication of circumcision
Intusssception	**Neurologic**
Reflux	Increased ICP
Constipation	Hydrocephalus
Anal fissure	**Metabolic**
Acute gastroenteritis	Electrolyte abnormality
Formula intolerance	Hypoglycemia
Colic	Inborn errors of metabolism
Toxins	
Drug withdrawal	
Medication exposure in breast milk	
Ingestion	

Source: From Refs. 7, 8.

physical examination begins the process of ruling out serous illness. One study found that the history alone directly led to the diagnosis in 20% of cases,[8] demonstrating the need for a comprehensive history. The physician needs to first rule out any possibility of a life-threatening infection such as sepsis, meningitis, encephalitis, or urinary tract infection. Any history of fever should prompt the physician to begin a full sepsis work-up. Also inquire about any possible causes leading to electrolyte disturbances such as normal feeding behavior and any recent deviation from normal feeding,

because electrolyte abnormalities or hypoglycemia are easily treated. Otherwise, a broad, detailed history about onset of symptoms, deviation from normal behavior, pregnancy and delivery history, medications, and previous medical history should be done.

PHYSICAL EXAMINATION

The physical examination may lead directly to or contribute to the diagnosis in 53% of infants.[8] As with any patient, the examination should be systematic and complete with a focus on specific areas. Life-threatening causes of crying such as infection, abuse, intussusceptions, intoxication, and metabolic diseases should be ruled-out quickly.

General Appearance

First, the general appearance of the baby may direct the physician in the work-up. Completely undress the neonate to expose any findings that might be hidden beneath clothing. Findings of increased crying with movement may point to meningitis or a musculoskeletal injury. An alert and fussy baby offers more reassurance than a fussy baby that is neither alert nor responsive to its surroundings. The vital signs can also give a general overview of the patient. An elevated temperature can point to an infectious etiology and point the work-up in that direction. Tachycardia may be secondary to supraventricular tachycardia (SVT), fever, discomfort, or dehydration. Tachypnea can be secondary to infection, neurologic, cardiac, or metabolic disorders.

Head

The head needs a thorough examination. The fontanelle and sutures may show signs of elevated intracranial pressure secondary to infection, congenital hydrocephalus, or trauma.[7] A funduscopic eye examination may reveal retinal hemorrhages (see Figure 1–3) suggestive of nonaccidental trauma. Excessive tearing can indicate glaucoma, a foreign body, or infection. The eyelids should be everted to inspect for foreign bodies. A fluorescein examination under a Wood's lamp can rule out corneal abrasion (Figure 2–2). Often, the application of tetracaine before the examination will calm the baby, signifying an abrasion and leading to its diagnosis and treatment. The ears should be examined for acute otitis media. Contusions around the ears may suggest trauma. Any signs of trauma merit a head CT looking for subdural hematomas. The mouth and hypopharynx

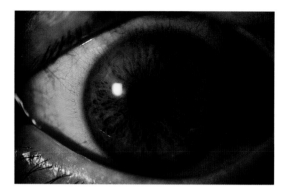

Figure 2–2. Corneal abrasion in a crying neonate. *Source:* From Knoop KJ, Stack LB, Storrow AB: *Atlas of Emergency Medicine,* 2nd ed. New York, NY: McGraw-Hill, 2002.

should be completely examined looking for burns, thrush, or stomatitis, which can be treated appropriately.

Chest & Abdominal Examination

A thorough lung and cardiac examination may reveal also a cause behind the crying. A high suspicion for SVT, congenital heart disease, and myocarditis may lead to a correct diagnosis of increased crying and fussiness.

The abdominal examination may reveal many different causes of crying. A full abdomen with easily palpated stool is significant for constipation when the history corresponds with an infant with hard, round stools. In a chronically constipated infant, consider a work-up and surgical consultation for Hirschsprung disease. A soft abdomen with the history of vomiting or diarrhea may suggest gastroenteritis and adequate hydration status should be assessed. A rectal examination may reveal anal fissures. Blood at the rectum suggests intussusception. A patent anus should be documented. Genitalia should be assessed for incarcerated hernias (Figure 2–3), hair tourniquets (Figure 2–4), and complications from a circumcision. Diaper rashes should be appropriately treated.

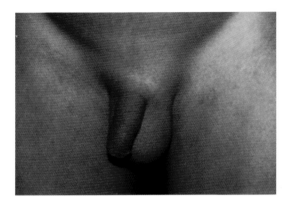

Figure 2-3. Inguinal hernia in a crying neonate.

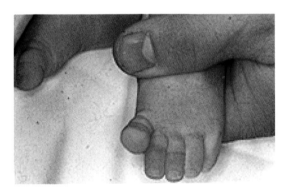

Figure 2-4. Hair tourniquet in a crying neonate.

Musculoskeletal Examination

A complete musculoskeletal examination may discover the etiology of crying. The long bones should be palpated for possible fractures or osteomyelitis. Any tenderness deserves a radiograph. Most fractures in the neonatal period are suspicious for abuse, and if found, a complete skeletal survey to search for other fractures must be done. However, a fractured clavicle found in the neonatal period may be due to shoulder dystocia after a difficult delivery. Red, swollen, or tender joints should lead the physician to look for septic joints. Hair tourniquets are an easily missed diagnosis. The physician should carefully examine each digit

for a hair or string wrapped around a digit and cutting off circulation. The skin should also be inspected for possible rashes, bruises, abrasions, or abscesses.

DIAGNOSTIC TESTS

Generally, the physician should not order screening laboratory or radiographic tests without a particular diagnosis in mind. A urinalysis and urine culture may be the only cost-effective screening tests.[8] Otherwise, tests should be chosen based on clinical suspicion of a particular diagnosis.

MANAGEMENT

Often, the history and physical examination will not direct the physician to a specific diagnosis. In fact, 40% of neonates worked-up for excessive crying will not yield a diagnosis at their initial presentation.[8] If the infant has an unrevealing history, a normal physical examination, and has reproducibly ceased crying during the initial assessment, the child may return home with prompt follow-up. On the other hand, if the infant continues to cry and cannot be consoled, further studies should be considered,[8] such as barium enema for intussusceptions, CT of the head to rule out trauma or increased intracranial pressure, blood tests and spinal tap to evaluate for infections, or a metabolic work-up including amino and organic acids, ammonia, lactate, pH, and urine-reducing substances. If no diagnosis is found for a continually fussy infant, they should be admitted for further work-up and observation.

The physician may entertain a diagnosis of colic only after ruling out all other serious illness. The definition of colic generally is accepted as recurrent, paroxysmal spells of excessive crying and fussiness lasting more than 3 hours a day for more than 3 days a week for over 3 weeks. It usually presents in the 2nd or 3rd week of life and lasts until the infant is 3 to 4 months old.[8] These infants are otherwise well. Often, parents will present within the first few days of crying before a definite pattern of crying becomes established. As discussed above, a thorough history and physical examination should first rule out a serious illness before giving a diagnosis of colic.

▶ THE HYPOTONIC NEONATE

Neonatal hypotonia, informally known as "floppy baby syndrome," occurs not uncommonly in the neonatal period. Decreased tone from a neurologic disorder usually becomes noticeable directly after birth or during early infancy. Hypotonia can be defined as a subjective decrease of resistance to passive range of motion, usually found in the limbs, trunk, and facial muscles (Figure 2–5). This differs from weakness, which is defined as a decrease in the power generated by the musculature. A neonate may or may not display weakness

associated with decreased tone. The presence or absence of weakness may even help lead to the underlying cause of hypotonia. The physician must find a quick diagnosis for the hypotonic neonate as there exist several medical conditions where a rapid diagnosis and treatment will affect the prognosis. A thorough history and physical exam should easily point to nonneurologic diseases requiring immediate attention such as sepsis, hypothyroidism, hypoglycemia, malnutrition, malrotation, toxin exposure, and congenital heart disease. If suspicious for one of these diseases, the appropriate laboratory evaluation and treatment should be quickly initiated.

DIFFERENTIAL DIAGNOSIS

When evaluating neonatal hypotonia, it often helps to approach the differential diagnosis in a systematic manner. Most diseases fall into two categories—those disorders affecting the upper motor neuron, or central disorders, and those disorders affecting the lower motor neuron, or

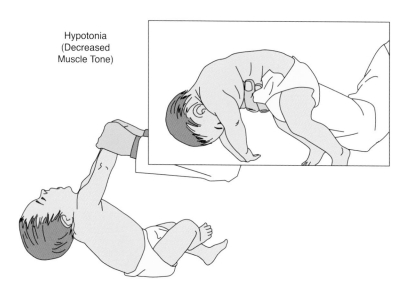

Figure 2–5. Examples of decreased neonatal tone.

▶ TABLE 2-6. **DIFFERENTIAL DIAGNOSIS OF HYPOTONIA**

Systemic	Central	Peripheral
Infection	Hypoxic ischemic encephalopathy	Anterior horn cells
Cardiac	Chromosome disorders	Spinal muscular atrophy I
Metabolic	Syndromes	Peripheral nerve
Hypoxia	Prader-Willi	Peripheral neuropathies
	Spinal cord injury	Guillian-Barré syndrome
		Neuromuscular junction
		Myasthenia syndromes
		Infantile botulism
		Muscle
		Pompe disease
		Congenital myopathies
		Congenital myotonic dystrophies
		Congenital muscular dystrophies
		Metabolic disorders

Source: From Refs. 11-14, 16.

peripheral disorders (Table 2–6).[11-13] Peripheral disorders can further be divided into those affecting each section of the neuromuscular unit. Delineating the disorder into one of these broad categories will help the physician arise at a correct diagnosis and tailor the work-up to avoid costly and timely diagnostic tests.

Central disorders generally affect the upper motor neuron—the brain and spinal cord. Approximately 66% of patients with hypotonia present with a central defect.[11] They usually display decreased strength with active motion in addition to hypotonia. In addition to multiple other symptoms, these patients more commonly present with seizures than do peripheral disorders. They often experience an altered level of consciousness. Many of these disorders are associated with spasticity and increased reflexes, but usually present in the neonatal period with hypotonia and weakness.

Several nonneurologic disorders resulting in central hypotonia exist and should quickly be ruled out.[11,14] As mentioned earlier, sepsis, encephalitis, GI disturbances, and cardiac failure also may present as lethargy and hypotonia. A toxic ingestion due to medical errors, exposure in breast milk, or intentional administration also may present with lethargy. Several metabolic disorders such as phenylketinuria, Zellweger syndrome, and galactossemia also present with hypotonia. Metabolic disorders usually present within the first 12 to 24 hours of life after enough toxic metabolites build up in the neonate's system, or when the infant becomes stressed by a febrile illness. A strong family predisposition suggests the diagnosis. Electrolytes, blood gas, lactate, and ammonia levels can be sent for a quick screening in the acutely ill child suspected of having a metabolic disorder. These all require prompt treatment because delayed treatment can have dire outcomes.

Direct Brain Insults

Direct insults to the brain often cause a central hypotonia.[15,14] Hypoxic ischemic encephalopathy from birth trauma or prolonged perinatal hypoxia can lead to decreased tone. Intracranial hemorrhage secondary to premature delivery, neonatal stroke, or nonaccidental trauma also often progress to hypotonia. In addition to injuries, defects in brain structure may lead to decreased tone. Lissincephaly, which literally means smooth brain, arises from defective neuronal migration causing absent or partially formed gyri and sulci in the cerebral cortex. These children display abnormal facies, failure to thrive, seizures, and mental retardation. Holoprosencephaly is a disorder of the forebrain or prosencephalon that divides it into two separate cerebral hemispheres and causes hypotonia with dysmorphic features of the midline face, seizures, and mental retardation. A head CT or magnetic resonance imaging (MRI) will diagnose causes of hypotonia due to changes in brain structure. Treatment consists of supportive care and developmental assistance.

Chromosomal Disorders

Several chromosomal disorders may cause central hypotonia.[11,14,16] Chromosomal disorders generally display characteristic dysmorphic features that aid in their diagnosis.[11] While many of these disorders will be suspected on clinical grounds based on a characteristic dysmorphic appearance, referral to a geneticist for karyotyping provides both a diagnosis and allows for discussions about future family planning. A few common diseases will be presented here, but many others exist.

Down syndrome or trisomy 21 is the most common chromosomal disorder and genetic cause of mental retardation. It results from a trisomy of the distal end of the long arm of chromosome 21. Found in 1 in 600 to 700 live births,[17] in addition to hypotonia, these infants display some variability of the well-known dysmorphisms of brachiocephaly, small ears, up slanted palpebral fissures, epicanthal folds, a flat midface, a single transverse crease, small nipples, and a central posterior hair whorl. Almost 40% of these patients have a congenital heart defect, most commonly an AV canal defect or a VSD. They also frequently have pulmonary hypertension, obstructive GI lesions, hypothyroidism, and increased susceptibility to infection. Trisomy 18, Edwards syndrome, and trisomy 13 also display hypotonia,

however, few of these infants survive beyond infancy.

Prader-Willi syndrome (PWS)[11,17] is another common chromosomal syndrome presenting with hypotonia. This arises in 1 of 12,000 to 15,000 live births from the paternal deletion of several genes on Ch15q. These patients present with hypotonia, feeding difficulties secondary to poor suck and swallow ability, and failure to thrive. This diagnosis may escape the physician in the hypotonic neonate as most physicians associate hyperphagia and obesity with PWS. These well-known symptoms actually do not develop until approximately 2 years of age, however. In addition, these patients display diamond-shaped eyes, a prominent nasal bridge, small hands and feet, lightly colored skin compared to their family, hypogonads, and developmental delay.

Spinal cord injuries may also cause central hypotonia.[14] These may occur when the fetus is delivered in the breech position with a hyperextended neck or during cervical presentations with the aggressive use of forceps. These complications are extremely rare occurring in 1 of 29,000 deliveries and usually present in the delivery room with severe respiratory distress. In addition, these patients will have hypotonia with asymmetry between the upper and lower extremities, depending on the location of the lesion. They may have bladder dysfunction, decreased rectal tone, and vasomotor instability. Most likely the diagnosis will be made soon after delivery with an MRI of the spinal cord. These patients may present to the emergency department if the newborn is intubated immediately in the delivery room for respiratory distress and assumed that all symptoms of hypotonia are attributed to hypoxic-ischemic encephalopathy (HIE). These patients may develop increased deep tendon reflexes and spasticity as a later progression of the injury.

Disorders of the peripheral nervous system present differently from disorders of the central nervous system.[15] In addition to hypotonia, these babies display generalized weakness. They usually appear alert and interactive. However, 28% of neonates with peripheral nerve disorders also sustain some degree of hypoxia secondary to birth complications, confounding the clear distinction between a central and a peripheral disease.[11] These disorders can be further grouped into disorders affecting each section of the motor-neuron unit: anterior horn cells, the peripheral nerve, the neuromuscular junction, and the muscle itself.

One example of a disorder affecting the anterior horn cell is spinal muscular atrophy (SMA) type I, or Werdnig-Hoffmann syndrome.[14,16] This autosomal recessive defect affects the SMN gene on chromosome 5. It usually presents in the first 6 months of life with 1/3 presenting in the neonatal period with weakness, hypotonia, and decreased reflexes. Often, the mother recalls a decrease in fetal movement, and the infant presents in a breech presentation. The disease generally progresses gradually, with symptoms often first noted after an exacerbation by a febrile illness. These infants have proximal, progressive weakness of the voluntary muscles with decreased movement of the extremities and the inability to lift the head. It weakens the bulbar muscles leading to poor suck and swallow mechanisms and poor secretion control. They feed poorly, display tongue fasciculations, and drool excessively. The disease weakens the respiratory muscles, and the child will display "paradoxical respirations" where the abdomen rises and the chest wall falls with each respiration. This leads to a bell-shaped chest wall, and respiratory weakness predisposes these infants to respiratory failure and pneumonia, the leading cause of death. Although these infants fail to meet developmental milestones, they are bright, inquisitive, and have alert facies. Without supportive care, 80% of these children will die by 8 months of age and all will die by 2 years of age. Other types of SMA syndrome with better prognoses exist, but these present after the neonatal period.

The diagnosis is suspected on clinical grounds and supported by an EMG and muscle biopsy. More recently, a genetic test has become available; it is a useful tool for making an accurate diagnosis and allows for genetic counseling when considering future pregnancies.

Disorders of the neuromuscular junction present with hypotonia, generalized weakness, ptosis, facial diplegia, feeding issues, and respiratory symptoms.[14,17] One common disorder is transient neonatal myasthenia gravis. This condition affects approximately 10% of children born to mothers with myasthenia gravis. It occurs when the mother's acetylcholine receptor antibody crosses over the placenta and binds to the neonate's acetylcholine receptors. These patients present with facial palsies, ptosis, decreased suck and swallow, a weak cry, and generalized weakness and hypotonia. They may encounter respiratory difficulties, especially during a concurrent illness. Although a strong suspicion in a child of a mother with myasthenia gravis may lead to the diagnosis, improvement in symptoms after administration of edrophonium or neostigmine provides confirmation. The symptoms normally resolve in 6 weeks once the infant's acetylcholine receptors regenerate into the synaptic membranes and the maternal antibody is no longer present. Until that time, cholinesterase inhibitors such as neostigmine or pyridostigme allow for better feeding and symptom control.

Infantile botulism also affects the neuromuscular junction.[17-20] It normally presents in infants between 6 weeks and 12 months of age but has been reported in an infant as young as 6 days old. Infantile botulism results from ingestion of spores from the gram-positive anaerobe *Clostridium botulinum*, which can be found in soil, contaminated foods such as home canning products, dust, and honey. Parents are instructed not to feed their children honey until they reach 1 year of age. This bacterium produces 7 different neurotoxins, 2 of which cause the symptoms described in infantile botulism. The neurotoxin binds irreversibly to cholinergic synapses, preventing the release of acetylcholine, and thus preventing effective nerve conduction. When toxin binds to over 70% of the presynaptic receptors, voluntary muscle movement and autonomic function begin to fail. When over 90% of the receptors are bound, diaphragmatic function begins to fail, placing the infant in danger of respiratory arrest.

Infantile botulism presents more commonly in the United States than elsewhere in the world, with 75 to 100 cases diagnosed each year.[18] These infants first present with only complaints of constipation. They progress to a descending flaccid paralysis and slowly progressive hypotonia with poor feeding, a head lag, and a weak cry. It may affect the cranial nerves with ptosis, poor extraocular movements, a poor suck, swallow, and gag, and areflexic and unreactive pupils. These patients remain alert throughout the illness. They progress to poor respiratory effort and failure secondary to weakness of the accessory muscles and the diaphragm. Laboratory testing for the toxin in a stool sample is diagnostic. An EMG also helps confirm the diagnosis. Affected infants require close monitoring and supportive care with a low threshold for mechanical ventilation. The hypotonia progresses over 2 to 10 days with a nadir at 1-2 weeks. Nutritional support often is needed, as these patients have difficulty feeding. Without treatment, full recovery will take approximately 4 to 6 weeks. There does exist a human-derived botulinum immunoglobulin, BabyBIG, shown to significantly decrease the length of hospital stay and supportive measures needed.[18,20]

Disorders affecting the peripheral nerve locally present with weakness and wasting in the distally involved muscle group.[13,15] Both hereditary and acquired disorders exist. One example is Guillain-Barré syndrome. This inflammatory demyelinating disorder occasionally occurs in neonates and sometimes even as congenital disease. Patients with a peripheral neuropathy are areflexic in addition to hypotonic. Other examples of peripheral neuropathies are Dejerine-Sottas syndrome and congenital hypomyelination syndrome. The diagnosis and treatment of all of these patients should be performed under the guidance of a pediatric neurologist.

Disorders affecting tone at the level of the muscle[12,14-17] also occur and include congenital muscular dystrophies, which are autosomal recessive genetic disorders presenting at birth with weakness and joint contractures. They are caused by a defect in the muscle structure leading to progressive weakness and wasting secondary to degenerative and fibrotic muscle changes. Congenital myopathies, on the other hand, are nonprogressive disorders, also presenting in neonates. These infants demonstrate hypotonia, proximal weakness, flabby muscles, and facial features such as a high, arched palate and the inability to fully close the mouth. Congenital myotonic dystrophies present with distal muscle group weakness, global developmental delay, and failure to thrive. This disorder actually arises from the muscles' inability to relax after contraction and symptoms worsen after long periods of rest. Twenty-five percent of these infants die from respiratory distress. These patients actually regain some muscle strength as they grow older and will survive if aggressive respiratory support is instituted.

Pompe disease, also known as acid maltase deficiency, is another example of a disease affecting muscle.[12-14,17] This autosomal recessive glycogen storage disease results in glycogen deposition in cardiac and skeletal muscle, liver, and brain tissue in about 1 of 138,000 live births. Initial symptoms normally appear at 1.6 months, but may present sooner, with feeding difficulty, failure to thrive, or cardiac failure. In addition, these patients display weakness, macroglossia, tongue fasciculations, decreased facial tone, wide-open eyes, poor oral secretion control, and ankle clonus. They may display an elevated respiratory rate, nasal flaring, and increased accessory muscle use due to weakness. Their muscles often feel rubbery on palpation, and they often have hepatosplenomegaly. Due to glycogen deposits in the cardiac muscle, they develop cardiomegaly and heart failure, and a murmur or a gallop may be heard on auscultation. Without mechanical support, these patients typically progress rapidly to death from cardiac or respiratory failure in their first year. Diagnosis was traditionally reached by finding muscular glycogen deposits in a biopsy sample, but genetic testing now provides more definite answers. Recently, an experimental enzyme replacement therapy was developed that may improve long-term functionality for these patients.

Benign congenital hypotonia is a concept fraught with controversy.[11,12,16,17] First described when fewer diagnoses of the neuromuscular unit were known, these patients display decreased tone from birth but have normal strength, reflexes, development, and, usually, intelligence. Often multiple family members will display similar symptoms without formal diagnosis after laboratory testing, imaging, and EMG studies. Often, the symptoms will resolve over time, but these patients will often develop joint laxity and hypermobility leading to easy joint dislocations as adults. Strictly a diagnosis of exclusion, a full negative work-up must be completed before the diagnosis is considered. As more genetic tests become available and more disorders become known, these patients may one day find an actual diagnosis.

HISTORY & PHYSICAL EXAMINATION

Discovering a diagnosis begins with a thorough history and physical examination.[11] Recent illness, fever, or acute onset of hypotonia leans toward nonneurological etiologies of hypotonia that require immediate diagnosis and treatment. However, these may also cause an exacerbation of a previously unknown or underlying disease causing hypotonia. After excluding patients needing immediate treatment for emergent causes of hypotonia or stabilizing those with chronic decreased tone, categorizing patients into either central or peripheral disease will guide further testing and treatment.[14] One study showed that after the history alone, 50% of patients easily fall into one of these two categories.[12]

The physician should determine the timing of onset of hypotonia. Hypotonia beginning in the first 12 to 24 hours of life strongly suggests an inborn error of metabolism. Other diseases present with progressive hypotonia, which may not be as noticeable in the young baby. The patient's level of consciousness, posture at rest and during activity, a progression or change in tone, and abnormal ocular movements should be pursued. A feeding history can give the physician a means of tracking the progression and severity of disease. A detailed prenatal history including maternal health and drug exposure should be known. Often mothers will notice decreased fetal movements in utero. A short umbilical chord or breech presentation often results from decreased fetal movements. A traumatic delivery or low APGAR score can point to a hypoxic brain injury now causing hypotonia. Up to one-third of all infants with hypotonia have a history of requiring resuscitation at birth.[16]

A history of early seizures, abnormal eye movements, fixed staring, and frequent apneas signify a recent brain injury. A detailed family history also is important. A detailed pedigree may aid in the diagnosis of a genetic disorder previously unknown to run in the family. Elevated parental age can predispose to certain chromosomal disorders as can consanguinity. Any affected siblings may direct further work-up. Sometimes, previously undiagnosed older siblings will be given a diagnosis when a new sibling arrives with similar and more pronounced symptoms.

A complete physical examination will also direct the physician in the work-up and diagnosis of neonatal hypotonia. Most patients with hypotonia will demonstrate full abduction and external rotation of their legs with flaccid extension of the arms while at rest. When the physician pulls the neonate to a sitting position by the neonate's arms, the neonate will demonstrate significant head lag. When holding the neonate's trunk upright between the physician's hands, the hypotonic baby will not support its own weight by its legs and easily slips through the physician's hands.

Central lesions of the upper motor neuron will produce a generally flaccid baby with mostly axial hypotonia but preserved strength during active motion. They may have either normal or increased reflexes and their level of consciousness may be depressed to the extent of being obtunded. Facial dysmorphisms characteristic of a particular syndrome are more often associated with central etiologies of hypotonia.

Peripheral or lower motor neuron defects display decreased tone along with often profound weakness. Decreased antigravitational movement will be observed. Different symptoms will manifest depending on what part of the neuromuscular unit is affected.[11,15] Neonates with defects of the motor neuron will be diffusely weak with sparing of the diaphragm, eyes and sphincters.

If the defect lies in the nerve, the distal muscle groups will be involved especially the intrinsic muscles of the hands and feet, leading to decreased palmar and solar creases. The neuromuscular junction defects will present with bulbar and oculomotor defects so affected patients will have ptosis, decreased extraocular movements, and poor suck and swallow. Finally, defects at the muscle itself will present with proximal weakness, flaccid diplegia, and diminished reflexes. Many diseases also have specific findings as discussed above; therefore, a thorough and complete examination is important in correctly identifying the disease. Remember that many patients may present with a mixed picture as a peripheral defect may predispose the baby to a difficult delivery

and perinatal hypoxia, creating an overlying central defect.

DIAGNOSTIC TESTS

The first priority when these patients present to the emergency department is to rule out life-threatening causes of decreased tone. These usually involve nonneurologic causes such as sepsis, hypoglycemia, metabolic disturbances, cardiac defects, trauma, or toxic exposures. A full sepsis work-up should begin if highly suspicious. Check a bedside glucose level and electrolytes as these abnormalities are easily treated. An EKG or chest radiograph may assist in diagnosing a congenital cardiac defect as a cause of hypotonia and lethargy. If trauma is suspected, quickly obtain a head CT. If the infant is sufficiently lethargic, a dose of Narcan (naloxone) 0.1 mg/kg given IV or IM will both diagnose and treat a toxic exposure to narcotics.

MANAGEMENT

If a neurologic cause of decreased tone is suspected, the first concern becomes supportive care. Carefully assess the patient's respiratory status. Respiratory rate, depth of inspiration, nasal flaring, and accessory muscle use require continuous monitoring. These patients usually have a poor respiratory effort at baseline, which any overlying illness can significantly worsen. Take the necessary measures to stabilize and maintain the airway and have a low threshold for admitting the patient with any signs of respiratory distress. Also evaluate the patient's ability to feed. If the patient is unable to protect its airway due to poor suck and swallowing mechanisms or cannot consume adequate calories for growth, the patient will need to be admitted for further interventions.

Besides immediate initial evaluation and interventions, the ED physician is unlikely to be involved in the complete work-up of a patient with neonatal hypotonia. Usually, further testing continues in the inpatient setting once the initial stabilization of the patient is completed and an underlying reason for the acute onset of illness needs to be found, or as an outpatient by a specialist or the patient's primary care doctor in a patient deemed stable enough to go home. However, the ED physician should initialize the work-up in the correct direction to avoid the necessity of expensive and painful laboratory procedures. A CT or MRI of the head may easily identify a hypoxic etiology or brain abnormality. Otherwise, guided by the history and physical examination, the physician should choose a testing modality appropriate for the most likely diagnosis, as discussed above.

▶ THE JITTERY NEONATE

Jitteriness in a neonate is often a normal finding. It can be defined as involuntary, rhythmic tremors of equal amplitude around a fixed axis and is one of the most common involuntary movements of the neonate.[21,22] Two-thirds of normal babies demonstrate tremors after the Moro reflex in the first week of life. Up to 44% of healthy term newborns display jitteriness with 23% having mild symptoms, 8% with moderate tremors, and 13% with severe jitteriness.[21,23] Behavioral states influence level of jitteriness, with increased movement in babies that are crying or stressed.[23] A normal, nonpathological tremor responds to outside stimulus. For example, as an extremity is held still, jitteriness decreases.[2] Also, a startle response to a loud noise often is accompanied by jitteriness. It normally begins to decrease during the second week of life.[23] The average age of complete resolution is 7.2 months of age, and 81% of neonates will no longer display tremors by their 9th month.[21]

However, jitteriness occasionally has a pathologic cause. Generally, tremors occurring

▶ **TABLE 2–7. DIFFERENTIATING JITTERINESS FROM SEIZURES**

	Jitteriness	Seizures
Frequency	Fast	Slow
Continues with stimulus	No	Yes
Automatisms	No	Yes
Abnormal eye movements	No	Yes

while the neonate is in a calm, alert state or during sleep signify a pathologic cause. Tremors beginning after the 3rd day of life also deserve further evaluation. Jitteriness should not be confused with seizures.

Jitteriness, as opposed to seizures, always ceases with a stimulus, such as holding an affected limb. Also, infants with benign tremors do not display gaze abnormalities or autonomic changes.[2,23,24] They remain alert and interactive throughout the abnormal movements (Table 2–7).

DIFFERENTIAL DIAGNOSIS

Metabolic Causes

Hypoglycemia commonly causes jitteriness.[21,22] In the fetus, glucose stores are laid down in the liver during the 3rd trimester. Newborns undergoing acute stress such as sepsis or hypoxia quickly utilize these stores and become hypoglycemic. Premature or intrauterine growth rate restricted (IUGR) infants will not have built up as large a store in utero and may deplete these stores more quickly in times of stress. Any infant with feeding intolerance can also become hypoglycemic. Gastroenteritis, with frequent vomiting and diarrhea, poses a significant threat. Parents should be questioned on how they are mixing the infant's formula, as a diluted mixture can lead to hypoglycemia and other electrolyte abnormalities. If the infant is tolerating feeds well and shows no signs of infection, inborn errors of metabolism should be considered as a cause of hypoglycemia. If an inborn error of metabolism is suspected, the appropriate work-up should begin.

Hypocalcaemia also causes jitteriness in neonates.[21,22,24] Decreased calcium causes neuromuscular irritability leading to jitteriness, tremors, overall irritability, and tetany. They may display systemic symptoms such as poor feeding, vomiting, and lethargy. In extreme cases, neuromuscular irritability can lead to laryngospasm or seizures, therefore appropriate evaluation and prompt treatment are important.

All neonates are susceptible to decreased calcium because of the normal process of building their calcium stores in utero. Maternal calcium is actively transported across the placenta by a pump regulated by maternal parathyroid hormone. Most of the fetal calcium stores are laid down during the 3rd trimester, making the last few months of gestation especially important for the neonate's calcium stores. The fetal calcium concentration actually rises above the mother's, making the calcium level of the newborn relatively high. This level rapidly falls after delivery with the disappearance of the placental calcium transport and then normalizes over the next 2 weeks.

Early neonatal hypocalcemia occurs during the first 2 to 3 days of life during this early transition to normalized calcium levels.[25] This transient exaggeration of the normal decrease in calcium reaches its nadir in about 24 hours. Several factors increase the risk of early hypocalcemia. Premature, IUGR, and low birth weight infants and infants with perinatal asphyxia have impaired opportunities to acquire adequate maternal calcium and, therefore, may exhibit an exaggerated decline in calcium levels. Infants of diabetic mothers also have an increased risk of hypocalcaemia the first 24 to 72 hours of life due to a decrease in maternal parathyroid hormone secretion leading to decreased transplacental calcium

transport. Twenty to 50% of babies born to diabetic mothers will experience hypocalcemia.[26] Other maternal factors, such as anticonvulsant medications, toxemia of pregnancy, and poor vitamin D status can lead to early hypocalcemia. Usually, early neonatal hypocalcemia resolves in several weeks. After the calcium level is acutely normalized, the infant may receive an oral supplement to maintain normal calcium levels.

Late neonatal hypocalcemia presents toward the end of the 1st week of life due to a variety of causes.[25,27] In the past, an increased phosphate load contained in infant formulas caused the suppression of parathyroid hormone release leading to hypocalcemia. Formula companies have since decreased the amount of phosphate in their formulas. DiGeorge syndrome, also known as velocardofacial syndrome, arises from the dysgenesis of the 3rd and 4rth pharyngeal pouches during embryogenesis. This results in absent parathyroid glands, cleft palate, cardiac defects, dysmorphic facies, thymus malformation, and renal defects. This arises from a microdeletion of CH22q11.2 in 1 in 4000 newborns. Sixty percent of these infants will present with hypocalcemia secondary to an absent parathyroid gland, often as the presenting symptom. Maternal hyperparathyroidism causes an increase in calcium transfer across the placenta. This leads to suppression of the neonate's secretion of parathyroid hormone, which continues after delivery and presents as hypocalcaemia in the 3rd week of life. Congenital hypoparathyroidism also leads to hypocalcemia. These patients have decreased calcium, increased phosphate, and low parathyroid hormone levels. This may easily be confused with pseudohypoparathyroidism, which is caused by a lack of response by target organs to parathyroid hormone. It presents like hypoparathyroidism with decreased calcium levels and increased phosphate levels, but the parathyroid hormone level is normal or elevated because the parathyroid gland continues to secrete hormone in response to low calcium levels.

Drug Exposures

Cocaine is the most common in utero drug exposure that can cause increased jitteriness in the newborn. Fifty to 59% of babies exposed to cocaine in utero display jitteriness in contrast to the 44% of unexposed infants.[23,28,29] In 1998, 2.8% of pregnant mothers used illicit drugs during their pregnancy with one-tenth of them using cocaine. Cocaine crosses the placenta and causes an increase in catecholamine levels in the developing fetus.[29] Elevated catecholamines alone are known to cause jitteriness.[30] Cocaine also causes vaso-oclusive changes contributing to fetal hypoxia and possible brain injury.[29-31] This leads to dysregulation of autonomic control and jitteriness. Maternal cocaine use increases the likelihood of spontaneous abortion or prematurity secondary to placental abruption from cocaine-induced constriction of the uterine arteries. They are more likely to be low birth weight and IUGR infants, with an increased risk for congenital brain malformations, intracranial hemorrhages, intestinal complications such as necrotizing enterocholitis, limb malformations, infections, and microcephaly.[6,29,30] They generally display poor feeding, sleep disturbances, difficulty with arousal modulation, and hypertonia in addition to a course tremor. Diagnosis is made by a positive urine toxicology screen from either the mother or the baby. Treatment is simply supportive care and developmental assistance in addition to treatment for other conditions caused by the maternal cocaine abuse.

Marijuana exposure in utero also causes jitteriness.[21,23] These babies show an increased startle response and a decreased visual response to stimulation in addition to the underlying tremor. This increased response may not appear directly after birth because of the effects of general anesthesia used during delivery, therefore a new tremor may begin only after discharge home. Babies exposed to alcohol or tobacco in utero will not display an increased tremor.[23] As marijuana is not thought to cause long-term effects on the newborn, these mothers may continue to breastfeed.[6]

Selective serotonin reuptake inhibitors (SSRIs) are another increasingly more common in utero drug exposure causing increased jitteriness. Depression affects 10-20% of pregnant mothers,[32] with 35% of these patients using medication during their pregnancy.[32,33] An increasing number of pregnant women are taking SSRIs for their favorable safety profile during pregnancy. These medicines work by inhibiting the reuptake of serotonin at the presynaptic junction. They cross the placenta and cause an increase in the serotonin levels in the fetus possibly causing jitteriness. They also have impaired behavioral state regulation, spend increased time in REM sleep, have increased autonomic dysregulation, and display increased motor activity. Further studies are being done on the safety profile of SSRIs during pregnancy as these new finding become clear. In a jittery baby whose mother was using SSRIs during her pregnancy, and who have a normal glucose and a negative urine toxicology screen, it may be assumed that the medications caused the jitteriness and only supportive care and education is needed. At this time, SSRIs are considered safe in breastfeeding.

Drug withdrawal also causes jitteriness in neonates.[21,34] Neonatal abstinence syndrome may occur after in utero exposure to opiates or benzodiazepine. These infants display tremors, hypertonia, increased high-pitched crying, irritability, yawning, sneezing, stuffiness, vomiting, diarrhea, poor sucking ability, and even seizures. Symptoms usually occur within hours of delivery. Many mothers are enrolled in a methadone program during their pregnancy. While helping mothers to wean off of their opiate addiction, this drug still leads to withdrawal symptoms in 60% to 80% of their babies.[23,34] As methadone has a longer half-life, symptoms will not appear until 24 to 48 hours after delivery. Infants exposed to narcotics will develop symptoms within 4 days of birth in 96% of cases.[6] If the drug was taken closer to delivery, symptoms will be delayed. Most hospitals use a neonatal abstinence scoring system to monitor severity of symptoms and guide treatment. Patients with mild symptoms, and therefore a lower score, need only supportive care in a low stimulus environment. The infants should be swaddled well and offered frequent, small, high calorie feedings. If symptoms progress, these infants need pharmacologic treatment to allow for adequate growth as the babies ability to feed declines and caloric need increases with increased tremors. Traditionally, these infants received paregoric, a mixture of alcohol, opium, benzoic acid, camphor, and glycerin. Morphine and methadone have become increasingly popular alternatives. Phenobarbital may be used with infants exposed to either multiple drugs or strictly benzodiazepines. The choice of medication often differs according to the practices of the treating institution. Generally, infants born to mothers known to use narcotics are monitored after until symptoms resolve or they require treatment. Once starting a medication, a weaning schedule can begin and the patients may be discharged home with a reliable caretaker. Symptoms may persist for 4 to 6 months with a mean treatment time of 17 days to several weeks.[34] Infants may breastfeed while their mother is on a methadone weaning schedule. If a neonate receiving treatment presents to the ED with increasing symptoms, the dose of the medication may need to be increased in consultation with the prescribing physician.[6,34]

HISTORY & PHYSICAL EXAMINATION

The differential diagnosis of pathologic jitteriness in a neonate focuses on a few broad categories making finding a possible cause relatively simple. A few aspects of the history will provide clues as to the necessity of a full work-up. A description of the actual tremor, including the baby's level of alertness, whether it occurs while the infant is awake or asleep, or if the tremor changes with stimulation, helps determine if this is a pathologic cause of jitteriness, as previously discussed. Any changes in temperature or possible signs of sepsis should alert the physician to an infections etiology. A birth history of prematurity, perinatal asphyxia, intracranial hemorrhage, IUGR, or maternal diabetes may signify an underlying disorder.[22] Any medications used by the mother, both during the pregnancy and currently being during mother breastfeeding, should be discussed. A complete feeding history will also provide important information.

The physical examination will also help determine if the jitteriness deserves further evaluation. As mentioned, jitteriness in a crying or startled baby is reassuring. Jitteriness while the baby is asleep or alert and quiet demands further evaluation. Normal eye movements with the infant focused and tracking appropriately also offers reassurance. The sucking-stimulus test may help to differentiate those with tremors from an underlying etiology.[22] A gloved finger placed in the infant's mouth should instantly cause the tremor to stop in patients with a nonpathologic cause of jitteriness. The tremor should resume after withdrawal of the finger from the patient's mouth. In patients in whom the tremor continues while the infant sucks on the finger, an underlying cause of jitteriness should be investigated.[31] A complete neurologic exam should also be completed.

MANAGEMENT

The management in the ED of the jittery neonate begins by ruling out severe, life-threatening illness. With any deviance of temperature from normal—either too high or too low—or any other signs of infection, a full sepsis work-up needs to begin. Next, a bedside glucose level should be obtained. If the glucose falls between 40 and 60 mg/dL in an alert and active infant, give an oral challenge of either formula or breast milk. The glucose should be checked again within 30 min for normalization. If the glucose does not improve to a level over 60, the baby cannot tolerate feeds, or initially falls below 40 mg/dL, an IV dose of .5 g/kg dextrose should be given. An infant generally cannot tolerate concentrated glucose formulations without central access as their small veins easily sclerose. Therefore, 4-5 cc/kg of 10% glucose solution should be given to meet the correct dosage. Again, the glucose should be rechecked in 30 min for resolution. A maintenance dose of 5-7 mg/kg/min should be given to maintain a constant glucose level. If the infant does not display signs of formula intolerance, vomiting, or dehydration as the source of hypoglycemia, an inborn error of metabolism should be suspected and the appropriate work-up begun.

If hypoglycemia is not found to be the cause of neonatal jitteriness and the history and physical examination do not suggest another cause, test the electrolytes, specifically looking for hypocalcemia. Ionized calcium should be tested in addition to a serum calcium level, as this may be falsely decreased secondary to hypoalbuminemia or changes in acid-base status. Symptomatic infants should be treated with 10% calcium gluconate, 100 mg/kg infused over 5 to 10 min. Calcium chloride 20 mg/kg may also be given. Use extreme caution in giving these in a peripheral IV as they can cause tissue necrosis after extravasation. They should never be infused through a scalp vein. If the calcium levels do not improve, give magnesium sulfate 25-50 mg/kg.[25] If the infant needs IV treatment for symptom control, they should be admitted for a complete work-up for hypocalcemia and referred to an endocrinologist.

If the history suggests an in utero drug exposure or drug withdrawal, the safety of the patient returning home needs evaluation. If the severity of the jitteriness prevents the infant from taking in enough calories for adequate growth, the patient needs to be admitted for growth monitoring and possibly medical treatment. The social situation of the infant should also be assessed. If it is deemed unsafe for the infant to return home, or the mother feels overwhelmed by an irritable baby, a short admission may be in order. However, as discussed, most infants will simply display normal, physiologic jitteriness. After ruling out all pathologic causes, reassure the parents that their infant displays normal behavior. As these babies have been shown to be more visually inattentive, and therefore less interactive and difficult to console, parental education becomes important to prevent frustration and facilitate bonding. Prompt follow-up with their primary physician should offer further reassurance and education and ensure appropriate resolution of symptoms.

▶ NEONATAL SEIZURES

Seizure is the most common neurologic emergency presenting to the ED during the neonatal period.[2] Of term newborns, 0.2% to 1.4 % present with seizures and 10% to 20% of premature babies experience a seizure.[35-37] Unlike a first seizure in older children, a new-onset seizure during the neonatal period is almost always associated with significant illness or underlying brain pathology, and, therefore, always deserves prompt work-up and intervention.[35-37]

Given that neonatal seizures have an underlying etiology, they must quickly be recognized and treated. Overall mortality of neonates with a seizure is as high as 15% in term infants with 2/3 developing sequelae such as mental retardation, cerebral palsy, and epilepsy. Prognosis ultimately depends upon the underlying etiology. Metabolic, subarachnoid hemorrhage, hypocalcemia, and familial disorders generally have a better prognosis, whereas patients with HIE, CNS malformations, and massive intracranial bleeds tend to fare poorly.[35,36] Ongoing or prolonged seizures lead to synaptic reorganization, cell death, a decrease in plasticity, and a predisposition to further seizures.[37] These infants become predisposed to cognitive, behavioral, and epileptic complications with 5.3 times the possibility of having mental retardation and 50 to 70 times the risk of developing cerebral palsy.[36]

The infant brain's structure and development makes it more susceptible to seizures not common in older children.[2,37,38] At delivery, the neonatal brain is still in the process of achieving cortical organization. The neonatal brain has relatively increased excitatory synapses and is still in the process of developing many inhibitory structures, such as the substantia nigra, making the seizure threshold much lower. The infant's brainstem and diencephalon are relatively more developed than the cortical structures, leading to distinctly unique seizure types.

HISTORY & PHYSICAL EXAMINATION

The neonate rarely presents with a generalized tonic-clonic seizure due to several differences in brain structure and development of the infant's brain when compared to the older child[2,35,38] (Table 2–8). The most common neonatal seizure is a clonic seizure. These are slow, rhythmic jerking movements of the facial, extremity, and axial musculature. It occasionally migrates but, due to the immature, disorganized brain, always migrates in a non-Jacksonian manner.[2] Tonic seizures consist of sustained posturing of either a single limb or, less often, of both of the upper and lower extremities. These occur much less

▶ **TABLE 2–8. SEIZURE TYPES**

Clonic	Most common
	Slow, rhythmic jerking
	Always non-Jacksonian
Tonic	Sustained posturing
	Involves either single limb or generalized
Myoclonic	Rapid jerking
	Flexor muscles
Subtle	Oral-buccal-lingual (lip smacking, chewing)
	Ocular movements (eye deviation, sustained eye opening)
	Autonomic dysfunction
	Stereotypical movements (pedaling, swimming, stepping)

frequently than they do in older children. Myoclonic seizures present as rapid jerks or twitches, mostly of the flexor muscle groups. When occurring during sleep or as isolated episodes upon waking, they are considered a benign occurrence. Lastly, infants may present with subtle seizures. These may include oral-buccal-lingual movements, ocular movements, autonomic dysfunction, or stereotypical movements.[38] Apnea may also rarely be attributable to a seizure, but only in the presence of other seizure movements. Many of these movements may occur in a normal neonate and should only be considered seizures if the movement does not respond to stimulus or involves an abnormal eye movement or autonomic symptoms.

DIFFERENTIAL DIAGNOSIS

Perinatal Asphyxia & Hypoxic-Ischemic Encephalopathy (HIE)

Perinatal asphyxia leading to HIE is the most common cause of neonatal seizures,[35] accounting for 2/3 of neonatal seizures. Most present within the first 24 hours of life with

60% occurring in the first 12 hours[2] making this an unusual cause for seizures seen in the ED. However, the anoxic event may occur at any time during gestation, and if the hypoxic insult occurred early in gestation, the infant may remain asymptomatic until a later time.[35] Risk factors for HIE include prolonged labor, fetal bradycardia, late decelerations, meconium staining, an APGAR score less than 6 at 1 and 5 minutes, and neonatal resuscitation. During the first few days of life, newborns with HIE will have acute encephalopathy with decreased level of consciousness, poor tone, difficulty feeding, apneas, and seizures. They often require ventilator support and close monitoring as the hypoxic event also can lead to multi-organ dysfunction. These infants slowly recover function over the next few days and weeks, but 15% to 30% will have long-term CNS dysfunction such as mental retardation, and motor and developmental delay. They are 2 to 5 times more likely to develop seizures than normal infants. These seizures will present as a variety of types, but commonly are focal secondary to focal areas of injury. Often, these are difficult to control with medication with overt status possible.[35] The seizures often are severe and occur frequently. Hypoxic ischemic encephalopathy in the setting of status epilepticus has a much worse prognosis that hypoxic ischemia alone.[37] A CT of the head may show areas of infarct or cerebral atrophy if the insult occurred early in utero.

Infections

Five to 10% of neonatal seizures occur secondary to intracranial infections or sepsis.[2,35,37,38] Seizures caused by bacterial infections usually occur toward the end of the 1st week of life. Nonbacterial TORCH infections may also present with seizures. Toxoplasmosis and congenital rubella will present around the 3rd day of life along with other related symptoms. Coxsackie and cytomegalovirus (CMV) also cause seizures.[2] Herpes simplex virus (HSV) usually presents after the 1st week with either seizures or encephalopathy. Have a strong suspicion for HSV in any neonate with seizure.[39] For any neonate presenting with a possible infection, a spinal tap needs to be done and appropriate antibiotics started. Acyclovir should be added if symptoms such as a vesicular rash, maternal history for HSV (although most cases of congenital HSV infection occur during the mothers primary, asymptomatic infection), or an increased spinal fluid WBC count without any findings on gram stain exist. A plasma clearance rate for HSV may be tested.

Electrolyte Abnormalities

Many electrolyte abnormalities cause neonatal seizures.[2,35-38] These occur after the first day of life after maternal regulation of electrolytes ceases. Abnormalities of sodium levels may cause seizures. Hyponatremia may result from water intoxication. A complete feeding history needs to be taken. Formula or breast milk will provide adequate free water, and a neonate should never receive supplemental fluids, even in states of dehydration. Specifically ask about teas, juices, or water that the infant receives. Specifically ask how the formula is mixed, possibly having the parents demonstrate how they prepare the formula. Other disorders such as syndrome of inappropriate antidiuretic hormone secretion (SIADH), CF, profuse diarrhea, and malabsorption may cause derangements in sodium levels. Adrenal or pituitary disorders such as congenital adrenal hypoplasia can also cause changes in sodium. Hypoglycemia can cause seizures. Infants who are LGA, SGA, or born to diabetic mothers have a higher likelihood of hypoglycemia. These infants may present with jitteriness, hypotonia, and apnea, in addition to seizures. Infants with gastroenteritis or other causes of feeding intolerance can also be hypoglycemic. Inborn errors of metabolism or endocrine disorders are also rarely found to be causes of persistent hypoglycemia. A bedside glucose level quickly offers both diagnosis and treatment for the seizure. Hypocalcemia should also be considered as a cause of seizures. These infants usually present with a focal seizure (Volpe) and often have accompanying jitteriness and neuromuscular irritability. Both hypoglycemia and hypocalcemia are more completely discussed in the section on neonatal jitteriness.

Metabolic Disorders

Inborn errors of metabolism are a set of rare causes of metabolic derangements leading to neurological sequelae and seizures.[2,35-38] Over 400 inborn errors of metabolism exist with more being discovered.[40] These autosomal recessive, single gene defects lead to decreased or absent activity of a particular enzyme causing either accumulation of a toxic metabolite or a decrease in an important metabolic end product.[41] Most of these patients are well at birth and present within the first 2 to 3 days as the toxic metabolites have a chance to build within the infant's system or with a sudden deterioration secondary to a stressor such as sepsis or gastroenteritis. These patients will display early signs of encephalopathy such as poor feeding, irritability, vomiting, poor weight gain, hypotonia, tachypnea, or tachycardia. Some parents may have noticed a strange odor such as sweet smelling urine (maple syrup urine disease) or sweaty feet (isovoleric academia). Some disorders will have characteristic dysmorphic features.

As the illness progresses, these neonates display persistent hypoglycemia, acidosis, dehydration, hypoperfusion, apnea, lethargy, arrhythmias, liver dysfunction, or seizures. A family history of affected siblings, consanguinity, developmental delay, mental retardation, or unexplained sudden perinatal death should alert the physician to underlying inborn errors of metabolism. Often, these babies are immediately assumed to be septic, and a diagnosis of inborn errors of metabolism fails to be considered.

The first priority with inborn errors of metabolism is to treat the seizures, as discussed at the end of this section. Quick laboratory evaluation can lead to both the diagnosis of the disorder and provide the means to treat the seizure. Nonspecific laboratory exams will point toward particular inborn errors of metabolism. Often, these infants present with persistent, recurrent hypoglycemia from a defect in carbohydrate metabolism or fatty acid oxidation within the first 48 to 72 hours of life.[40] Others present with metabolic acidosis from organic acidemias or pyruvate oxidation defects. All states perform newborn screening on all babies but each state tests for a different number of disorders. However, many infants present before the results become available, and many more inborn errors of metabolism exist than are tested for. Glucose, electrolytes, ammonia, lactate, liver function tests, and serum amino acid levels along with urine glucose and ketones should be sent in the initial evaluation for inborn errors of metabolism. These infants will likely need admission for further treatment and extensive workup.[40,41]

Intracranial Hemorrhage

Intracranial hemorrhage also causes seizures in neonates.[2,35,37,38] This occurs more frequently in premature infants in the form of intraventricular hemorrhage, but is possible for a variety of reasons in the term neonate. Infants with intracranial hemorrhage usually present with lethargy, altered mental status, vomiting, and seizures. They may be unresponsive and apneic with no history of any inciting event. Although rare, birth trauma can cause parenchymal bleeding and occasionally intraventricular hemorrhage. A more common etiology is nonaccidental trauma. A direct blow to the head or shaken baby syndrome can cause subarachnoid hemorrhage, subdural hemorrhage, and multiple skull fractures. Often, the infant presents with no visible signs of trauma, so any intracranial hemorrhage should raise suspicion for abuse, and a skeletal survey and referral to ophthalmology to document retinal hemorrhages should quickly proceed. Hemorrhagic disease of the newborn can also cause intracranial bleeding. This occurs after home births when vitamin K is not administered after delivery. These infants present with mucosal bleeding from the nose, GI tract, and circumcision site, in addition to intracranial hemorrhage.

Congenital Brain Malformations

Congenital brain malformations also present with neonatal seizures.[2,35,37,38] These may occur any time after birth. The seizure type is unpredictable with a variable presentation. These patients may have dysmorphic features or microcephaly according to their underlying disorder. Several disorders, such as tuberous sclerosis or neurofibromatosis, will have cutaneous findings. A CT of the head is a useful screening tool in the ED looking for gross malformations. Likely, the neonate will need an MRI in the future to look for more subtle findings.

Pyridoxine Deficiency

Pyridoxine deficiency is a rare cause of neonatal seizures, occurring in only 1 of 400,000 to 750,000 infants,[2,35,36,42,43] but is important to remember because it is easily treatable. An autosomal recessive defect in pyridoxine metabolism leads to decreased GABA synthesis, an important inhibitory neurotransmitter. The mother may report episodic, recurrent staccato movements during the pregnancy, often thought to be hiccups. Usually within hours of delivery, the infant presents with a variety of different seizure types. These infants may be encephalopathic with temperature instability, vomiting, respiratory distress, and metabolic acidosis. They appear agitated and hyperexcitable. Traditional seizure medications will have no effect. Any neonate continuing to seize

after receiving a complete course of antiseizure medication deserves a trial of pyridoxine. Diagnosis is traditionally made when seizure activity on EEG monitoring stops after receiving an IV dose of pyridoxine. However, many patients require several weeks of oral pyridoxine before complete resolution. Pyridoxine can cause respiratory and neurologic depression, so close monitoring for several days is required.

Benign Idiopathic Neonatal Convulsions

Several seizure or seizure-like conditions with no long-term sequelae or developmental issues exist.[2] Benign idiopathic neonatal convulsions,[2,38] or the "fifth day fits," present as focal clonic or occasionally tonic self-limited seizures each lasting 1 to 3 min. Eighty to 90% of these will occur on the 4th through 6th day and may recur over the next 24 to 48 hours. Between seizures, the infant has a normal neurologic examination. The diagnosis can only be made in term infants with an uneventful antenatal history, normal APGARs, no family history of seizure disorders, and after a full work-up yields no other etiologies. These infants subsequently develop normally with no increased incidence of seizures or developmental delay.

Benign familial neonatal seizures[2,38] are a similar disorder presenting during the first week of life with 10 to 20 seizures per day with normal interictal periods (Volpe). Again, all diagnostic studies must remain negative. This is an autosomal dominant disorder with variable penetrance. The seizures generally cease by 3 to 6 months of age with an 11% to 16% chance of these patients developing a seizure disorder later in life but otherwise normal development. Benign neonatal sleep myoclonus[2,44] occurs in the first week of life with either bilateral or unilateral myoclonus of both the upper and lower extremities occurring only during active sleep. It persists for approximately 2 months with no sequelae. Hyperkerkplexia[2] or "stiff-man syndrome" is an exaggerated startle response. These infants have an abnormal response to both auditory and visual stimuli with a sustained tonic spasm. These patients may progress to apnea, bradycardia, and even death during an episode. This disorder will respond to benzodiazepines, and all patients will outgrow it by 2 years of age.

DIAGNOSTIC TESTS

Laboratory studies should cast a broad net in order to exclude all possible causes of neonatal seizures.[45] Complete a sepsis workup with a CBC, urinalysis and urine culture, and spinal tap and begin appropriate antibiotics as meningitis has significant morbidity and mortality if not diagnosed and treated promptly. In addition to culture of the spinal fluid, also perform studies for HSV, as this may present as seizure in the 1st months of life. Electrolytes, if not already obtained, need to be checked along with the acid-base status of the patient. A urine toxicology screen may be useful if there are findings of concern on history or physical examination. Send serum amino acids, lactate, and ammonia for the diagnosis of an inborn error of metabolism.[40] Neonates with seizure need a screening CT of the head to discover hemorrhage, intracranial calcifications secondary to TORCH infection, a late infarct, or gross brain abnormalities.[38] An MRI may be more useful in diagnosing more subtle brain abnormalities, but as this study is often difficult to obtain in a timely manner and requires sedation, evaluation may begin with a MRI obtained after the patient is admitted for further evaluation.[38]

MANAGEMENT

Treatment should focus on the acute, rapid treatment of the seizure and then identification

▶ **TABLE 2-9. TREATMENT OF NEONATAL SEIZURES**

ABCs: Ensure airway, IV access, cardiac monitoring
If hypoglycemic: Glucose 10% 4 mL/kg IV, then appropriate maintenance fluids
If hypocalcemia: Calcium gluconate 10% 4 mL/kg IV
Phenobarbital: 20 mg/kg IV given over 1-2 mg/kg/min, may repeat up to 40 mg/kg
Phenytoin: 20 mg/kg IV given over 1 mg/g/min
Lorazepam: .05-.1 mg/kg IV, may be repeated up to .15 mg/kg
Pyridoxine: 100 mg IV, may be repeated up to total 500 mg

of the underlying etiology[2,35,37] (Table 2-9). The first priority when treating a seizing neonate is to secure adequate ventilation and perfusion. While evaluating and securing the airway, obtain IV or intraosseous access and check a quick bedside glucose level. Blood should also immediately be sent for electrolytes—specifically sodium, calcium, and magnesium. If the infant is hypoglycemic, give a quick bolus of 2-4 mL/kg of a 10% glucose solution to deliver .5 g/kg. This should be followed by 5-7 mg/kg/min of maintenance glucose after the initial correction. Remember that an infant's small veins are easily sclerosed, so use nothing with a higher concentration of glucose than 10% through a peripheral IV. Treat other electrolyte abnormalities as they become known.

The first line of therapy for a neonatal seizure is phenobarbital.[36,37] An IV loading dose of 20 mg/kg given at a rate of 1-2 mg/min should raise the serum levels to within the therapeutic range of 20-40 mg/L. The dose may be repeated up to 40 mg/kg if no response. If IV access is difficult to obtain, this drug may be given IM. This drug may cause apnea and hypotension, so ensure close cardiovascular monitoring with resuscitation equipment available. Some controversy surrounds this medication as only 1/3 to 1/2 of infants will actually respond, with a better response in neonates not in status epilepticus and with mild to moderate background EEG abnormalities.[37] Babies responding to phenobarbital generally have a better prognosis than babies that require further therapy.[37] Phenobarbital may also offer a false reassurance as it causes an electrical dissociation so that the seizure will appear to stop when, in reality, the infant is only sedated and has underlying EEG abnormalities.

The next line of therapy if phenobarbital fails is phenytoin.[36,37] This is given IV as a 15 to 20 mg/kg dose over 1-2 mg/min. It may not be given IM as it causes tissue necrosis. As a first-line agent, approximately 45% of neonates respond.[46] However, its side effect profile of hypotension and cardiac arrhythmias secondary to the propylene glycol diluents make this the second-line therapy in neonates. Fosphenytoin at a dose of 30 mg/kg IV or IM is becoming more popular in the treatment of neonatal seizures due to its better safety profile.

Benzodiazepines, while the mainstay of treatment in older children and adults, are the third line of therapy in neonates.[36,37] If the infant continues to seize, give lorazepam .05-.1 mg/kg IV over 2 to 5 min. This may be repeated up to a total dose of .15 mg/kg. Diazepam has also been used at .25 mg/kg over 2 to 5 minutes. This may be an excellent choice either in the field by EMS or when an IV cannot be promptly obtained as rectal dosing at .5 mg/kg offers seizure control. Remembered that all of these medications can cause respiratory depression and the infant needs close monitoring. For seizures refractory to the above treatments with no other underlying cause, give pyridoxine. Administer an initial loading dose of 100 mg IV and repeat up to a total of 500 mg. Traditionally, only one dose was attempted in refractory seizures and the diagnosis made if the infant acutely responded with cessation of seizures with EEG monitoring. However, some infants will not respond to the first dose and require up to several weeks of oral treatment with 5 mg/kg/day of oral pyridoxine.

Once the acute seizure desists, a diligent work-up is necessary as neonatal seizures are rarely idiopathic. Often the timing of the seizure can give clues as to the etiology (Table 2–10).[35] The history should cover pregnancy, including maternal infections, substance abuse, and medications, labor and delivery, and the initial hospital course. Current issues such as feeding, including what the infant eats and how it is prepared, sleep patterns, level of alertness, and activity, should be assessed. Family history of seizures should be covered. Any signs of infection should immediately prompt a

► TABLE 2–10. **TIMING OF PRESENTATION**

Days 1 and 2	Days 2 to 4	Day 4 to 6 Months
Infection	Infection	Infection
Intracranial hemorrhage	Hypoglycemia	Hypocalcaemia
Hypoxia	Inborn errors of metabolism	Hyponatremia
Hypoglycemia	Drug withdrawal	Hypernatremia
Hypocalcaemia	Cerebral malformation	Inborn errors of metabolism
Cerebral malformations	Trauma	Cerebral malformation
Trauma	Neonatal epilepsy syndromes	Neonatal epilepsy syndromes
Pyridoxine deficiency		

Source: From Ref. 35.

suspicion for sepsis. Any history of neuromuscular instability should be noted. The mother may have noticed a strange smell or taste to the child. The physical examination, in addition to a complete neurologic examination, should include looking for any signs of brain malformations such as dysmorphic features. A bruit auscultated through the anterior fontanelle represents an arterial-venous malformation. Any signs of trauma in a neonate are abnormal and need further investigation. Cutaneous findings such as café au lait spots, herpetic vesicles, or ash leaf spots may also suggest a particular syndrome.

REFERENCES

1. Lowe MC, Jr, Woolridge DP. The normal newborn exam, or is it? *Emerg Med Clin North Am.* 2007;25:921-946, v.
2. Volpe JJ. *Neurology of the Newborn.* 3rd ed. Philadelphia, PA: W.B. Saunders Company; 1995.
3. Hamrick SE, Miller SP, Leonard C, et al. Trends in severe brain injury and neurodevelopmental outcome in premature newborn infants: the role of cystic periventricular leukomalacia. *J Pediatr.* 2004;145:593-599.
4. Futagi Y, Toribe Y, Ogawa K, Suzuki Y. Neurodevelopmental outcome in children with intraventricular hemorrhage. *Pediatr Neurol.* 2006;34:219-224.
5. Bassan H, Limperopoulos C, Visconti K, et al. Neurodevelopmental outcome in survivors of periventricular hemorrhagic infarction. *Pediatrics.* 2007;120:785-792.
6. Thureen PJ, ed. *Assessment and Care of the Well Newborn.* 1st ed. W.B. Saunders Company; 1999.
7. Herman M, Le A. The crying infant. *Emerg Med Clin North Am.* 2007;25:1137-1159, vii.
8. Poole SR. The infant with acute, unexplained, excessive crying. *Pediatrics.* 1991;88:450-455.
9. Brazelton TB. Crying in infancy. *Pediatrics.* 1962;29:579-588.
10. Reijneveld SA, van der Wal MF, Brugman E, Sing RA, Verloove-Vanhorick SP. Infant crying and abuse. *Lancet.* 2004;364:1340-1342.
11. Richer LP, Shevell MI, Miller SP. Diagnostic profile of neonatal hypotonia: an 11-year study. *Pediatr Neurol.* 2001;25:32-37.
12. Paro-Panjan D, Neubauer D. Congenital hypotonia: Is there an algorithm? *J Child Neurol.* 2004;19:439-442.
13. Howell RR, Byrne B, Darras BT, Kishnani P, Nicolino M, van der Ploeg A. Diagnostic challenges for pompe disease: an under-recognized cause of floppy baby syndrome. *Genet Med.* 2006;8:289-296.
14. Stiefel L. Hypotonia in infants. *Pediatr Rev.* 1996;17:104-105.
15. Crawford TO. Clinical evaluation of the floppy infant. *Pediatr Ann.* 1992;21:348-354.
16. Birdi K, Prasad AN, Prasad C, Chodirker B, Chudley AE. The floppy infant: retrospective analysis of clinical experience (1990-2000) in a tertiary care facility. *J Child Neurol.* 2005;20:803-808.
17. Prasad AN, Prasad C. The floppy infant: contribution of genetic and metabolic disorders. *Brain Dev.* 2003;25:457-476.
18. Clemmens MR, Bell L. Infant botulism presenting with poor feeding and lethargy: a review of 4 cases. *Pediatr Emerg Care.* 2007;23:492-494.
19. Cox N, Hinkle R. Infant botulism. *Am Fam Physician.* 2002;65:1388-1392.
20. Committee on Infectious Diseases, AAP. *Red Book: 2006 Report of the Committee on Infectious Diseases.* 27th ed. USA: American Academy of Pediatrics; 2006.
21. Uddin MK, Rodnitzky RL. Tremor in children. *Semin Pediatr Neurol.* 2003;10:26-34.
22. Armentrout DC, Caple J. The jittery newborn. *J Pediatr Health Care.* 2001;15:147-149.
23. Parker S, Zuckerman B, Bauchner H, Frank D, Vinci R, Cabral H. Jitteriness in full-term neonates: Prevalence and correlates. *Pediatrics.* 1990;85:17-23.
24. Rosman NP, Donnelly JH, Braun MA. The jittery newborn and infant: a review. *J Dev Behav Pediatr.* 1984;5:263-273.
25. Haynes S. A neonate with persistent twitching. patient report. *Clin Pediatr (Phila).* 2007;46:458-459.
26. Donati-Genet PC, Ramelli GP, Bianchetti MG. A newborn infant of a diabetic mother with refractory hypocalcaemic convulsions. *Eur J Pediatr.* 2004;163:759-760.

27. Manzar S. Transient pseudohypoparathyroidism and neonatal seizure. *J Trop Pediatr.* 2001;47:113-114.

28. Ebrahim SH, Gfroerer J. Pregnancy-related substance use in the united states during 1996-1998. *Obstet Gynecol.* 2003;101:374-379.

29. Singer LT, Arendt R, Minnes S, Farkas K, Salvator A. Neurobehavioral outcomes of cocaine-exposed infants. *Neurotoxicol Teratol.* 2000;22:653-666.

30. Bauer CR, Langer JC, Shankaran S, et al. Acute neonatal effects of cocaine exposure during pregnancy. *Arch Pediatr Adolesc Med.* 2005;159:824-834.

31. Sims M, Artal R, Quach H, Wu PY. Neonatal jitteriness of unknown origin and circulating catecholamines. *J Perinat Med.* 1986;14:123-126.

32. Santos RP, Pergolizzi JJ. Transient neonatal jitteriness due to maternal use of sertraline (zoloft). *J Perinatol.* 2004;24:392-394.

33. Zeskind PS, Stephens LE. Maternal selective serotonin reuptake inhibitor use during pregnancy and newborn neurobehavior. *Pediatrics.* 2004;113:368-375.

34. Ebner N, Rohrmeister K, Winklbaur B, et al. Management of neonatal abstinence syndrome in neonates born to opioid maintained women. *Drug Alcohol Depend.* 2007;87:131-138.

35. Hill A. Neonatal seizures. *Pediatr Rev.* 2000; 21:117-121; quiz 121.

36. Wirrell EC. Neonatal seizures: To treat or not to treat? *Semin Pediatr Neurol.* 2005;12:97-105.

37. Rennie JM, Boylan GB. Neonatal seizures and their treatment. *Curr Opin Neurol.* 2003;16:177-181.

38. Mizrah EM. Neonatal seizures and neonatal epileptic syndromes. *Neurol Clin.* 2001;19:427-463.

39. Young Infants Clinical Signs Study Group. Clinical signs that predict severe illness in children under age 2 months: a multicentre study. *Lancet.* 2008;371:135-142.

40. Colletti JE, Homme JL, Woodridge DP. Unsuspected neonatal killers in emergency medicine. *Emerg Med Clin North Am.* 2004;22:929-960.

41. Burton BK. Inborn errors of metabolism in infancy: A guide to diagnosis. *Pediatrics.* 1998;102:E69.

42. Gospe SM, Jr. Pyridoxine-dependent seizures: new genetic and biochemical clues to help with diagnosis and treatment. *Curr Opin Neurol.* 2006;19:148-153.

43. Gospe SM, Jr. Current perspectives on pyridoxine-dependent seizures. *J Pediatr.* 1998;132:919-923.

44. Paro-Panjan D, Neubauer D. Benign neonatal sleep myoclonus: experience from the study of 38 infants. *Eur J Paediatr Neurol.* 2008;12:14-18.

45. Scarfone RJ, Pond K, Thompson K, Fall I. Utility of laboratory testing for infants with seizures. *Pediatr Emerg Care.* 2000;16:309-312.

46. Painter MJ, Scher MS, Stein AD, et al. Phenobarbital compared with phenytoin for the treatment of neonatal seizures. *N Engl J Med.* 1999;341:485-489.

CHAPTER 3

Respiratory Emergencies

Jennifer Mackey, MD

▶ NORMAL LUNG DEVELOPMENT

In utero, the fetal lungs are filled with fluid and gas exchange occurs via the placenta. Fetal lung fluid and fetal breathing movements are two important factors in the development of healthy newborn lungs.[1] There are 5 stages of lung development; embryonic, pseudoglandular, canalicular, saccular, and alveolar.[1] The alveolar stage continues up to 2 years of age where the alveoli are continuing to septate and multiply.[2] Lung development continues into young adulthood with enlargement of the terminal bronchioles and alveoli. If there is an arrest in development in any one of the stages of development, congenital pulmonary diseases may result. For example, the failure of normal division of airway structures at the pseudoglandular stage may lead to pulmonary hypoplasia or sequestration, cystic adenomatoid malformation, and, crucially, failure of the pleuro-peritoneal membrane to close, which may result in congenital diaphragmatic hernia.[2] Preterm infants born during the time of surfactant production (the canalicular and saccular stages) have surfactant deficiency and chronic lung disease of prematurity. Surfactant decreases the surface tension of the alveoli and prevents alveolar collapse.

TRANSITION AT DELIVERY

In the term newborn, hormonal influences and chest wall squeeze during labor expel fluid from the lungs. Lack of chest compression during caesarian delivery predisposes the infant to the development of transitional delay and transient tachypnea. The first breaths open the alveoli, which should not collapse with adequate surfactant levels. The stretch on the type II pneumocytes stimulates surfactant production as well and pulmonary blood flow is increased. The combination of drying of the lung fluid and decreased pulmonary vascular resistance results in a well-oxygenated baby.

▶ NORMAL NEWBORN BREATHING

The normal neonatal respiratory rate is between 40 and 50 breaths per minute. Tachypnea would therefore be a respiratory rate greater than 60 breaths per minute. Many parents will be concerned about sneezing and nasal congestion, both of which are normal in newborns. It is typical for newborns to frequently sneeze, even without a respiratory infection. Due to their small nasal passages, newborns frequently sound congested. When evaluating a newborn with congestion, as long as the newborn does not have cyanotic episodes, poor feeding, or tachypnea, the congestion is benign and can be treated with saline nose drops and nasal suction.

Parents are frequently distressed by irregular breathing in their newborns and present with a chief complaint of "funny breathing." A good history and physical examination will help to decipher whether this breathing may be periodic breathing. Periodic breathing, due to a newborn's immature respiratory center, is a normal irregular breathing pattern. It typically involves faster breathing that is shallow and almost like panting followed by a slowing of the respiratory rate. Periodic breathing can also be associated with cessation of respiration but is not worrisome unless there is cyanosis, pallor, or decreased tone. A complete history and observation will ensure that the neonate does not have true apnea.

▶ ABNORMAL BREATHING

SIGNS OF RESPIRATORY DISTRESS

There are many clinical signs of respiratory distress in the neonate; tachypnea, grunting, wheezing, retractions, stridor, cough, and cyanosis are the most common. These signs may or may not indicate a respiratory etiology. For example, a neonate with tachypnea may have bronchiolitis, pneumonia, or exacerbation of bronchopulmonary dysplasia. Another neonate with tachypnea may be in shock and compensating for the associated acidosis. A wheezing neonate may have bronchiolitis or heart failure associated with pulmonary edema. It is, therefore, imperative that a complete history and physical examination be performed on all neonates with respiratory distress to aid in the correct diagnosis. Associated symptoms of respiratory distress include poor feeding, dehydration, and lethargy.

An initial approach to any neonate in respiratory distress must always begin with an evaluation of airway, breathing, and circulation. The neonate should be placed on a monitor to evaluate the cardiac rate and rhythm, respiratory rate, oxygenation, and blood pressure. Oxygen should be supplied as needed. Cyanosis may or may not be associated with respiratory distress. If oxygen fails to improve the hypoxemia, one must consider a cardiac etiology of the respiratory distress. The hyperoxia test can be helpful in this delineation as well as a cardiac examination, chest radiograph, and ECG. All neonates in respiratory distress should have a chest radiograph. When evaluating a neonatal chest radiograph, the thymus is expected to appear as a triangular- shaped mass in the right upper lung field. This is called a "sail sign" (Figure 3–1).

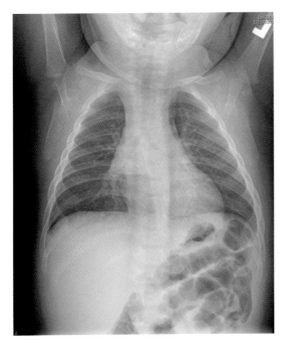

Figure 3–1. Normal neonatal chest x-ray demonstrating the thymic shadow ("the sail sign").

▶ APNEA

The definition of apnea is the cessation of airflow for 20 seconds or longer. This definition can be altered to include cessation of airflow of any length of time associated with cyanosis. Apnea must be differentiated from normal newborn breathing patterns including periodic breathing. There are three types of apnea: central, obstructive, and mixed.

1. *Central:* No airflow and no respiratory effort (no chest wall movement)
2. *Obstructive:* No airflow and respiratory effort (chest wall movement)
3. *Mixed:* Components of both central and obstructive

Apnea in the neonate should always be considered abnormal, and an etiology should be determined. The most common cause of apnea in the neonatal period is apnea of prematurity, which frequently persists beyond term gestation in infants delivered at 24 to 28 weeks of gestational age.[3] It is not uncommon to evaluate premature newborns in the emergency department (ED) whose parents report having the alarm sound on their home monitor, alerting parents of a potential problem. In that clinical scenario as well as in any evaluation of an apneic child, a complete history is crucial to be sure that the neonate was truly apneic. The parent should be able to recount what the child looked like during the alarm to exclude an inappropriate alarm. For example, if the newborn was pink during the alarm, this was likely a false alarm. Parents may be unable to accurately estimate the amount of time elapsed during breathing cessation. The presence of central cyanosis regardless of the time involved is true apnea.

CLINICAL MANIFESTATIONS

Many neonates in the first few days of life may have acrocyanosis, which is a benign finding. Acrocyanosis is a peripheral, as opposed to central, cyanosis that includes the hands and feet of the newborn and is caused by peripheral vasoconstriction and vascular instability. Central cyanosis refers to blue or purple discoloration of the tongue and lips, which indicates hypoxemia. Hypoxemia needs to be corrected promptly with supplemental oxygen and or assisted ventilation to prevent the development of bradycardia.

The differential diagnosis in the apneic neonate is vast; a thorough history can be helpful in determining the etiology. Fever or hypothermia may suggest an infectious etiology. Lip smacking, eye rolling, increased tone, or shaking of one or more extremity may suggest seizure as the etiology. For a complete list of causes of apnea in the neonate see Table 3–1. On physical examination close attention should be given toward the cardiopulmonary and neurologic systems.

▶ **TABLE 3-1 CAUSES OF NEONATAL APNEA**

Respiratory
  Viral illnesses
    Respiratory syncytial virus
    Adenovirus
    Influenza
    Parainfluenza
    Enteroviridae
    Rhinovirus
  Pertussis
  Pneumonia
  Congenital pulmonary lesions
    Congenital diaphragmatic hernia
    Cystic adenomatoid malformation

Cardiac
  Arrhythmias
  Congenital cyanotic heart defects
    Patent ductus arteriosus

Neurologic
  Hydrocephalous
    Meningitis/encephalitis
    Seizure
  Intracranial injury (abuse)
    Subdural/subarachnoid bleed
    Cerebral edema

Gastrointestinal
  Gastroesophageal reflux
  Aspiration

Hematologic
  Anemia

Metabolic
  Hyponatremia
  Hypoglycemia

DIAGNOSTIC TESTING

After a complete history and physical examination, and if the parent clearly has witnessed apnea or the clinican suspects apnea from the history, the following diagnostic tests may be helpful in determining a diagnosis: bedside dextrostick; basic electrolytes; complete blood count as hypoglycemia, electrolyte disturbances and anemia can cause apnea; and chest x-ray and ECG to evaluate for possible pneumonia, congenital pulmonary lesions, heart size, and rhythm disturbances.

Apnea can be a sole presentation of serious bacterial illness in the neonate; therefore, unless there is another clear reason for the apnea (eg, subdural hemorrhage in an abused infant, respiratory syncytial virus [RSV] bronchiolitis), a complete sepsis evaluation must be performed. A complete sepsis evaluation includes a complete blood count and differential, blood culture, urinalysis, urine Gram stain, urine culture, and spinal fluid studies and culture. Other studies to consider on a case-by-case basis would include a nasal wash for RSV and influenza especially between November and March, CT scan of the brain (suspected abuse, abnormal neurologic exam, or possible herpes encephalitis), and EEG. Further imaging such as an MRI of the brain may be needed during hospital admission if there is concern of seizure.

MANAGEMENT

Many patients seen in the ED will have apnea by history, and therefore continuous monitoring of the heart rate, respiratory rate, oximetry, and blood pressure are essential. If a neonate becomes apneic while in the ED, gentle stimulation may resolve the event. If stimulation does not induce spontaneous breathing then oxygen and bag mask ventilation should be used as needed. Intubation may be required for patients with recurrent apneic episodes, or one prolonged episode at discretion of the treating physician. Prompt correction of hypoxemia is essential as prolonged hypoxemia will cause bradycardia. For patients who develop bradycardia with a heart rate <60 beats per minute, cardiopulmonary resuscitation should be initiated. Neonates with apnea should be admitted to the hospital for observation and other diagnostics tests that may be indicated.

▶ TACHYPNEA

A respiratory rate greater than 60 breaths per minute in a neonate is considered tachypnea, or fast breathing. Tachypnea can be caused by respiratory and nonrespiratory etiologies. Nonrespiratory etiologies of tachypnea broadly include metabolic, cardiac, neurologic, or infectious causes. Always consider sepsis as a cause of tachypnea. Tachypnea is a sign of respiratory distress, and may or may not be associated with cyanosis. Retractions, or use of accessory muscles of respiration, may be associated with tachypnea. The respiratory causes of tachypnea can be parenchymal or nonparenchymal. In the evaluation of a tachypneic neonate, adventitious breath sounds are diagnostically helpful.

The tachypneic, wheezing neonate may have bronchiolitis; if the infant was premature and has a history of bronchopulmonary dysplasia with the same presentation, the episode may be an exacerbation of the existing chronic respiratory disease. Tachypnea and wheezing may allude to a cardiac diagnosis; palpate for an enlarged liver and listen for a murmur to exclude heart failure and myocarditis. For a complete list of causes of neonatal tachypnea, see Table 3–2. All neonates with tachypnea should have a chest radiograph to assist in diagnosis.

▶ WHEEZING

Wheezing is a musical noise heard on expiration that indicates a lower airway obstruction. A lower airway obstruction can be caused by bronchoconstriction, edema, or airway compression. Keep in mind that if the obstruction is severe and air entry is minimal, one may not hear wheezing; a prolonged expiratory phase may be heard instead. Neonates have very compliant chest walls due to their cartilaginous rib cage and, therefore, the use of accessory muscles can be dramatic on examination. Retractions of the supraclavicular, suprasternal, intercostals, subcostal, and subxiphoid areas all indicate increased work of breathing. Head bobbing can be seen when neonates use accessory muscles in the neck. Wheezing is associated with tachypnea. The most common causes of wheezing in the neonate are bronchiolitis and bronchopulmonary dysplasia in those that were premature.

▶ BRONCHIOLITIS

EPIDEMIOLOGY

Bronchilolitis is a lower respiratory tract infection, most commonly caused by RSV that occurs mostly commonly between December and March in epidemic numbers.[4] Neonates are particularly susceptible to respiratory distress and apnea with RSV as well as other bronchiolitis-causing viruses. RSV infection leads to more than 90,000 hospitalizations annually.[5] Transmission occurs by direct or close contact with respiratory secretions.[6] The incubation period of the disease is 4-6 days, and viral shedding may take place for as long as 4 weeks.[6] RSV is the most common but not the only cause of bronchiolitis. Other bronchiolitis-causing viruses

▶ **TABLE 3–2. RESPIRATORY CAUSES OF NEONATAL TACHYPNEA**

Parenchymal	Nonparenchymal
Bronchopulmonary dysplasia	Pleural effusion
Bronchiolitis	Pneumothorax
Pneumonia	
Pulmonary edema	
Pulmonary hypoplasia	
Congenital diaphragmatic hernia	
Congenital cystic adenomatoid malformation	

include: influenza, parainfluenza, human metapneumovirus, and adenovirus, as well as many other respiratory viruses.

CLINICAL MANIFESTATIONS

Neonates with bronchiolitis may present with rhinorrhea, cough, tachypnea, wheezing, crackles, and retractions to different degrees. Lethargy, irritability, poor feeding, and apnea may also be presenting signs of bronchiolitis.[6] Premature infants and those with congenital heart disease are the most vulnerable to severe disease. The pathophysiology of bronchiolitis can explain the wheezing and increased work of breathing. The virus infects the bronchioles creating edema and secretions in these lower airways, which decreases the airway diameter and hence causes wheezing. Some neonates may have a degree of bronchospasm, although the majority do not. Bronchiolitis may or may not be associated with fever.

When assessing a patient with bronchiolitis, the most important aspects of the examination are the infant's work of breathing, aeration, oxygen saturation, and hydration status. The differential diagnosis includes myocarditis, cardiac failure, pneumonia, and sepsis. On physical examination hepatomegaly and a murmur may be indicative of a cardiac etiology.

DIAGNOSTIC STUDIES

Virologic tests for RSV demonstrate a high predictive value.[6] Many institutions have the capability to perform a rapid antigen detection test for RSV and influenza. Nasal secretions can also be collected for viral culture. Determining the viral etiology of bronchiolitis will not change the patient management, although it may be necessary for admission and patient cohorting, as well as isolation.

Current evidence does not support the use of routine radiography in children with bronchiolitis.[5] A chest x-ray would typically

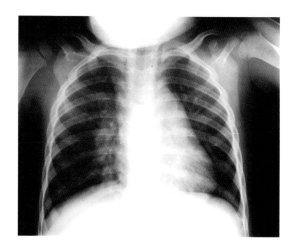

Figure 3–2. Typical chest x-ray seen in brochiolitis.

show hyperinflation and atelectasis due to mucous plugging (Figure 3–2). Two studies suggest that the presence of consolidation and atelectasis on a chest radiograph is associated with increased risk for severe disease.[5,7,8] A chest radiograph should be performed at the physician's discretion and may be potentially helpful if the diagnosis is unclear.

Many neonates with bronchiolitis have fever. Neonates with fever typically have complete sepsis evaluations including a complete blood count, blood culture, urine studies, and lumbar puncture. A study by Titus and Wright demonstrated a low risk of serious bacterial infection in infants less than 8 weeks of age with documented RSV in comparison to a control group of non-RSV infants. It has been suggested that examination of the urine in RSV-positive patients be performed as they found a clinically relevant rate of concomitant urinary tract infection with RSV.[9] The author does recommend a complete sepsis evaluation in the toxic-appearing neonate with RSV bronchiolitis.

MANAGEMENT

The treatment of patients with bronchiolitis is supportive. Oxygen should be administered as needed. Intravenous hydration should be initiated for the clinically dehydrated or poor-feeding infant. The patient should be placed on respiratory droplet and contact precautions to prevent nosocomial spread. A designated patient stethoscope should be used to decrease spread by fomites. Neonates are obligatory "nasal breathers" and typically have copious amounts of nasal discharge with this infection. Many times nasal suction with a flexible catheter can relieve some of the increased work of breathing, and is recommended. There have been many randomized controlled studies (RCTs) of bronchodilator use in bronchiolitis that do not demonstrate consistent benefit. A Cochrane review found 8 RCTs involving 394 children.[10-17] The studies involved both beta and alpha agonists. Overall, results of the meta-analysis indicated that approximately 1 in 4 patients treated with bronchodilators might have a transient improvement.[5]

It is the author's opinion that a trial of a nebulized beta agonist accompanied by a pre- and post-administration chest examination for signs of improvement in respiratory effort, wheezing, and oxygen saturation is appropriate. Bronchodilators should continue as needed if an improvement is noted clinically. For severe disease, inhaled racemic epinephrine may be helpful due to the alpha effects on airway edema. The use of steroids has not been shown to be useful in the treatment of bronchiolitis. Chest physiotherapy can be performed to assist in aerating areas of atelectasis and expulsion of mucoid material. Hospital admission is recommended for all neonates with bronchiolitis as they have an increased risk of apnea and severe disease.

▶ BRONCHOPULMONARY DYSPLASIA

EPIDEMIOLOGY

Bronchopulmonary dysplasia (BPD), also known as chronic lung disease (CLD), is not exclusive to but is most common in premature infants born less than 30 weeks of gestation. BPD is a clinical diagnosis, defined by oxygen dependence for a specific period of time after birth and accompanied by characteristic radiographic findings that correspond to anatomic abnormalities.[18] In 1967 Northway first described BPD as developing in premature infants exposed to mechanical ventilation and oxygen supplementation.[19] BPD is not a diagnosis to be made in the ED setting. The diagnosis will be typically made shortly after birth in the neonatal intensive care unit. It is important to review BPD in this setting as one may see patients presenting to the ED with an exacerbation of this disease. Accepted definitions of BPD are an oxygen requirement at 28 postnatal days[20,21] or an oxygen requirement at 36 weeks postmenstrual age.[22,23]

Approximately 60,000 infants under 1500 g (1.5% of all newborns) are born in the United States each year,[24] and bronchopulmonary dysplasia develops in about 20% of them.[25] BPD is a multifactorial illness. Other risk factors besides low birth weight and prematurity include a patent ductus arteriosus, postnatal sepsis, antenatal maternal infection (eg, chorioamnionitis), and maternal or neonatal colonization with *Ureaplasma histolyticum*.[18]

CLINICAL MANIFESTATIONS

The diagnosis of BPD, as mentioned above, is clinical and diagnosed typically in the neonatal intensive care unit. When a patient presents to the ED, the parents will likely be aware of the diagnosis. The patient may be on oxygen at home or use inhaled steroids or bronchodilators routinely. If the history is unclear a review of the neonatal admission record can be helpful.

The neonate with an exacerbation of BPD will present with one or more of the following; tachypnea, retractions, wheezing, and crackles. These clinical exacerbations can

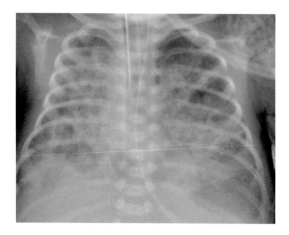

Figure 3–3. Chest x-ray in a 2 month old with brochopulmonary dysplasia (BPD).

occur in association with pulmonary edema, superimposed infection, or right heart failure.[18] Patients with severe BPD may have pulmonary hypertension, which may lead to right-sided heart failure. A thorough history including the presence or absence of fever, cold symptoms, cough, cyanosis, or increased oxygen requirement may help to determine the etiology of the exacerbation.

A chest radiograph will show varying amounts of bilateral haziness representing atelectasis and potentially pulmonary edema (Figure 3–3). In severe BPD, there may be hyperinflation of the lung fields. A comparison chest radiograph if available can be helpful as a baseline as which to compare.

DIAGNOSTIC STUDIES

BPD is not a diagnosis made in the ED, although the etiology of the exacerbation will be. A viral etiology should be considered as a possible exacerbating factor; therefore, depending on the time of year, a nasopharyngeal wash for RSV, influenza, and general viral culture should be done as clinically relevant. Upper respiratory tract infections may also cause increased lower airway brochospasm and exacerbation.

If the exacerbation is associated with fever, a chest radiograph could be helpful in evaluating for pneumonia. Other findings on chest radiograph that can be diagnostically helpful are heart size (seen in right-heart failure), or evidence of pulmonary edema. An ECG can be helpful in the acute exacerbation if pulmonary hypertension is suspected.

MANAGEMENT

The treatment is largely supportive during an exacerbation of BPD. Oxygen should be administered to maintain oxygen saturations ≥92%. A nasal cannula or oxyhood may be used at the physician's discretion. Intravenous hydration should only be used as needed without over hydration, as subsets of patients with BPD have baseline pulmonary edema. Many patients with BPD may be maintained on bronchodilators. Established BPD is associated with increases in airway resistance, decreased dynamic compliance, and wheezing.[26] The use of bronchodilators or beta agonists should be used in an acute exacerbation of BPD. A pre- and postexamination will be helpful in determining the clinical response. Given the lack of reliable evidence to support (or refute) bronchodilator use for the prevention and treatment of BPD, it may be reasonable to restrict bronchodilator therapy to infants with clinical signs of bronchial obstruction or increased work of breathing for improving lung function.[26]

Many neonates with bronchopulmonary dysplasia may be currently taking routine inhaled steroids. Continuation of the inhaled steroids during an exacerbation may decrease inflammatory changes in the lungs and reduce lower airway obstruction. The use of oral or intravenous corticosteroids such as prednisolone in a short 5-day course may be helpful in the treatment of an exacerbation of BPD. Diuretics may be helpful if the patient clinically or radiographically has evidence of pulmonary edema. If the patient is currently taking a diuretic for BPD or an addition is made during an exacerbation, examination of electrolytes particularly sodium, potassium, and calcium is prudent.

▶ NEONATAL PNEUMONIA

EPIDEMIOLOGY

Pneumonia, as defined as inflammation and infection of the lung, is a unique disease in the neonatal population. Pneumonia contributes to between 750,000 and 1.2 million neonatal deaths annually, accounting for 10% of global child mortality.[27] The greatest risk of death from pneumonia in childhood is in the neonatal period.[28] Neonatal pneumonia can be acquired early or late. Early-onset neonatal pneumonia, presenting within the first week of life, is acquired by aspiration of infected amniotic fluid at birth. Risk factors for early-onset pneumonia include maternal fever, evidence of chorioamnionitis, positive Group B streptococcal status in the mother and a history of sexually transmitted diseases. Late-onset pneumonia in the neonate can be nosocomial from infected individuals or hospital equipment. Neonates may develop nosocomial pneumonia, particularly if they required prolonged intubation.[29]

CLINICAL MANIFESTATIONS

Neonates with pneumonia may present with signs of systemic illness including hyper- or hypothermia, jaundice, hepatosplenomegaly, lethargy, irritability, anorexia, vomiting, or abdominal distension.[30] Respiratory signs may appear at the onset or later in the illness. Respiratory signs include tachypnea (heart rate >60), cough, use of accessory muscles of respiration (suprasternal, supraclavicular, intercostal, or subcostal retractions), nasal flaring, crackles on auscultation, cyanosis, and

▶ **TABLE 3–3. CAUSES OF NEONATAL PNEUMONIA**

Bacterial	Viral
Group B streptococcus	RSV
Listeria monocyto-genes	Human meta-pneumovirus
Escherichia coli	Influenza
Klebsiella	Parainfluenza
Proteus	Herpes simplex
Staphylococcus aureus	Cytomegalovirus
Pseudomonas	Human immuno-deficiency virus
Group A streptococcus	
Neisseria meningitidis	

Atypical	Fungal
Chlamydia trachomatis	*Candida albicans*
Mycoplasma	
Mycobacterium spp.	

apnea. In severe illness neonates may present in respiratory failure or shock.

In viral pneumonias associated with bronchiolitis (eg, RSV), the patient may present with wheezing or with apnea alone. A comprehensive list of causes of neonatal pneumonia can be found in Table 3–3.

DIAGNOSTIC TESTING

A chest radiograph should be obtained in any neonate with suspected pneumonia. The chest radiograph findings may be varied depending on the organism. Potentially one may see increased localized densities and air bronchograms, peribronchial cuffing, effusions, and/or pneumatoceles. Pleural effusions, abscess cavities, and pneumatoceles are frequent in infants with staphylococcal infections, but may occur in pneumonia caused by Group A *Streptococcus, Escherichia coli,* or *Klebsiella pneumoniae.*[30] The offending organism may be isolated from the blood; therefore, it is recommended to obtain a complete blood count and blood culture. A urine culture and lumbar puncture should also be performed on any neonate with a suspicion of bacterial pneumonia, as hematogenous spread of the organism is not uncommon.

On physical examination, if any skin lesions are noted, particularly pustules worrisome for *Staphylococcus* or *Streptococcus*, they should be cultured. Vesicular lesions should be examined and fluid sent for herpes simplex polymerase chain reaction (PCR). *Chlamydia* pneumonia may be associated with conjunctivitis; therefore, if signs of conjunctivitis are present, the eyes should be swabbed keeping in mind that *Chlamydia* is an intracellular organism and that swab should involve the conjunctiva itself as well as the discharge.

In winter months consider RSV and influenza as possibilities. A nasopharyngeal swab can be sent for rapid antigen detection or viral culture. Pertussis should be suspected if there is a family history of chronic cough particularly in adolescents and adults, or if there is apnea, cyanosis, or the classic paroxysmal cough.

MANAGEMENT

Management is largely supportive with oxygen and intravenous fluid as needed. One should anticipate the possibility of respiratory failure and be prepared to secure a definitive airway. If the patient's hemodynamic status permits, a complete blood count with differential, blood culture, urinalysis, Gram stain, urine culture and spinal fluid studies should be obtained prior to broad antibiotic coverage. Antibiotic coverage should be determined by the local resistance patterns. Ampicillin and a third-generation cephalosporin are the typical agents used initially until organism identification can be made. Consider the addition of acyclovir to cover herpes simplex. All neonates with pneumonia should be admitted to the hospital for close observation, supportive care, and intravenous antibiotic therapy. Intensive care admission should be considered.

► PERTUSSIS

EPIDEMIOLOGY

Pertussis is a life-threatening illness in neonates. Despite global immunization practices, there is a waning of immunity that occurs in adolescence and adulthood that results in an increased rate of exposure to young infants. Pertussis is a disease in which infants are at the greatest risk for death or serious complications.[31] A history of a chronic cough in an adult or adolescent in the home should raise suspicion of the disease.

Since the early 1980s, reported cases of pertussis have increased, with cyclical peaks occurring every 3 to 4 years.[32] In the years 2004 and 2005, pertussis was at an all time high with 25,827 and 25,616 cases, respectively, on a national level.[33] There was a decrease in 2006 to 15,632 cases nationally.[33] This decrease in incidence likely represents the cyclical nature of the disease. Pertussis is caused by *Bordetella pertussis*, a gram-negative rod. The bacterium infects the lower respiratory epithelium causing edema and cellular debris. The transmission of the disease is by respiratory droplets.

CLINICAL MANIFESTATIONS

The classic presentation in neonates includes chronic cough in paroxysms that may include cyanosis, difficulty feeding due to choking or gagging, and apnea. Posttussive emesis is also frequently seen. The cough is episodic with multiple coughs in series ending with an inspiration. Neonates do not typically generate enough force to create an inspiratory "whoop"; therefore, its absence should not eliminate the diagnosis. Examination of the pharynx with a tongue depressor may stimulate the cough, which can be helpful in diagnosis.

Affected neonates are typically afebrile. In a retrospective study by Mackey et al to predict pertussis in a pediatric emergency population, there were 4 variables that were highly predictive of pertussis: age less than 2 months, history of cough or choking associated with cyanosis, cough in the ED, and rhonchi on auscultation.[34] If all 4 of these predictors are present, pertussis should be high on the differential diagnosis and the patient should placed on droplet precautions. Additional clinical findings seen in pertussis may include facial and truncal petechiae and subconjunctival hemorrhages due to the forceful cough. Complications of pertussis among infants include pneumonia (22%), seizures (2%), encephalopathy (<0.5%), and death.[35] On the basis of cases reported to local and state health departments (1990-1999), the case fatality rate was approximately 1% in infants younger than 2 months of age.[35]

There are typically three phases of the disease; catarrhal, paroxysmal, and convalescent.

Catharral

The initial 1 to 2 weeks of the illness consists of "cold-like" symptoms of rhinorrhea and nasal congestion. There may be a mild cough that progresses.

Paroxysmal

In the next 2 to 6 weeks, the cough is quite distinctive and consists of coughing in episodes where there are multiple coughs in sequence with an inspiration at the end of the paroxysm. While coughing the neonate may become cyanotic, dusky, or very red. There also may be choking and gagging involved and posttussive emesis.

Convalescent

Over the next several weeks the cough will start to subside with less frequent paroxysms of cough. Pertussis literally translates to "100 day cough"; therefore, parents can expect a long course.

DIAGNOSTIC STUDIES

There are no rapid diagnostic studies for pertussis; therefore, one needs a high clinical suspicion for the disease. The initial diagnosis may be presumed by history and character of the cough. There are studies that may support the diagnosis of pertussis including a predominant lymphocytosis on a complete blood count and the classic chest x-ray finding of a "shaggy right heart border" (Figure 3–4). The existing diagnostic studies available are culture, direct fluorescent antibody, and PCR. The pertussis PCR has a high sensitivity and specificity for the disease (93.5% and 97.1%, respectively) and is widely available.[36] A nasopharyngeal swab in charcoal agar is sent for the PCR sample.

MANAGEMENT

Supportive management is the mainstay of treatment. Many patients require oxygen and intravenous fluid therapy. The patient should be placed on droplet precautions as soon as a diagnosis of pertussis is entertained to prevent

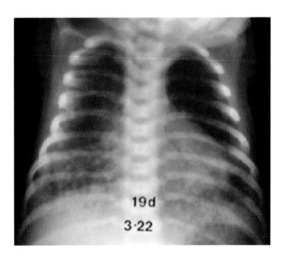

Figure 3–4. The shaggy right heart border seen in pertussis.

nosocomial spread of the disease. Because of the severity of this disease in the neonatal period, it is recommended that all neonates with pertussis or presumed pertussis should be hospitalized; intensive care may be necessary.

Antimicrobial agents are recommended for the patient and any close contacts including all family members living with the patient. The antimicrobial agent will decrease the transmissibility of the disease but does not generally decrease the course of the illness. Azithromycin is currently the drug of choice, and an appropriate dose per age should be given.

► CONGENITAL ANOMALIES OF THE LUNG

Neonates may present after discharge from the nursery with congenital pulmonic anomalies. Typically they will present with respiratory

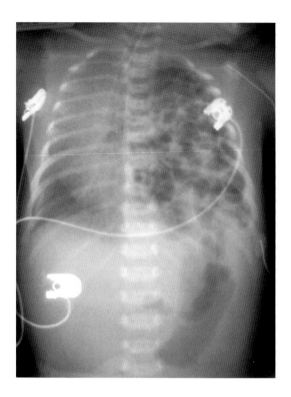

Figure 3–5. Chest x-ray demonstrating a diaphragmatic hernia. *Source:* From Brunicardi FC, Andersen DK, Billiar TR. *Schwartz's Principles and Practice of Surgery,* 8th ed. New York, NY: McGraw-Hill; 2005.

distress (tachypnea or grunting). The anomalies be realized on a chest radiograph but may also be discovered as incidental findings. The lesions are not exclusive to but include congenital cystic adenomatoid malformation, congenital lobar emphysema, bronchogenic cysts, and pulmonary hypoplasia due to a congenital diaphragmatic hernia. Table 3–4 reviews these lesions (Figure 3–5). All of these anomalies require a surgical consultation.

► STRIDOR

Stridor is a high-pitched respiratory noise caused by an obstruction in the upper airway.

► TABLE 3–4. **CONGENITAL ANOMALIES OF THE LUNG**

Congenital cystic adenomatoid malformation:
- Hamartoma consisting of cystic and adenomatous lesions
- Incidence: 1 in 25,000-35,000 pregnancies[37]

Congenital lobar emphysema:
- Hyperinflated pulmonary lobe(s)[38,39]
- Incidence: 1 in 20,000-30,000[40]

Bronchogenic cysts:
- Abnormal budding of the tracheal diverticulum
- Potentially may become infected

Congenital diaphragmatic hernia:
- Failure of diaphragmatic closure resulting in migration of abdominal contents into the chest, causing pulmonary hypoplasia due to compression
- Incidence: 1 in 5,000 live births[41]

The management of these lesions is supportive. Patients with congenital diaphragmatic hernias may benefit from a nasogastric tube to decompress the bowel located in the chest.

The obstruction causes a turbulence of airflow resulting in a sound that can be heard on inspiration or expiration. The upper airway can be divided into two regions: the extrathoracic and intrathoracic areas. The extrathoracic airway refers to the airway from the nasopharynx to the thoracic inlet. The extrathoracic area is further divided into the supraglottic and subglottic areas. The supraglottic area refers to the anatomic areas from the nasopharynx to the false vocal cords. On inspiration, a negative intraluminal pressure is established that causes collapse of the airway, thus causing stridor. The supraglottic airway does not have much cartilaginous support and is more susceptible to collapse. The subglottic area includes the vocal cords and the trachea up to point where the trachea meets the thoracic inlet. This portion of the upper airway has more cartilaginous support and therefore can be more rigid; the stridor may be heard on inspiration and expiration when located in this area. The intrathoracic airway refers to the distal trachea located within the thorax and the main stem bronchi. Obstruction in this area may be heard as expiratory stridor due to the increase in intrathoracic pressure during expiration.

In neonates with stridor, the clinician must consider congenital anomalies of the upper airway as highly suspect. In a study by Zoumalan et al where 202 patients less than 1 year of age were examined for the etiology of stridor, 170 (84%) of patients had a diagnosis of a congenital anomaly.[42] Of the congenital causes of stridor, laryngomalacia is the most common and accounts for 75%.[43] The second most common cause is vocal cord paralysis.[43,44] The most common cause of congenital expiratory stridor is tracheomalacia.[43] For a complete list of etiologies of neonatal stridor, see Table 3–5.

► **TABLE 3–5. ETIOLOGIES OF NEONATAL STRIDOR**

Extrathoracic	Intrathoracic
Supraglottic	Vascular rings
Nasal deformities	Mediastinal tumors:
Craniofacial	Lymphoma
anomalies	Teratoma
Tumors:	Granuloma
Papillomas	Cystic hygroma
Hemangiomas	Rhabdomyosarcoma
	Lymphadenopathy
Subglottic	
Laryngomalacia/	
tracheomalacia	
Laryngeal webs	
Laryngeal cysts	
Vocal cord paralysis	
Subglottic stenosis	
Congenital	
Acquired	
Croup	
Bacterial tracheitis	
Epiglottitis	

Other causes
Gastroesophageal reflux
Angioedema
Hypocalcemia
Hydrocephalous
Compression of the recurrent laryngeal nerve

► **LARYNGOMALACIA/ TRACHEOMALACIA**

EPIDEMIOLOGY

Laryngomalcia is the most common cause of congenital stridor. In the Zoumalan study of causes of stridor, of all of the laryngeal causes, laryngomalacia accounted for 94% of the diagnoses. Laryngomalacia results from the collapse of supraglottic structures (such as the arytenoids cartilages and epiglottis) during inspiration.[45] This effect results in inspiratory stridor. Tracheomalacia also refers to a "floppy" airway but in the location of the intrathoracic trachea.

CLINICAL MANIFESTATIONS

A neonate with laryngomalacia typically presents within the first few days or weeks of life with intermittent stridor. Typically the stridor worsens when the infant is supine and agitated, and improves in the prone position. The neonate may demonstrate supraclavicular, intercostal, and sternal retractions. Placing the infant in the prone position may diminish the stridor because gravity pulls laryngeal structures anteriorly, improving the patency of the glottis.[45] Upper respiratory tract infections and gastroesophageal reflux may worsen the stridor. In severe cases neonates may have failure to thrive due to the increase in metabolic requirements. Lastly, the intermittent stridor does not generally cause a life-threatening obstruction.

Tracheomalacia is similar to laryngomalacia in that it is caused by a weakness of the airway cartilage, specifically of the trachea in the intrathoracic area. On expiration the increase in intrathoracic pressure collapses the trachea and creates a high-pitched noise on expiration, which creates a wheeze. This wheeze may be difficult to differentiate clinically from other causes of neonatal wheezing. The wheeze heard in tracheomalacia often is central, low-pitched, and homophonous.[45] Placing an infant with tracheomalacia in a prone position may also alleviate the symptoms.

DIAGNOSTIC STUDIES

The diagnosis of laryngomalacia and tracheomalacia are typically made by history and physical examination. If there is clinical concern regarding a mediastinal mass or any external airway compression, a chest radiograph may be helpful. Patients with the typical presentation of laryngomalacia where the stridor is intermittent and improves with positioning and there are no growth concerns can be followed by the primary care physician. If the clinical picture is atypical or if the stridor is accompanied by poor feeding, failure to gain weight, or episodes of cyanosis, apnea, or hoarseness, the child requires further evaluation by an otolaryngologist.[46]

MANAGEMENT

Ensure appropriate oxygenation and ventilation in all patients with laryngomalacia and tracheomalacia. Supine positioning should be attempted if there is respiratory distress. If the diagnosis of laryngomalacia is certain from the history and if the neonate is acutely worsening and appears to have an upper respiratory tract infection, a trial of racemic epinephrine may help to decrease the inflammation and alleviate some of the work of breathing. Beta-agonists have not been shown to alleviate the wheezing in tracheomalacia.

▶ SUMMARY

Respiratory complaints in the neonatal period can present in many different ways. Signs of increased respiratory effort include tachypnea, cough, retractions, wheezing, and stridor. All patients should be initially approached in the same manner with examination of the airway, breathing, and circulation. When an intervention is needed, initiation should be prompt to avoid persistent hypoxemia and respiratory fatigue. Hydration status should be considered as many neonates in respiratory distress may have poor feeding due to respiratory rate or effort.

Keep in mind that all respiratory complaints may not indicate a respiratory etiology. A chest radiograph should be examined for any patient with respiratory distress, which may aid in diagnosis. A low threshold for hospital admission is necessary as is the case in many respiratory illnesses. It is the neonate who may be at highest risk for complications such as RSV and pertussis.

REFERENCES

1. Kotecha S. Lung growth for beginners. *Paediatr Respir Rev.* 2000;1:308-313.
2. Joshi S, Kotecha S. Lung growth and development. *Early Hum Dev.* 2007;83:789-794.
3. Eichenwald EC, Aina A, Stark AR. Apnea frequently persists beyond term gestation in infants delivered at 24 to 28 weeks. *Pediatrics.* 1997;100:354-359.
4. Mullins JA, Lamonte AC, Bresee JS. Substantial variability in community respiratory syncytial virus season timing. *Pediatr Infect Dis J.* 2003;22:857-862.
5. Lieberthal AS, Baucher H, Hall CB, et al. Diagnosis and management of bronchiolitis. Subcommittee on diagnosis and management of bronchiolitis. *Pediatrics.* 2006;118:1774-1793.
6. American Academy of Pediatrics. Respiratory syncytial virus. In Pickering LK, Baker CJ, Long SS, McMillan JA, eds. *Red Book: 2006 Report of the Committee of Infectious Diseases.* 27th ed., Elk Grove Village, IL: AAP, 560-563.
7. Wang EE, Law BJ, Stephens D. Pediatric Investigators Collaborative Network on Infections in Canada (PICNIC) prospective study of risk factors and outcomes in patients hospitalized with respiratory syncytial viral lower respiratory tract infection. *J Pediatr.* 1995;126:212-219.
8. Shaw KN, Bell LM, Sherman NH. Outpatient assessment of infants with bronchiolitis. *Am J Dis Child.* 1991;145:151-155.
9. Titus MO, Wright SW. Prevalence of serious bacterial infections in febrile infants with respiratory syncytial virus infection. *Pediatrics.* 2003;112:282-284.
10. Kellner JD, Ohlsson A, Gadomski AM, Wang EE. Bronchodilators for bronchiolitis. *Cochrane Database Syst Rev.* 2000;(2):CD001266.
11. Lowell DI, Lister G, Von Koss H, McCarthy P. Wheezing in infants: the response to epinephrine. *Pediatrics.* 1987;79:939-945.
12. Alario AJ, Lewander WJ, Dennehy P, Seifer R, Mansell AL. The efficacy of nebulized metaproterenol in wheezing infants and young children. *Am J Dis Child.* 1992;146:412-418.
13. Henry RL, Milner AD, Stokes GM. Ineffectiveness of ipratropium bromide in acute bronchiolitis. *Arch Dis Child.* 1983;58:925-926.
14. Klassen TP, Rowe PC, Sutcliffe T, Ropp LJ, McDowell IW, Li MM. Randomized trial of salbutamol in acute bronchiolitis. *J Pediatr.* 1991;118:807-811.
15. Lines DR, Kattampallil JS, Liston P. Efficacy of nebulized salbutamol in bronchiolitis. *Pediatr Rev Commun.* 1990;5:121-129.
16. Mallol J, Barrueo L, Giradi G, et al. Use of nebulized bronchodilators in infants under 1 year of age: analysis of four forms of therapy. *Pediatr Pulmonol.* 1987;3:298-303.
17. Tal A, Bavilski C, Yohai D, Bearman JE, Gorodischer R, Moses SW. Dexamethasone and salbutamol in the treatment of acute wheezing infants. *Pediatrics.* 1983;71:13-18.
18. Vaucher YE. Bronchopulmonary dysplasia: an enduring challenge. *Pediatr Rev.* 2002;23:349-358.
19. Baraldi E, Filippone M. Chronic lung disease after premature birth. *N Engl J Med.* 2007;357:1946-1955.
20. Kraybill EN, Runyan DK, Bose CL, Khan JH. Risk factors for chronic lung disease in infants with birth weights of 751 to 1000 grams. *J Pediatr.* 1989;115:115.
21. Sinkin RA, Cox C, Phelps DL. Predicting risk for bronchopulmonary dysplasia: selection criteria for clinical trials. *Pediatrics.* 1990;86:728.
22. Shennean At, Dunn MS, Ohlsson A, Lennox K. Abnormal pulmonary outcomes in premature infants: prediction from oxygen requirement in the neonatal period. *Pediatrics.* 1988;82:527.
23. Marshall DD, Kotelchuck M, Young TE, et al. Risk factors for chronic lung disease in the surfactant era: a North Carolina population—based study of very low birth weight infants. *Pediatrics.* 1999;104:1345.
24. Martin JA, Hamilton BE, Sutton PD, Ventura SJ, Menacker F, Munson ML. *Births: Final Data for 2003.* Hyattsville, MD: National Center for Health Statistics, Centers for Disease Control and Prevention, 2005.
25. Lemons JA, Bauer CR, Oh W, et al. Very low birth weight outcomes of the National Institute of Child health and human development neonatal research network, January 1995 through December 1996. *Pediatrics.* 2001;107(1):e1.
26. Pantalitschka T, Poets CF. Inhaled drugs for the prevention and treatment of bronchopulmonary dysplasia. *Pediatr Pulmonol.* 2006;41:703-708.

27. The Child Health Research Project. *Reducing Perinatal and Neonatal Mortality: Report of a Meeting.* Vol 3. Baltimore, MD: Author. 1999;6-12.

28. Duke T. Neonatal pneumonia in developing countries. *Arch Dis Child Fetal Neonatal Ed.* 2005;90:F211-F219.

29. Gaston B. Pneumonia. *Pediatr Rev.* 2002;23:132-140.

30. Klein JO, Barnett ED. Neonatal pneumonia. *Semin Pediatr Infect Dis.* 1998;9:212-216.

31. Colletti JE, Homme JL, Woodbridge DP. Unsuspected neonatal killers in emergency medicine. *Emerg Med Clin North Am.* 2004;22:721-728.

32. Karras DJ. Update on emerging infections: news from the Centers for Disease Control and Prevention. *Ann Emerg Med.* 2002;40:115-119.

33. Centers for Disease Control and Prevention (CDC). Summary of notifiable diseases, United States, 2008. *MMWR Morb Mortal Wkly Rep.* 2008;55:1-94.

34. Mackey JE, Wojcik S, Long R, Callahan JM, Grant WD. Predicting pertussis in a pediatric emergency department population. *Clin Pediatr.* 2007;46:437-440.

35. American Academy of Pediatrics. Respiratory syncytial virus. In Pickering LK, Baker CJ, Long SS, McMillan JA, eds. *Red Book: 2006 Report of the Committee on Infectious Diseases.* 27th ed., Elk Grove Village, IL: AAP, 498.

36. Loeffelholz MJ, Thompson CJ, Long KS, et al. Comparison of PCR, culture, and direct fluorescent-antibody testing for detection of *Bordetella pertussis.* *J Clin Microbiol.* 1999;37:2872-2876.

37. Laberge JM, Flageole H, Pugash D, et al. Outcome of the prenatally diagnosed congenital cystic adenomatoid lung malformation: a Canadian experience. *Fetal Diagn Ther.* 2001;16:178.

38. Kravitz RM. Congenital malformations of the lung. *Pediatr Clin North Am.* 1994;41:453.

39. Stanton M, Davenport M. Management of congenital lung lesions. *Early Hum Dev.* 2006;82:289.

40. Thakral CL, Maji DC, Sajwani MJ. Congenital lobar emphysema: experience with 21 cases. *Pediatr Surg Int.* 2001;17:88.

41. Behrman RE, Kliegman RM, Jenson MD. *Nelson Textbook of Pediatrics.* 16th ed. Philadelphia, PA: W.B. Saunders; 2000, p. 1231.

42. Zoumalan R, Maddalozzo J, Holinger L. Etiology of stridor in infants. *Annals of Otology, Rhinology & Laryngology.* 2007;116(5):329-334.

43. Baren JM, Rothrock SG, Brennan JA, Brown L. *Pediatric Emergency Medicine.* Philadelphia, PA: W.B. Saunders; 2008, p. 314.

44. De Jong Al, Kuppersmith RB, Sulek M, Friedman EM. Vocal cord paralysis in infants and children. *Otolaryngol Clin North Am.* 2000;33:131-149.

45. Vincencio AG, Parikh S. Laryngomalacia and Tracheomalacia: Common dynamic airway lesions. *Pediatr Rev.* 2006;27:e33-e35.

46. Adam HM. Comment on Vincencio AG, Parikh S. Laryngomalacia and Tracheomalacia: Common dynamic airway lesions. *Pediatr Rev.* 2006;27:e35.

CHAPTER 4

Cardiac Emergencies

Jahn Avarello, MD

This chapter is meant to be a guide to evaluating the neonate who is thought to have cardiac disease. Although management of the different presentations is discussed, all providers who feel they are dealing with neonatal cardiac disease process should consult a pediatric cardiologist and intensivist as soon as possible to ensure the best possible outcome for the patient.

▶ EPIDEMIOLOGY

The overall incidence of congenital heart disease in the United States is approximately 8 per 1000 live births.[1] The incidence of severe cases requiring expert cardiology care is approximately 2.5 to 3 per 1000 live births with moderately severe forms accounting for another 3 per 1000 live births. Although the majority of children born with congenital heart disease are diagnosed either in utero or during their newborn hospital stay, some will present

after the newborn period with initial signs and symptoms ranging from subtle (mild congestive heart failure and/or cyanosis) to profound shock. Presentations after the newborn period have become more prevalent given the recent trend of earlier discharge after delivery. In many cases, it is up to the emergency provider to be the first to make a diagnosis of heart disease in the neonate. Parents may have one or many of an assortment of chief complaints, and the patients may have varying signs and symptoms. It is often a difficult task to identify the subtle signs and symptoms of cardiac disease; therefore it is imperative that providers know the various presentations of the neonate with cardiac disease.

▶ PATHOPHYSIOLOGY OF NEONATAL CIRCULATION

In order to conceptualize neonatal congenital cardiac disease, it is essential to understand the

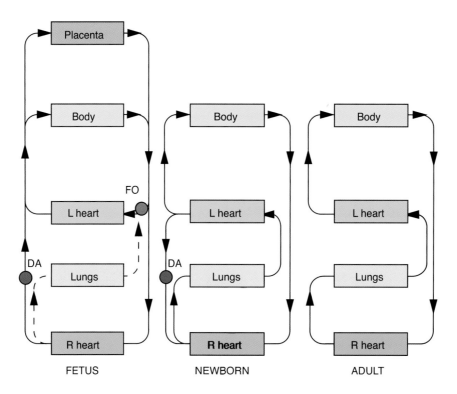

Figure 4–1. Circulation in fetus, newborn, and adult. *Source:* From Ganong WF. Review of Medical Physiology, 22nd ed. New York, NY: McGraw-Hill; 2005.

normal pathophysiologic circulatory changes that take place after delivery (Figure 4–1).[2-4] In utero, fetal blood is oxygenated by the placenta and bypasses the lungs due to the high pulmonary vascular resistance (PVR) of the fetus. Blood enters the placenta via the umbilical arteries, is oxygenated, and returns to the fetus via the umbilical vein. From the umbilical vein about half of the blood enters the ductus venosis and bypasses the liver. The oxygenated blood then enters the right atrium (RA) via the inferior vena cava (IVC), where approximately 33% is shunted into the left atrium (LA) through the foramen ovale while the rest mixes with deoxygenated blood from the superior vena cava (SVC) and enters the right ventricle (RV). From the LA, the oxygenated blood enters the left ventricle (LV), where it is ejected into the aorta and is preferentially distributed to the fetal coronary, cerebral, and upper torso circulations. The deoxygenated blood that has entered the RV from the IVC and SVC enters the pulmonary artery (PA) but because of the elevated PVR, approximately 90% of the blood is shunted through the ductus arteriosus and enters into the aorta mixing with oxygenated blood from the LV. So, in all, there are 3 major normal anatomic shunts of the fetal circulation: the ductus venosis, the foramen ovale, and the ductus arteriosus.

With the delivery of the fetus comes the generation of increased negative pressure as the baby takes his or her first breath. The more negative intrathoracic pressure expands the lungs and augments the elimination of fluid from the lungs. Under the influence of multiple factors, the pulmonary vasculature dilates, therefore leading to a reduction in the PVR and an increase in pulmonary blood flow (PBF), resulting in a rise in the PaO_2 (arterial partial pressure of oxygen). The increased PaO_2 assists in the closure of the ductus venosis, ductus arteriosus, and the umbilical vessels. Blood flow to the lungs increases by 4- to 10-fold shortly after birth and subsequently increases venous return to the left atrium, increasing the left atrial pressure and thus encouraging the closure of the foramen ovale. This closure prevents clinically significant right-to-left shunting. As the ductus arteriosus functionally closes over the first 24 hours, the pulmonary and systemic circulations are effectively separated leading to a reduction in mean pulmonary artery pressures. The ductus arteriosus usually does not reach complete anatomic closure until 2 to 3 weeks after birth.

At delivery, fetal circulation transitions from one dependent upon placental oxygenation and shunts both at the intra- and extracardiac level, to one dependent upon oxygenation in the lungs devoid of the need for shunting. Unless the fetus undergoes a perinatal traumatic event or has an underlying anatomic or physiologic abnormality, the transition from fetal to newborn circulation should occur smoothly and without the need for medical intervention.

► DUCTAL DEPENDENT LESIONS AND PVR

Some congenital heart defects (CHD) are dependent upon the ductus arteriosus remaining patent to: 1) sustain systemic blood flow (ie, hypoplastic left heart syndrome, critical aortic stenosis, and interrupted aortic arch); 2) ensure adequate PBF (ie, pulmonary atresia, critical pulmonary stenosis, and tricuspid atresia); or 3) ensure adequate mixing between the systemic and pulmonary circulations (ie, transposition of the great arteries). Depending

upon the degree of the lesion, the open ductus may be the only source of flow between the pulmonary and systemic circulations. Patients with ductal dependant lesions usually present in the first 3 weeks of life as the ductus arteriosus closes. That being said, it is imperative to remember that in the face of the acutely decompensating infant with cyanosis and/or shock in the first few weeks of life, there is a potential for the ductus arteriosus to be reopened with the use of prostaglandin E_1 (PGE_1).

As discussed above, a series of events leads to a rapid drop in the PVR after birth (Figure 4–2). This reduction of the PVR along with the rise in systemic arterial pressure and functional closure of the ductus arteriosus allows for an increase in PBF. Because the PVR drops more than PBF increases, the mean pulmonary artery pressure falls rapidly after birth as well.

As the PVR continues to drop over the first few weeks to months after birth, lesions

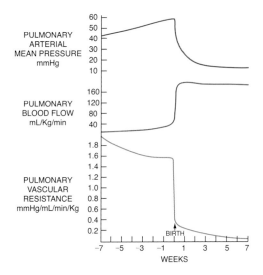

Figure 4–2. Changes in total pulmonary arterial pressure, pulmonary blood flow, and pulmonary vascular resistance (PVR) in the prenatal period. *Source:* From Rudolph's Pediatrics, 21st ed. New York, NY: McGraw-Hill, 2003, p. 1752.

with left-to-right shunting (ie, VSD, AV canal, and PDA) will have an increasing amount of blood entering the pulmonary circulatory system, often causing the child to present with signs and symptoms of congestive heart failure.

GENERAL ASSESSMENT

History

During the newborn period, the presentation of CHDs is often acute and life threatening, and therefore does not initially allow time for an in depth history. There is a higher incidence of CHDs in the presence of certain maternal medical conditions, infections, and medications taken throughout pregnancy (ie, maternal diabetes, systemic lupus erythematosis, and drug use such as lithium). There may be a family history of CHD as well as findings on prenatal ultrasounds suggestive of CHD. The child may have developed particular symptoms of which a caretaker would be unaware unless specifically questioned. A summary of a focused history can be found in Table 4–1.

▶ **TABLE 4–1. FOCUSED HISTORY IN THE NEONATE WITH SUSPECTED CHD**

Prenatal	Maternal medications
	Maternal infections
	Maternal medical conditions
	Ultrasound findings
Perinatal	Risk factors for infections or persistent pulmonary hypertension
	Gestational age
	Delivery (route and course)
Postnatal	Feeding difficulties
	Breathing difficulties
	Excess weight gain
	NICU stay and why

Examination

The initial evaluation starts with the physician's first glance of the newborn. Often it can be determined whether a patient has a life-threatening emergency based on an observational first impression even before a physical examination. The pediatric assessment triangle (PAT) is an tool to help establish the severity of illness or injury and to determine the urgency of intervention.[5] The PAT is based on the 3 categories of observations and can help rapidly answer some pertinent questions.

Appearance: Does the baby have good tone or is he/she limp and listless? Does the child appear to be alert and responding appropriately to the environment? Does he or she appear consolable, or irritable and inconsolable? If there is a cry, is it weak or vigorous?

Work of Breathing: Is the baby breathing at a normal rate; if not, does breathing appear too slow or too fast? Are there any abnormal airway sounds such as stridor, wheezing, or grunting? Are there any retractions, nasal faring, or head bobbing?

Circulation to the Skin: Is there any pallor, mottling or cyanosis?

After the general observational assessment has been made, a brief, focused examination needs to be done. First, ensure that the baby is breathing and maintaining his/her own airway. Count the respiratory rate and auscultate for abnormal breath sounds and a heartbeat. Palpate the pulses to assess the heart rate and quality, and note any discrepancy between the brachial pulses as well as weak femoral pulses, which may indicate an aortic arch abnormality. Look for mottling or cyanosis and assess the capillary refill. Palpate the precordium for hyperactivity and/or thrills while simultaneously looking for any surgical scars suggestive of cardiothoracic surgery.

Auscultate the head, chest, and abdomen to listen for any abnormal sounds such as bruits, murmurs, or gallops. Palpate the abdomen to assess for hepatomegaly. Finally, ensure that the child is attached to a cardiorespiratory monitoring system and has blood pressures evaluated in all limbs with oxygen saturations determined in at least the right arm and a lower limb to evaluate the pre- and postductal circulation.

COMMON PRESENTATIONS OF CONGENITAL HEART DISEASE

The age at which a child presents with signs and symptoms of a CHD is dependent upon the severity of the anatomic defect, patency of any shunts, and the PVR (Table 4–2). Children

Diagnosis	% of Patients
0-6 days	
D-transposition of the great arteries	19
Hypoplastic left heart	14
Tetralogy of Fallot	8
Coarctation of the aorta	7
Ventricular septal defect	3
Others	49
7-13 days	
Coarctation of the aorta	16
Ventricular septal defect	14
Hypoplastic left heart	8
D-transposition of the great arteries	7
Tetralogy of Fallot	7
Others	48
14-28 days	
Ventricular septal defect	16
Coarctation of the aorta	12
Tetralogy of Fallot	7
D-transposition of the great arteries	7
Patent ductus arteriosus	53
Others	

with CHD will present with cyanosis, congestive heart failure (CHF), or shock, or with an asymptomatic heart murmur.[6]

Cyanosis seen in the child with CHD is secondary to the shunting of deoxygenated blood from the right to the left side of the heart. The shunting may take place through an atrial and/or ventricular septal defect, as well as though a patent ductus arteriosus. Depending on the lesion, there may be cyanosis with increased PBF or with decreased PBF. Common etiologies of cyanotic CHD include:

1. Tetralogy of Fallot (TOF)
2. Total anomalous pulmonary venous return (TAPVR)
3. Transposition of the great arteries (TGA)
4. Tricuspid atresia
5. Truncus arteriosus
6. Pulmonary atresia or stenosis
7. Ebstein anomaly

Neonates presenting with cyanosis must first be categorized into having either central cyanosis or peripheral cyanosis (acrocyanosis). Acrocyanosis is a bluish discoloration of the hands, feet, and sometimes the circumoral area that is commonly seen in the newborn period. It is secondary to peripheral vasoconstriction rather than arterial oxygen desaturation, and is most evident when the child is exposed to cold temperatures. Although mostly a benign finding, acrocyanosis can be accentuated if the child is in distress from a general illness or has poor perfusion from a shock state. Central cyanosis is a bluish discoloration involving the lips, tongue, skin, nailbeds, and mucous membranes that always reflects a pathologic cause. The presentation of cyanosis can be secondary to cardiac, respiratory, or hemoglobin disorders.

Differentiation between the cyanosis from a cardiac disorder vs that from respiratory or hemoglobin disorders can be quickly assessed by utilizing the hyperoxia test (oxygen challenge test).[7] The test is done by first obtaining

▶ **TABLE 4–3. EXAMPLES OF HYPEROXIA TEST RESULTS (OXYGEN CHALLENGE TEST)**

	FiO$_2$ = 0.21 PaO$_2$ (% saturation)		FiO$_2$ = 1.00 PaO$_2$ (% saturation)	PaCO$_2$
Normal	70 (95)		>200 (100)	35
Pulmonary disease	50 (85)		>150 (100)	50
Neurologic disease	50 (85)		>150 (100)	50
Methemoglobinemia	70 (85)		>200 (85)	35
Cardiac disease				
Separate circulation[a]	<40 (<75)		<50 (<85)	35
Restricted PBF [b]	<40 (<75)		<50 (<85)	35
Complete mixing without restricted PBF[c]	50 (85)		<150 (<100)	35
Persistent pulmonary hypertension	Preductal	Postductal		
PFO (no R-to-L shunt)	70 (95)	<40 (<75)	Variable	35-50
PFO (R-to-L shunt)	<40 (<75)	<40 (<75)	Variable	35-50

[a]D-transposition of the great arteries with intact ventricular septum

[b]Tricuspid atresia with pulmonary stenosis or atresia; pulmonary atresia or critical pulmonary stenosis with intact ventricular septum; or tetralogy of Fallot

[c]Truncus, total anomalous pulmonary venous return, single ventricle, hypoplastic left heart, D-TGA with ventricular septal defect, tricuspid atresia without pulmonary stenosis or atresia.

Abbreviations: PBF, pulmonary blood flow; PFO, patent foramen ovale.

Source: From the Harriet Lane Handbook, 7th ed., 2005, p. 194.

a preductal (right radial) blood gas while the child is breathing room air (FiO$_2$ = 0.21) and then repeating the test after the child has inspired 100% oxygen (FiO$_2$ = 1) for a period of 10 to 15 minutes. With pulmonary disease, PaO$_2$ usually rises to >150 mm Hg. When there is significant right-to-left shunting, the arterial PaO$_2$ usually does not exceed 150 mm Hg, and the rise is usually not more than 10 to 30 mm Hg. It is possible for the PaO$_2$ to be as low as 50 mm Hg yet have a pulse oximetry reading in the 90s; therefore, the use of pulse oximetry, while being a reasonable screening test, should not be relied upon for final interpretation. In the scenario of methemoglobinemia, the patient appears cyanotic and the pulse oximetry routinely registers in the mid 80s both before and after the patient receives 100% oxygen (Table 4–3).

It is possible to have a cyanotic congenital heart defect in the face of anemia and not actually be able to clinically detect cyanosis. In order to calculate the hemoglobin oxygen saturation, divide the saturated hemoglobin (g/dL) by the total hemoglobin (g/dL). It takes 3 to 5 g/dL of desaturated hemoglobin to detect cyanosis. In normal newborn with, let's say 18 g/dL of hemoglobin, it would take an oxygen saturation of 86% (18 g/dL–3 g/dL of desaturated hemoglobin divided by 18 g/dL) to detect cyanosis. If the same newborn were anemic with a hemoglobin of 9 g/dL, it would take an oxygen saturation of 67% (9 g/dL–3 g/dL of desaturated hemoglobin divided by 9 g/dL) to detect cyanosis. It can be seen, then, that in an anemic patient with a cardiac lesion causing a hemoglobin oxygen saturation in the 70s, it is possible to be acyanotic.

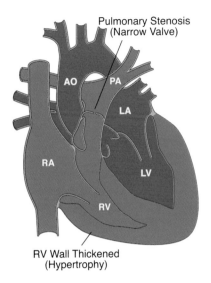

Figure 4–3. Pulmonary stenosis.

Differential Diagnosis

Decreased PBF

Pulmonary atresia and severe pulmonary stenosis can be isolated intracardiac anomalies or concur with other anomalies such as a VSD (Figure 4–3). When seen with a VSD and a normal tricuspid valve, pulmonary atresia may be considered a severe form of TOF. Both pulmonary atresia and severe pulmonary stenosis are dependent upon both flow across the septum and the PDA for systemic flow; therefore, they usually present with cyanosis fairly early in the neonatal period.

With pulmonary atresia, the murmur heard is usually the machine-like murmur of the PDA and possibly a soft, systolic blowing murmur heard at the lower left and right sternal borders representing tricuspid insufficiency. The murmur of pulmonary stenosis is dependent upon the severity of the lesion; often, a loud ejection murmur is heard best at the left-upper sternal border and is sometimes associated with a thrill. The pulmonic component of the second heart sound may be delayed with severe pulmonary stenosis and absent with pulmonary atresia. Left ventricular hypertrophy and a mild

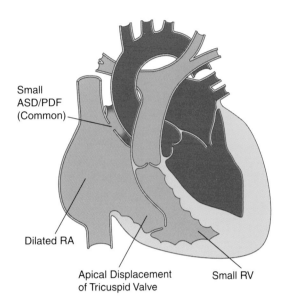

Figure 4–4. Ebstein anomaly.

left QRS axis are usually seen with pulmonary atresia. Pulmonary stenosis is usually associated with right ventricular hypertrophy, right atrial enlargement, and a mild left QRS axis as well. Chest x-ray can show varying cardiomegaly with decreased pulmonary vascularity.

Ebstein anomaly is an abnormality of the tricuspid leaflet(s) and secondary right ventricular defects (Figure 4–4). It is characterized by varying degrees of inferior displacement of the proximal attachments of the septal and posterior leaflets of the tricuspid valve from the atrioventricular ring, and is commonly associated with other cardiac defects.[8] There has been an association with first trimester use of lithium; overall, Ebstein anomaly represents <1% of all congenital heart disease. The more severe forms have insufficient tricuspid valves, reduced right ventricular cavity size, and right ventricular outflow tract obstruction resulting in severe cyanosis, which is a common presentation in the neonatal period. Although the rate has decreased from a number of years ago, neonates presenting with cyanosis still have a high mortality rate.[9]

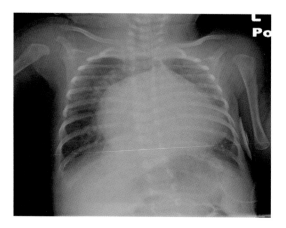

Figure 4–5. Chest x-ray in Ebstein anomaly. *Source:* From Chen MY, Pope TL, Ott DJ, et al. Basic Radiology. New York, NY: McGraw-Hill; 2004.

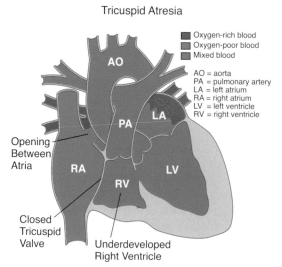

Figure 4–6. Tricuspid atresia.

Ebstein anomaly has a fairly typical murmur, chest x-ray, and ECG. On auscultation, a systolic murmur that increases in intensity with inspiration can be heard and may be associated with a mid-diastolic murmur. A triple or quadruple gallop associated with widely split first and second heart sounds are characteristic. Chest x-ray shows an enormous cardiomegaly ("wall to wall heart") with diminished pulmonary vascularity (Figure 4–5).[10] The classical ECG findings are right bundle branch block, large P waves, right axis deviation, and PR prolongation. A Wolff-Parkinson-White pattern may be present and will have a left bundle branch pattern. Some patients may present with a re-entrant SVT because of the accessory pathways that are commonly associated with the lesion.

Tricuspid atresia (TA) represents approximately 1% to 2% of all congenital heart disease in the first year of life, and results from agenesis of the tricuspid orifice without direct right AV communication (Figure 4–6). Pulmonary blood flow is dependent on intra-atrial communication and an associated VSD and/or PDA. Without a VSD, pulmonary atresia and a hypoplastic right ventricle will likely be present. Approximately 30% of cases are associated with transposition of the great vessels and a large VSD (often presenting with a CHF picture), but overall there is normal artery anatomy more than half the time.

Unless the VSD and right ventricular outflow tract are widely patent, these neonates often present with severe cyanosis as the PDA closes. The severity of the cyanosis is indirectly related to the amount of pulmonary blood flow. The quiet precordium distinguishes tricuspid atresia from other forms of cyanotic congenital heart defects with the exception of hypoplastic right heart syndrome. Auscultation usually reveals a single S2, a machine-like murmur indicating the presence of a PDA, and a systolic murmur indicative of a VSD. The systolic murmur is best heard at the left lower sternal border and can range from soft to harsh depending upon the size of the VSD. Neonates with TA and a large VSD may have long and harsh pansystolic murmurs. Without transposition of the great vessels, chest x-ray will likely show a normal-sized heart with decreases in pulmonary vascularity. With transposition there will likely be mild cardiomegaly with increased pulmonary vascularity. An ECG may

Tetrology of Fallot

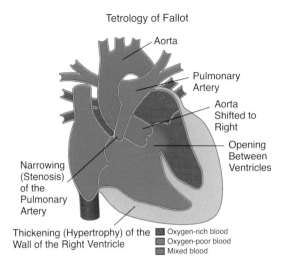

Figure 4–7. Tetralogy of Fallot.

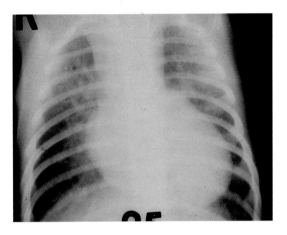

Figure 4–8. Boot-shaped heart in tetralogy of Fallot.

show left ventricular hypertrophy, right atrial hypertrophy with prominent P waves in limb lead II, left QRS axis deviation, and a short P-R interval.

Tetralogy of Fallot (TOF) represents approximately 10% of all congenital heart disease and is one of the most common forms of CHDs in the neonatal period.[11] It is defined as having 4 anatomic abnormalities: 1) VSD, 2) right ventricular outflow obstruction, 3) overriding aorta, and 4) right ventricular hypertrophy (Figure 4–7). Clinical presentations vary depending on the numerous anatomic variations that exist. The severity of right ventricular outflow obstruction is directly related to the degree of cyanosis seen. Because of the large VSD associated with TOF, the pressure in the right ventricle is nearly equal to that of the left ventricle. Neonates may have an acute hypoxic episode ("hypercyanotic spell" or "tet spell") with any action that results in a reduction of systemic vascular resistance, therefore leading to a right-to-left shunting of deoxygenated blood. Once the right-to-left shunting begins, a viscous cycle of increased systemic venous return and increased right-to-left shunting

follows, resulting in hypoxia, hypercapnea, and acidosis.[12] Following is a list of factors that may precipitate a tet spell:

1. Crying
2. Straining (ie, defecation)
3. Feeding
4. Fever
5. Hypovolemia (ie, gastroenteritis)

Most neonates who present after the newborn period with a sudden onset of cyanosis, irritability, and deep rapid respirations (hyperpnea) will likely have one of the above events in their immediate history. The hyperpnea during the event helps distinguish a tet spell from other disease processes that produce tachypnea (ie, respiratory tract infections). Their physical examination includes a prominent right ventricular impulse on precordial examination. There may be a single S2, an ejection click, and loud systolic ejection murmur. The chest x-ray classically shows a boot-shaped heart with normal heart size and normal to decreased pulmonary vascular markings (Figure 4–8). The ECG is likely to show right ventricular hypertrophy and right axis deviation.

Increased PBF

Total anomalous pulmonary venous return (TAPVR) is characterized by pulmonary venous drainage into the right atrium or the systemic veins that ultimately drain into the right side of the heart. Although TAPVR represents a small percentage of patients with CHDs, close to half of patients will develop symptoms during the first month of life.[13] There are 4 different subtypes:

1. Supracardiac (50%)
2. Cardiac (20%)
3. Infracardiac and subdiaphagmatic (20%)
4. Mixed (10%)

The common denominators of the 4 subtypes of lesions are an increase in systemic venous return, increased pulmonary blood flow, and a right-to-left shunt.

A right-to-left shunt at the atrial level (PFO, ASD) is always seen with this diagnosis and approximately one-third of patients have other associated defects such as a PDA, VSD, TGA, heterotaxy syndrome, and aortic arch anomalies (Figure 4–9). Neonates who have an obstruction of the pulmonary venous return will almost always present shortly after birth with severe cyanosis and respiratory distress requiring emergent surgical intervention. Obstruction is most commonly seen in the infracardiac and subdiaphragmatic subtype as the vessels make their way through the diaphragm to the portal system. The more common nonobstructive pattern may not be present until the PVR starts to drop and blood flow increases to the lungs causing signs and symptoms of CHF. Right-to-left shunting will increase, causing a noticeable cyanosis

Most neonates with a nonobstructed TAPVR will present with signs of CHF and mild-to-moderate cyanosis.[14] Heart sounds may be normal early in the neonatal period but later on a gallop rhythm with a soft ejection murmur (left sternal border) and a midi-astolic rumble (lower left sternal border and

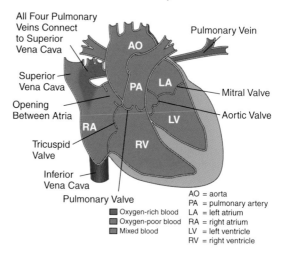

Total Anomalous Pulmonary Venous Return

AO = aorta
PA = pulmonary artery
LA = left atrium
RA = right atrium
LV = left ventricle
RV = right ventricle

■ Oxygen-rich blood
■ Oxygen-poor blood
■ Mixed blood

Figure 4–9. Total anomalous pulmonary venous return.

apex) may be heard. The chest x-ray may show cardiomegaly with pulmonary vascular engorgement. The classic "snowman sign" on chest x-ray is not usually seen in the neonatal period. TAPVR that has pulmonary venous obstruction can have a very mean appearing chest x-ray that can be misinterpreted as diffuse interstitial pneumonia. The ECG may show RAD, RAH, and RVH.

d-Transposition of the great arteries (d-TGA) is the most common of the many varieties of aortic malposition. It is also the most common cause of cyanotic heart disease in the neonatal period with an incidence of 3 to 4 /10,000 live births. In d-TGA, the aorta originates from the right ventricle and the main pulmonary artery from the left ventricle, giving the neonate 2 separate circulations that run in parallel instead of in series (Figure 4–10). One could conceptualize that if the blood returning from the systemic circulation was put directly back into the systemic circulation, and the blood returning from the lungs was put directly back into the lungs, that this would be incompatible with life unless there was a congenital anomaly connecting the 2 parallel

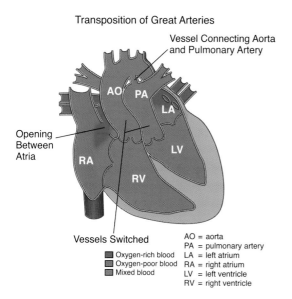

Figure 4–10. Transposition of the great arteries.

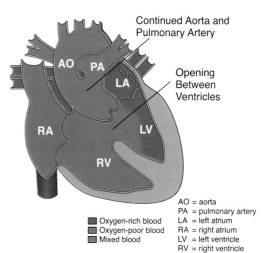

Figure 4–11. Truncus arteriosus.

systems. With VSD occurring in only 20% to 40% of patients with d-TGA, and ASD being a rare coexistence, most newborns rely on the ductus arteriosus and/or the foramen ovale to remain patent. Unfortunately, the ductus usually closes fairly soon in these patients, and the increase in pulmonary vascular return occurring as a result of the anomaly cause the foramen to close soon after birth. For this reason a majority of these patients become severely cyanotic and critically ill within hours after birth and require an emergent atrial septostomy. Those who have a connection between the 2 systems (ie, VSD, ASD) will likely present within the first few weeks of life with cyanosis and signs and symptoms of CHF. The severity of cyanosis can vary with the size of the shunt.

The auscultory examination may only reveal a grade 2 to 3/6 ejection murmur, heard best at the middle of the left sternal border, and a loud single S2. If there is a VSD, a loud, harsh systolic murmur may be heard. The chest x-ray can vary from almost normal to severely abnormal. Neonates with larger VSDs are more likely to have cardiomegaly and increased pulmonary vascular markings. The characteristic "egg on a string" finding on the chest x-ray is diagnostic if present, and represents a narrow superior mediastinum, small thymic shadow, and an egg-shaped heart. The ECG may show RVH and RAD, which are normal findings in the first week of life.

Truncus arteriosus is characterized by the supply of systemic, pulmonary, and coronary arteries from a single arterial trunk that originates from the ventricular chambers (Figure 4–11). The truncus has a single valve with between 2 and 5 leaflets and, except in rare cases, is associated with a VSD. The lesion occurs in approximately 1 per 10,000 live births.

The truncal root supplies both oxygenated and deoxygenated blood to the systemic and pulmonary circulations at systemic pressures, with the flow to either of those circulations depending upon the resistance of each system. The presentation of a neonate with truncus arteriosus is dependent upon the PBF. In most cases, PBF is increased and patients have mild cyanosis with signs and symptoms of CHF. If the PVR is elevated or if there is a restriction at the level of the pulmonary arteries, the patient will have more pronounced cyanosis and less of a CHF picture.

On clinical examination, the precordium may be hyperdynamic with a fairly typical loud, pansystolic murmur that is often heard at the lower-left sternal border, radiating to the entire precordium. A blowing, diastolic high-pitched murmur or rumble may be heard along the left sternal border. The second heart sound is usually single and loud. With 2 to 6 leaflets on the single valve of the truncal root, 1 or many ejection clicks may be heard as well. The ECG may show biventricular hypertrophy. The chest x-ray usually shows cardiomegaly with increased pulmonary vascular marking but is dependent on the amount of PBF. Thirty to 50% of patients may have a right aortic arch.

Management

The initial focus on any sick neonate is to evaluate and manage the ABCs. Oxygen (non-rebreather at 10-15 L/min) should be placed on the patient immediately and the airway controlled accordingly. The patient should be hooked up to a cardiopulmonary monitor, vital signs obtained with pre- and postductal pulse oximetry measurements as well as upper (right) and lower extremity blood pressures. An ECG and chest x-ray must be done but should not interfere with the initial patient stabilization. IV access should to be obtained as soon as possible (unless the patient is a known TET with a hypercyanotic spell [see the next section], then calming may be the first approach) with blood drawn for labs (CBC, electrolytes, bedside glucose, blood culture) and urine sent for analysis and culture. If an ABG is going to be done as part of the hyperoxia test, it should be obtained from the right arm (preductal) with the patient breathing room air. For patients who seem lethargic and/or have respiratory distress, consider elective intubation as

neonates tire quickly and rapidly progress to respiratory failure.

Sepsis can present as cyanosis, so once blood and urine are obtained, broad-spectrum antibiotics should be given as soon as possible. It is not necessary to evaluate the cerebrospinal fluid prior to treatment with antibiotics, but an attempt should be made once the child is stabilized and if the diagnosis of CHD has not been confirmed.

As stated above, patients with cyanotic heart disease will either have increased PBF or decreased PBF associated with their lesion with a PDA being the means of blood flow between the systemic and pulmonary circulations.[6] If the immediate confirmatory diagnosis of CHD is not available (echocardiography) but there is suspicion of CHD, infusion of PGE1 should be initiated at 0.05 to 0.1 µg/kg to maintain ductal patency. For those with increased PBF (ie, d-TGA), the ductus allows oxygenated blood to flow from the pulmonary arteries into the pulmonary circulation. In those with decreased PBF (ie, pulmonary stenosis), opening the ductus provides increased blood flow to the lungs with a subsequent increase in return of oxygenated blood to the systemic circulation. Apnea as a side effect of PGE1 is of most concern (Table 4–4) and elective intubation should be strongly considered, especially if the patient is going to be transported to another facility.

If the patient becomes unstable after PGE1 infusion is initiated, there may be a rare lesion that has obstructed blood flow out of

▶ TABLE 4-4. **PGE1 SIDE EFFECTS**

Apnea
Hypotension
Fever
Tachycardia
Diarrhea
Seizures
Pulmonary congestion
Hypoglycemia

the pulmonary veins (ie, obstructed TAPVR) or left atrium (ie, hypoplastic left heart syndrome, severe mitral stenosis) and the PGE1 infusion should be immediately discontinued. In these instances, echocardiography and interventional catheterization or surgery arrangements must be made immediately.

A pediatric cardiologist should be immediately consulted, as there are certain lesions that may be rapidly stabilized with interventional catheterization and others that may need emergent surgery. For instance, D-TGA with restrictive atrial shunting can be temporarily stabilized with balloon atrial septostomy while critical valvar pulmonary stenosis may be amenable to balloon dilation of the pulmonary valve.

▶ TET (HYPERCYANOTIC) SPELLS

In any neonate presenting with a hypercyanotic spell in which the diagnosis is unknown the initial aim should be to focus on the ABCs then initiate prostaglandin E_1 (PGE1) therapy, as there may be a ductal dependant lesion. If there is a known diagnosis or high suspicion of TOF, then treatment should be targeted on breaking the hypercyanotic viscous cycle. Overall, the goal is to increase SVR and reduce the amount of right-to-left shunting across the VSD. Some neonates will respond to calming and being placed in the knees-to-chest position. Neonates who do not respond to positioning should immediately have an IV placed for administration of IV fluids (10-20 mg/kg of normal saline) and medications. A bolus of IV fluids will maximize preload and may be somewhat protective of the potential hypotension seen with medications used during the spell. Morphine may be given IM, SC, or IV (0.1-0.2 mg/kg/dose). Morphine is thought to suppress the respiratory center responsible for the hyperpnea portion of the viscous cycle, although caution should be taken, as it has the

potential to further decrease SVR. IV sodium bicarbonate (1 mEq/kg IV) may lessen the acidosis, potentially reducing the stimulation of the respiratory center. Ketamine can be given either IV or IM (1-2 mg/kg/dose) to provide sedation and potentially increase SVR. If none of the previous maneuvers break the cycle, then consideration should be given to start of IV phenylephrine (5-20 μm/kg/dose via IV bolus) for its alpha agonist effects in elevating SVR. Lastly, paralysis and intubation should be considered if none of the previous medical interventions have shown effect. Paralysis may be obtained with the use of IV vecuronium (0.1-0.2 mg/kg/dose IV) or rocuronium (0.6-1 mg/kg/dose IV). Make certain to provide sedation if paralysis and intubation is going to be performed.

▶ PROFOUND SHOCK

Neonates who present with signs of poor systemic circulation need to be rapidly evaluated and categorized as having CHD or other diagnosis such as sepsis or metabolic disease, as these can have very similar presentations. Neonates with congenital obstructive left heart syndromes or left ventricular outflow tract obstructive disorders will usually present in the first few weeks of life as their ductal dependant systemic circulation becomes compromised with the closure of the PDA. As the PDA closes and systemic circulation becomes compromised, shock will surely ensue; however, in the interim, they can present with signs and symptoms that crossover with left-to-right shunting physiology.

DIFFERENTIAL DIAGNOSIS

Hypoplastic Left Heart Syndrome

Hypoplastic left heart syndrome (HLHS) is the most common cause of neonatal death secondary to CHD.[15] It is characterized by the

▶ **TABLE 4–5. FINDINGS IN NEONATES WITH CARDIOGENIC SHOCK**

Tachycardia
Hypotension
Diaphoresis
Poor perfusion (dusky, mottled)
Oliguria
Acidosis

underdevelopment of the left side of the heart. The lesions include atresia or stenosis of the mitral and aortic valves, left atrial and ventricular hypoplasia, and hypoplasia of the ascending aorta. The right side of the heart must support both systemic and pulmonary circulations through a patent ductus arteriosus resulting in marked hypertrophy and dilation. The driving force of flow through the PDA is a combination of high PVR and low SVR pre- and antenatally. At birth the SVR dramatically increases and the PVR starts to decline ultimately resulting in a compromise of systemic flow across the PDA.

Those newborns that did not get diagnosed in utero will usually present in the first days to weeks of life with signs of CHF and profound shock (Table 4–5). Neonates presenting with HLHS often have a grayish pallor and poor peripheral pulses. Precordial examination may reveal a prominent right ventricular impulse. On auscultation there will usually be a single second heart sound (P2) heard best at the upper-left sternal border. Although not prominent, a soft midsystolic murmur, midiastolic rumble, and systolic ejection click may be heard. ECG will usually show RVH, LVH, and decreased left-sided forces. Cardiomegaly and pulmonary congestion may be prominent on chest x-ray, especially after the first few days of life.

Critical Aortic Stenosis

Neonates with critical aortic stenosis have a defect that is either valvar, supravalar, or subvalvar.[15] Their age of presentation depends on the degree of stenosis. Many cases that present in the neonatal period have coexisting anomalies such as mitral valve anomalies, aortic coarctation, and hypoplastic left ventricle. Neonates with critical aortic stenosis are dependent on right-to-left shunting and will present with profound shock if that shunt is compromised (ie, PDA closure). Prior to PDA closure they may present with CHF. Depending on the left ventricular output, a systolic thrill as well as a systolic murmur may be heard but are absent with greatly reduced cardiac output. When present, the murmur is best heard at the mid-left sternal border. There is often an early systolic ejection click. ECG will likely show right axis deviation in the neonatal period and chest x-ray usually reveals marked cardiomegaly and pulmonary venous congestion.

Coarctation of the Aorta

Coarctation of the aorta is a narrowing of the upper thoracic aorta caused by posterior infolding or indentation opposite the insertion of the ductus arteriosus and occurs in approximately 4 per 10,000 live births. As the aorta narrows, systemic flow becomes dependant on a PDA (Figure 4–12). Depending on the severity of the coarctation and the degree of

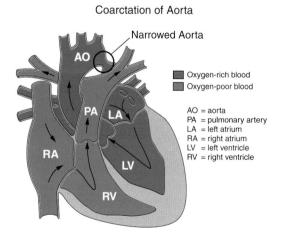

Figure 4–12. Coarctation of the aorta.

ductal closure presentation can vary from profound shock to slowly progressing CHF. If the ductus closes completely, the patient has no means of systemic circulation and will present with profound shock.

Although there is no specific murmur associated with aortic coarctation, murmurs from associated lesions (ie, VSD) may be heard. If the PDA has not yet closed then a machine-like murmur may be heard. ECG may show right axis deviation and right ventricular hypertrophy. Chest x-ray may show marked cardiomegaly and pulmonary venous congestion.

Interrupted Aortic Arch

Complete interrupted aortic arch is characterized by a disconnect of the transverse aortic arch and the descending thoracic aorta. Blood flow to the descending aorta is supplied by a patent ducts arteriosus. Most cases have an associated ventricular septal defect.

The clinical presentation and findings are very similar to that of an aortic coarctation and such are determined by ductal patency. The coexistence of a VSD may add a murmur to the clinical examination.

With a disconnection of the upper and lower body systemic circulation, as seen in severe aortic coarctation and interrupted aortic arch, differential cyanosis may be appreciated. Differential cyanosis is when the upper part of the body is pink and the lower is cyanotic (or vice versa). Some patients will have this finding on examination of skin color, while in others it will only be detected by pulse oximetry. To detect it, oxygen saturation must be measured from both a preductal site (preferably the right arm) and a post-ductal site (lower extremity).

MANAGEMENT

When managing the neonate who presents with profound shock it is imperative to ensure a stable airway, as they can quickly tire and become apneic. Immediately place the patient on oxygen and cardiopulmonary monitoring, and be sure to have a bag-valve-mask at bedside with an appropriately sized mask and oxygen already flowing. Vital signs should include pre- (right arm) and post- (lower extremity) ductal pulse oximetry and blood pressures. Two IV/IO access points need to be immediately obtained. When concerned about cardiogenic shock only 10 mL/kg of crystalloid should initially be given, as a larger bolus may lead to fluid overload. An ECG and portable chest x-ray should be done as soon as possible; labs to be done initially should include a bedside glucose, CBC, BMP, blood culture, and an ABG. The hyperoxia test will assist in the diagnosis but may not be ideal when in the midst of stabilizing a neonate in shock.

The mainstay of treating a neonate who presents with shock and is thought to have a ductal dependant lesion is to immediately start an infusion of PGE1 (0.05-0.1 μ/kg) to re-open/maintain the ductus. As mentioned above, apnea is a major side effect of PGE1 infusion and elective intubation should be strongly considered. Although it would be ideal to have a definite diagnosis of a ductal-dependent lesion prior to staring the infusion, it is not necessary as starting the PGE1 infusion as soon as possible could be a life-saving intervention. Because it is often difficult if not impossible to immediately rule out septic shock, antibiotics should be given as soon as possible, with plans for a lumbar puncture as soon as the patient is stabilized.

A pediatric cardiology consult and echocardiogram should be obtained as soon as possible and, if available, a pediatric intensivist should be notified and included in the patient stabilization. Should the shock state progress to a rhythm disturbance, then the resuscitation should continue following the PALS guidelines for rhythm disturbances.

▶ CONGESTIVE HEART FAILURE

CHF is a result of excessive PBF and/or insufficient systemic blood flow (ie, myocarditis). The presentation of infants with left-to-ight shunting physiology is relatively dependent upon the PVR and the size of the shunt (the larger the size of the shunt means the less resistance to flow across it). As the PVR drops over the first weeks to months of life, the increase in left-to-right shunting causes excessive PBF leading to signs and symptoms of CHF.

Within the spectrum of CHF, it is important to include other etiologies such as those secondary to acquired heart disease. Diagnoses to consider are myocarditis, endocrine and metabolic disorders, endocarditis, and dysrhythmias. Common causes of CHF from left to right shunting are[16,17]:

1. Ventricular septal defect
2. Atrioventricular septal defect
3. Patent ductus arteriosus
4. Large atrial septal defect

With the presentation of CHF often being subtle, patients can be mistaken for having a viral respiratory infection such as bronchiolitis (Table 4–6). Even if a child tests positive for a virus such as respiratory syncytial virus (RSV), it is important to remember that such a clinical picture can exacerbate the symptoms of CHF, adding to the confusion. Infants with CHF can present with various combinations of signs and symptoms.

DIFFERENTIAL DIAGNOSIS

Ventricular Septal Defect

The most common of all congenital heart defects, ventricular septal defects (VSDs) occur in approximately 3.6 per 1000 live births (Table 4–7).[18] The anomaly may be isolated or associated with other heart defects. The defects vary in size and as such determine the timing and overall clinical presentation. Small defects in the muscular septum account for the majority of lesions and usually spontaneously close. To the contrary, larger lesions may consist of nearly complete absence of the interventricular wall creating a common ventricle that can lead to CHF and pulmonary hypertension (Figure 4–13).

Neonates with larger VSDs may present with signs and symptoms of CHF and varying cyanosis. A thrill may be appreciated on

▶ **TABLE 4–6. PRESENTATION OF INFANTS WITH CHF**

History	Physical Exam	Chest X-ray
Sweating (especially with feeds)	Tachypnea	Cardiomegaly
Difficulty feeding	Tachycardia	Pulmonary venous
Failure to thrive	Murmur	congestion
	Respiratory distress	Hyperinflation
	Wheeze or rales	
	Peripheral edema	
	Cyanosis (usually responds to oxygen)	
	Hepatomegaly	
	Gallop rhythm	
	Shock	

Source: Modified from Fuhrman: Pediatric Critical Care. St. Louis, MO: Mosby/Elsevier, p. 401.

▶ TABLE 4–7. PRESENTATIONS OF SPECIFIC CHDS

Presentation	Exam	Findings	
		ECG	Chest X-ray
Cyanotic			
↓PBF			
Pulmonary atresia (intact VSD)	No P2, soft blowing M (TI), machine-like M (PDA)	Mild left QRS axis, LVH	Heart size varies, ↓PVM
Severe pulmonary stenosis	Prolonged P2, ejection click, machine-like M (PDA)	Mild left QRS axis, RVH, RAH	CM, ↓PVM
Ebstein anomaly	Triple or quadruple gallop; systemic and mid-diastolic M	RBBB, large P waves, right axis deviation and PR prolongation	Enormous CM
Tricuspid atresia	Single S2, machine like-M (PDA), systolic M	LVH, RAH, left QRS, short P-R	Normal to mild CM; usually ↓
Tetralogy of Fallot	Single S2, ejection click, loud systolic ejection M	RVH,RAD	Boot-shaped heart
↑PBF			
TAPVR (unobstructed)	Soft-ejection M, mid-diastolic R	RAD, RAH, RVH	↑PVM, cardiomegaly
D-TGA	VSD-related ejection M if any	RAD, RVH	"Egg on a string"
Truncus arteriosus	Pansystolic M, diastolic R; 1 or many ejection clicks	RVH, LVH	Typically cardiomegaly and ↑PVM (varies depending upon PBF)
Profound Shock			
Hypoplastic left heart	Midsystolic M and midiastolic R[a]	RVH, LVH	CM, PC
Critical aortic stenosis	Systolic murmur[b]	RAD	CM,PC
Coarctation of the aorta	From other defects	RAD, RVH	CM,PC
Interrupted aortic arch	VSD related	RAD,RVH	CM,PC
CHF			
VSD	Grade 2-5/6 holosystolic M with thrill	RVH, LVH, RAH	CM, ↑PVM
AV septal defect	Holosytolic M, thrill, mid-diastolic rumble	LAD, LVH, RBBB, prolonged PR interval	
PDA	Machine-like M	LVH, RVH	
Large ASDs	Systolic ejection M	RAD, RVH	

[a]Not prominent. [b]If present.

Abbreviations: CHD, congenital heart disease; CM, cardiomegaly; PC, pulmonary venous congestion; RAD, right axis deviation; RVH, right ventricular hypertrophy; RAH, right atrial hypertrophy; M, murmur; LAD, left axis deviation; PVM, pulmonary vascular markings; M, murmur; RBBB, right bundle branch block; VSD, ventricular septal defect; LVH, left ventricular hypertrophy; PDA, patent ductus arteriosus; TI, tricuspid insufficiency.

Ventricular Septal Defect

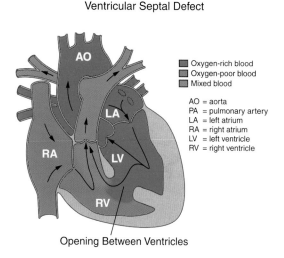

Figure 4–13. Ventricular septal defect.

Atrioventricular Canal Defect

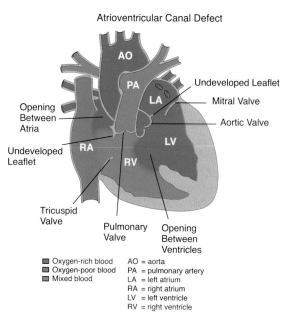

Figure 4–14. Atrioventricular septal defect.

precordial examination and a systolic murmur of varying degrees will likely be heard. The murmur of a VSD is usually a grade 2 to 5/6 holosystolic murmur, heard best at the left-lower sternal border and may radiate throughout the precordium. The ECG of larger VSDs may show LVH, RVH, and LAH. Chest x-ray may show cardiomegaly and increased pulmonary vascular markings.

Atrioventricular Septal Defect

Atrioventricular septal defects are also known as complete AV canal defects and endocardial cushion defects. They account for approximately 3% to 5% of all congenital heart disease and are found in approximately 15% to 20% of newborns with Down syndrome. The defect involves the following:

1. Atrial septal defect
2. Ventricular septal defect
3. Atrioventricular valve defects

The defect has 3 subtypes: complete, incomplete (or partial), and transitional (Figure 4–14). The difference between a complete and incomplete defect is that the ventricular septum is intact in the incomplete subtype. In the transition type, the leaflets of the common AV valve are stuck to the ventricular septum. The common ground for all of the subtypes is a left-to-right shunt at varying degrees with subsequent volume overload. Neonates can present with CHF and cyanosis, with the more complex defects presenting earlier in life.

The precordial examination will likely reveal a hyperactive heart with an associated thrill. Auscultory examination can vary with the most consistent murmur being th at of a VSD. A midiastolic rumble may also be heard. ECG may show left axis deviation, P-R interval prolongation, RBBB, and LVH. Chest x-ray will likely show marked cardiomegaly with the pulmonary vasculature dependent on the level of shunting and the amount of AV valve regurgitation.

Patent Ductus Arteriosus

Vessel Connecting
Aorta and
Pulmonary Artery

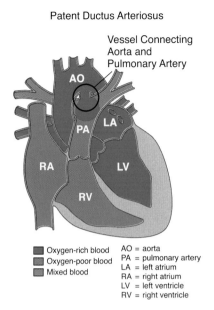

Oxygen-rich blood
Oxygen-poor blood
Mixed blood

AO = aorta
PA = pulmonary artery
LA = left atrium
RA = right atrium
LV = left ventricle
RV = right ventricle

Figure 4–15. Patent ductus arteriosus.

Atrial Septal Defect

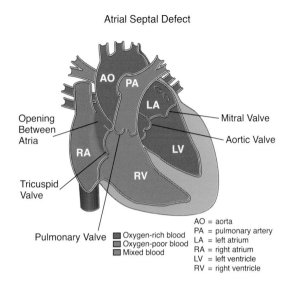

Opening
Between
Atria

Mitral Valve

Aortic Valve

Tricuspid
Valve

Pulmonary Valve

Oxygen-rich blood
Oxygen-poor blood
Mixed blood

AO = aorta
PA = pulmonary artery
LA = left atrium
RA = right atrium
LV = left ventricle
RV = right ventricle

Figure 4–16. Atrial septal defect.

Patent Ductus Arteriosus

The ductus arteriosus may remain patent as an isolated lesion that is often idiopathic or as a means of maintaining communication between the pulmonary and systemic circulation in a CHD that would otherwise separate the 2 systems (ie, d-TGA) (Figure 4–15).[18] In the former, the higher systemic pressure directs ductal flow toward the pulmonary circulation (unless there is underlying pulmonary hypertension) and, depending on the amount of blood entering the pulmonary artery, can lead to signs and symptoms of CHF in the neonatal period. That being said, the vast majority of neonates with a PDA will be free of CHF symptoms and diagnosed after an asymptomatic murmur is heard on examination.

As stated above, when the PDA is large, the neonate may present with signs and symptoms of CHF. Assuming a large PDA, precordial examination may reveal a thrill that is best felt in the left second intercostals space. A machine-like (or rolling-thunder) murmur that reaches maximum intensity at the end of systole is classic. The pulse pressure may be wide with associated bounding pulses. Depending upon the amount of blood returning to the left atrium, a mid-diastolic may be heard due to increased blood flow across the mitral valve. ECG may show RVH and LVH with larger PDAs, but otherwise is normal with smaller lesions. Chest x-ray will show cardiomegaly and increased pulmonary vascular markings with larger lesions.

Large ASD

An ASD is a rare cause of CHF in any neonate unless there are other defects or if the defect is large; even then, the presentation is usually after the first month of life. With large ASDs accompanied by significant left-to-right shunting, oxygenated blood enters the pulmonary circulation with increasing overload as the PVR drops (Figure 4–16). This overload of the pulmonary circulation leads to signs and symptoms of CHF.

If a neonate does present with CHF because of a significant ASD-related left-to-right shunt, they may have a widely split S2 and a systolic murmur secondary to an increased amount of blood through the right ventricular outflow tract and pulmonary valve. ECG may show right axis deviation/right ventricular hypertrophy and possibly and a mild right ventricular conduction delay. Chest x-ray may show cardiomegaly and increased pulmonary vascular markings.

MANAGEMENT

The initial focus is on evaluating and stabilizing the ABCs followed by the correction of any metabolic supply and demand mismatches.[19] Neonates may have CHF secondary to volume overload, excess afterload, decreased contractility, rhythm abnormalities, or any combination of the aforementioned, and should be treated accordingly. If there is decreased cardiac contractility and subsequent volume overload, then the focus will be to remove excess fluid (ie, furosemide) and increase cardiac contractility (ie, dopamine and dobutamine).[20] On the other hand, if the failure is secondary to excess afterload, then the focus is to decrease the afterload with a vasodilating agent such as nitroprusside or milrinone.

With the initial ABCs, include O_2 support via a nonrebreather and early IV access. Elevation of the head to 30 to 45 degrees is optimal. Vital signs should include pre- (right extremity) and postductal pulse oximetry as well as upper (right) and lower extremity blood pressures. If the patient is having significant respiratory distress or failure, then a definitive airway should be placed.

Tertiary evaluation should include a chest x-ray and ECG, as well as blood sent for CBC, electrolytes, blood culture, and brain natriuretic peptide (BNP).[21] The chest x-ray will help determine heart size and whether or not there

is any pulmonary edema. ECG may augment the diagnosis by revealing ventricular hypertrophy, ST changes, and/or T wave abnormalities. The CBC and electrolytes will aid in evaluating for anemia, acidosis, and any electrolyte imbalances that may need correction to maximize cardiac contractility. Evaluation of the BNP has been a well-known marker of CHF in adults and now appears to be a helpful indicator when there are clinical signs of heart failure in children. An important point when evaluating a BNP level in the neonate is that a level of 232 pg/mL is normal at birth and decreases to approximately 48 pg/mL by the end of the first week, and to less than 33 pg/mL by 2 weeks of age. Although the mainstay of diagnosis is echocardiography and should be done as soon as possible, it is not always immediately obtainable and the use of clinical judgment with the available ancillary data must be relied upon to make the initial diagnosis of CHF.

When treating a neonate with clinically significant CHF, diuretics and inotropes are the usual drugs of choice.[20] In patients with volume overload, the goal is to remove excess fluid from the circulation to decrease preload. A loop diuretic such as furosemide can be given at a dose of 0.5-1 mg/kg IV. When contractility is an issue, there are a few inotropic agents that may be used. Dopamine (5-10 µg/kg/min) can be given to increase contractility but will not have a major effect on reducing the afterload. Caution needs to be taken as higher doses (>10-15 mcg/kg/min) have known vasoconstrictor and chronotropic properties. Neonates do not have large catecholamine stores; therefore, because its pharmacologic effects are secondary to indirect stimulation of the β_1 receptor by release of norepinephrine, dopamine may have decreasing efficacy over time in this age group. When reduction of afterload as well as inotropy is the desired effect, dobutamine and milrinone are good agents. Dobutamine directly stimulates β_1 and β_2 receptors leading to increased contractility and a reduction in SVR. It is given at a dose of 2.5-20 µg/kg/min and is titrated to effect. Milrinone is a phosphodiesterase inhibitor that acts by increasing intracellular cyclic adenosine monophosphate (cAMP). It can be considered an "ino-dilator" in that it produces positive inotropy and causes systemic and pulmonary vasodilation. It is dosed via an initial loading dose of 50 µg/kg over 15 minutes followed by a maintenance dose of 0.35-75 µg/kg/min.

If there is a sudden cardiovascular collapse, then the neonate should be carefully re-evaluated and further investigation into other cardiovascular and medical causes should be done. It is unlikely that the sudden collapse would be due to an isolated left-to-right shunt (ie, VSD, PDA, AV canal, large ASD).

Asymptomatic Murmur

It is far more likely that a pediatric provider will encounter a neonate with an asymptomatic heart murmur rather than with signs and symptoms of a structural defect. That being said, it is pertinent to know the qualities of a physiologic murmur in order to weed out the pathologic entities. Overall, heart murmurs in the first 6 months of life are more likely to reflect a structural defect than an innocent process, with exception being in the newborn period where it has been reported that 60% of healthy newborns have an audible murmur.[22,23]

Generally speaking, innocent murmurs are always heard in systole (usually early in systole), have a short duration, a low intensity (grade 1 or 2), and a vibrating (or musical) quality. There will never be a diastolic component (except for a venous hum) and there are no extra or absent heart sounds. The most common innocent murmur heard in the neonatal period is the physiologic peripheral pulmonic stenosis murmur (PPPS) that is usually a grade I-II/IV soft ejection murmur best heard at the left-upper sternal border. It is characteristically heard at the bilateral axillae and the back. The murmur is caused by the relatively small size of the pulmonary artery branches compared to the large main pulmonary artery, as well as the sharp angle created as they branch from the main pulmonary artery. Most murmurs related to PPPS should disappear by 6 months as the vessels grow in diameter.

In contrast to an innocent murmur, pathologic murmurs are usually longer and louder than innocent murmurs and often obscure heart sounds. Heart sounds may be abnormally split, excessive (ie, S4), or absent. They are usually grade 3 or higher and may be associated with thrills and/or extra sounds such as clicks. All pansystolic and diastolic murmurs, with the exception of a venous hum, are pathologic.

If a pathologic murmur is detected, further testing should be done (ie, ECG, chest x-ray, CBC, BMP) and a pediatric cardiologic consultation should be arranged. For neonates with asymptomatic murmurs that are thought to be ductal dependent, immediate cardiac consultation should be obtained.

▶ CLASSIC ARRHYTHMIAS

The heart rate in the first month of life ranges between 90 and 180 bpm depending upon whether the patient is awake, sleeping, or crying. There are many variations of normal arrhythmias, the most common being sinus arrhythmia.[24] It can be very pronounced and sound very abnormal on auscultation and is the autonomic reflex associated with respiration. Pauses will come with the patient's inspirations. In sinus arrhythmia, one of the keys is to note that the P-wave morphology and the P/QRS relationship is constant even though the distance between the two vary. Patients can have tachycardias or bradycardias from secondary causes that are not indicative of cardiac disease. The most common scenario that any pediatric practitioner will see is the infant with sinus tachycardia secondary to fever or crying.

Premature atrial contractions (PAC) are extremely common in the first weeks of life and are almost always benign. Sometimes the premature atrial contractions are blocked and sometimes they are conducted. They have narrow complex QRS waves associated with them. Sometimes the physician may see a newborn with atrial bigeminy (every other atrial beet blocked) and the baby may appear bradycardic, but this is usually a benign process and should break with time. In general, PACs, either blocked or conducted, are very common in the newborn period. Premature beats can come from the junction (AV node), which is a narrow complex, but there is no P wave in front of them. They are relatively rare but usually benign.

Premature ventricular contractions (PVCs) come from the ventricle and they cause a wider complex QRS. PVCs are not uncommon in the newborn period and in fact have been found in up to 18% healthy neonates. Polymorphic and frequent PVCs are more likely to be significant. That being said, neonates with PVCs found on an ECG should undergo a full cardiac evaluation to ensure the absence of other underlying electrophysiologic and congenital abnormalities.

The neonate with a dysrhythmia can present with any of the following:

1. Irritability
2. Difficulty feeding
3. Sweating
4. Vomiting
5. Respiratory distress
6. Shock

The approach to any arrhythmia should be systematic. First, an effort should be made to obtain a 12-lead ECG. Determine whether the rhythm is to fast or to slow; then evaluate the QRS complex to establish if it is wide or narrow and if every P wave has a QRS that follows it, and if every QRS complex has a preceding P wave. If the QRS complex is narrow and is not associated with P waves, then the physician is most likely dealing with a form of supraventricular tachycardia (SVT) (Figure 4–17). Rhythms originating in the

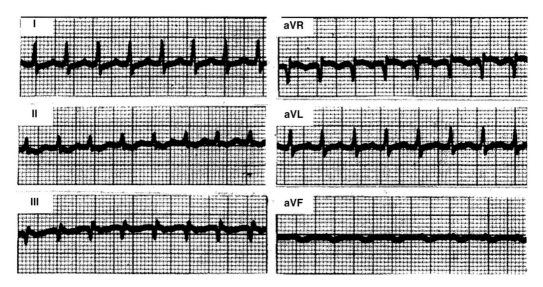

Figure 4–17. Supraventricular tachycardia. *Source:* From McPhee SJ, Papadakis MA: *Current Medical Diagnosis and Treatment*, 48th ed. New York, NY: McGraw-Hill; 2009.

ventricle are usually wide complexes, bizarre in configuration and randomly associated with P waves.

BRADYARRHYTHMIAS

The most common reason that a neonate will be bradycardic is sinus bradycardia secondary to respiratory failure and subsequent hypoxia. This is crucial to recognize because rapid correction of the hypoxia will likely correct the sinus bradycardia and avoid cardiac arrest.

First degree is a prolonged PR interval; second degree has 2 types, Mobitz I (Wenckebach) and Mobitz II. Mobitz I has progressive PR prolongation followed by a nonconductive beat (Figure 4–18). First degree and Mobitz I are usually benign. Mobitz II has intermittent loss of atrioventricular (AV)

conduction without preceding PR prolongation and commonly progresses to complete block (third degree) but is uncommon in the neonatal period. Thirddegree heart block or complete heart block is a form of AV dissociation. It is sometimes difficult to differentiate Mobitz type I and complete heart block. One way to differentiate is that the R-R interval is constant in complete heart block, whereas in second degree Mobitz I the R-R interval varies. The most common causes are maternal collagen vascular disease such as maternal lupus, congenitally corrected L-transposition of the great vessels, and myocarditis. Cardiac surgery for such pathologies as VSD, transposition, subaortic stenosis, and endocardial cushion defects can cause third-degree heart block as well. Symptoms can be subtle and include poor feeding, shortness of breath, and signs and symptoms of CHF. If the patient is symptomatic or if the rate is

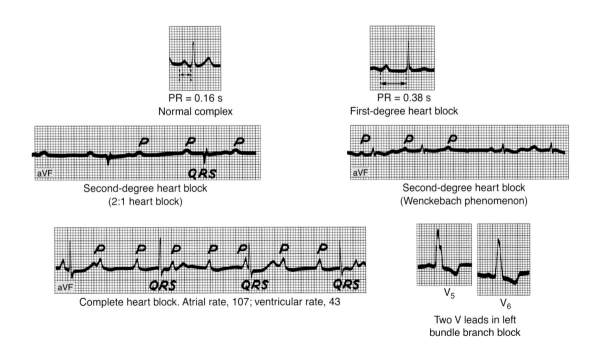

Figure 4–18. Types of heart blocks. *Source:* From Ganong WF. Review of Medical Physiology, 22nd ed. New York, NY: McGraw-Hill; 2005.

less than 60 bpm in the infant then pacing is needed.

TACHYARRHYTHMIAS

As stated above, most neonates who are tachycardic will have a sinus tachycardia secondary to crying or an existing fever. Although it is possible for a neonate with sinus tachycardia to have a rate in the lower 200s, extreme caution must be taken, as supraventricular tachycardia must first be ruled out.

Abnormal tachycardias consist of SVT, junctional tachycardia, and ventricular tachycardia. Atrial flutter and atrial fibrillation are included in SVT—SVT simply refers to any tachyarrhythmia that has its origin above the level of the ventricles.

The majority of SVTs in children are reciprocating (reentry) AV tachycardias (RAVT) rather than a single foci that is rapidly firing. Most cases are narrow-complex tachycardias with absent P waves and heart rates greater than 220 bpm. Unstable patients need cardioversion with 0.5-1 j/kg and 2 j/kg if the first attempt is unsuccessful. The treatment of the stable patient is IV adenosine 0.1-0.3 mg/kg; because adenosine has less than a 10-sec half-life, it needs to be pushed as a rapid infusion with a rapid 5-10 cc bolus of normal saline after administration. Adenosine blocks the AV node, hence terminating AV reciprocating tachycardias. Vagal maneuvers such as ice to the face or rectal stimulation may work but should not slow down the process of preparing for IV adenosine or cardioversion. Digoxin does have some utility in the patient with RAVT but is not recommended for the patient with Wolff-Parkinson-White (WPW) syndrome and therefore should not be used unless in conjunction with expert pediatric cardiac consultation. Verapamil should not be used for the treatment of SVTs in the first year of life, particularly in the first month of life. Calcium channel blockers are potent negative inotropes that can further decompensate the ventricular function in a neonate who has already sustained prolonged tachycardia and may already have ventricular compromise. There have been reports of neonates treated with a calcium channel blocker that had sudden death.

Twenty-five to 50% of infants with SVT have WPW; 80% have a normal heart and 20% an abnormal heart (eg, L-TGA, Ebstein anomaly, and hypertrophic cardiomyopathy). In WPW there is a normal AV node as well as another accessory pathway for electricity to move between the atria and the ventricles. The ECG in a pre-exited heart will have a delta wave when the patient is in normal sinus rhythm (Figure 4–19). The diagnosis of WPW should be heavily considered when the ECG (while in sinus rhythm) has a short PR interval and an up slurring of the QRS (delta wave).

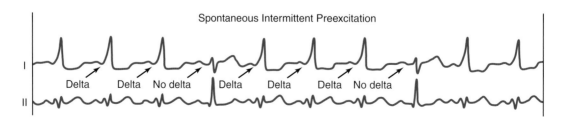

Spontaneous Intermittent Preexcitation

Figure 4–19. ECG in Wolff-Parkinson-White syndrome. *Source:* From Hay WW, Levin MJ, Sondheimer JM, Deterding RR. Current Diagnosis and Treatment, 19th ed. New York, NY: McGraw-Hill; 2009.

Atrial fibrillation and atrial flutter are rare events in the neonatal period and when present are usually secondary to a congenital heart defect or post intra-atrial surgery. Post surgical sick sinus syndrome is the usual culprit and can lead to a multitude of other arrhythmias including:

1. Profound sinus bradycardia
2. Sinoatrial exit block
3. Sinus arrest with junctional escape
4. Paroxysmal atrial tachycardia

Ventricular dysrhythmias are far less common than SVT in the neonatal period. There is a wide QRS complex and the heart rate is usually between 150 and 200 bpm. Causes include but are not limited to the following:

1. Electrolyte imbalances
2. Metabolic disturbances
3. Systemic infections
4. Sympathomimetic agents
5. Cardiac tumors
6. Drug toxins
7. Congenital cardiac disease
8. Acquired cardiac disease
9. Post cardiac surgery
10. Prolonged Q-T syndrome

Topical anesthetics, such as dibucaine and others that may be used for teething, can cause deadly ventricular tachycardias with a very small ingestion. These infants may also be hypoxic and cyanotic secondary to the oxidant effects of the anesthetic inducing methemoglobinemia. Aggressive treatment with sodium bicarbonate and an antidysrhythmic such as lidocaine should be given in this scenario.

Accelerated idioventricular rhythm is the most common ventricular tachycardia in the neonate. It is caused by an autonomic mechanism that arises from the right ventricular outflow tract. The ventricular rate is the same or faster than the atrial rate (usually within 12-20 beats) and there is often AV dissociation during the tachycardia. There may be an association with anesthetics given the higher prevalence in neonates who were delivered by cesarean section. The patients are usually asymptomatic and the dysrhythmia usually resolves spontaneously over weeks to months.

Regardless of the origin of the ventricular tachycardia, the unstable patient should be treated following PALS guidelines. In neonates with wide complex tachycardias who have pulses but poor perfusion, synchronized cardioversion should be attempted (under sedation if possible) followed by the administration of antidysrhythmics if needed. If the patient is pulseless (with a shockable rhythm), then immediate defibrillation should be attempted (Figures 4–20 & 4–21).

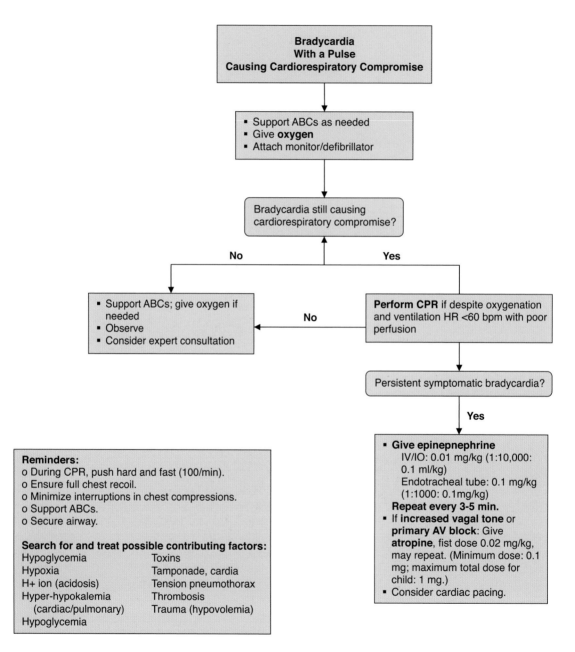

Figure 4-20. Treatment of bradycardia. *Source:* Pediatric Advanced Life Support Textbook, American Heart Association, 2009.

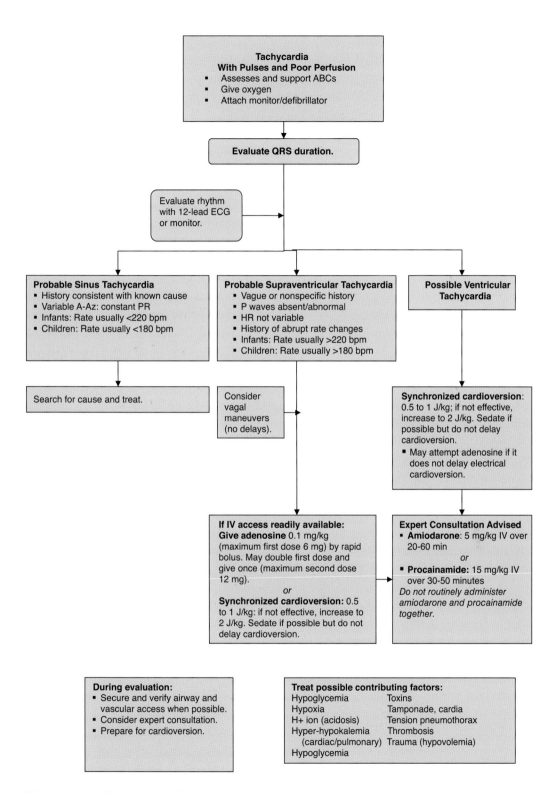

Tachycardia
With Pulses and Poor Perfusion
- Assesses and support ABCs
- Give oxygen
- Attach monitor/defibrillator

Evaluate QRS duration.

Evaluate rhythm with 12-lead ECG or monitor.

Probable Sinus Tachycardia
- History consistent with known cause
- Variable A-Az: constant PR
- Infants: Rate usually <220 bpm
- Children: Rate usually <180 bpm

Probable Supraventricular Tachycardia
- Vague or nonspecific history
- P waves absent/abnormal
- HR not variable
- History of abrupt rate changes
- Infants: Rate usually >220 bpm
- Children: Rate usually >180 bpm

Possible Ventricular Tachycardia

Search for cause and treat.

Consider vagal maneuvers (no delays).

Synchronized cardioversion: 0.5 to 1 J/kg; if not effective, increase to 2 J/kg. Sedate if possible but do not delay cardioversion.
- May attempt adenosine if it does not delay electrical cardioversion.

If IV access readily available:
Give adenosine 0.1 mg/kg (maximum first dose 6 mg) by rapid bolus. May double first dose and give once (maximum second dose 12 mg).
or
Synchronized cardioversion: 0.5 to 1 J/kg: if not effective, increase to 2 J/kg. Sedate if possible but do not delay cardioversion.

Expert Consultation Advised
- **Amiodarone:** 5 mg/kg IV over 20-60 min
  or
- **Procainamide:** 15 mg/kg IV over 30-50 minutes
Do not routinely administer amiodarone and procainamide together.

During evaluation:
- Secure and verify airway and vascular access when possible.
- Consider expert consultation.
- Prepare for cardioversion.

Treat possible contributing factors:
Hypoglycemia   Toxins
Hypoxia   Tamponade, cardia
H+ ion (acidosis)   Tension pneumothorax
Hyper-hypokalemia   Thrombosis
  (cardiac/pulmonary) Trauma (hypovolemia)
Hypoglycemia

Figure 4–21. Treatment of tachycardia. *Source:* Pediatric Advanced Life Support Textbook, American Heart Association, 2009.

REFERENCES

1. Hoffman J, Kaplan D. The incidence of congenital heart disease. *J Am Coll Cardio.* 2002;39:1890-900.

2. Friedman A, Fahey J. The transition from fetal to neonatal circulation: Normal responses and implications for infants with heart disease. *Semin Perinatol.* 1993;17:106-121.

3. Oishu P, Hoffman J, Fuhrman P, Fineman J. Regional circulation. In: *Pediatric Critical Care.* 3rd ed. Philadelphia: Mosby; 2006:225-250.

4. Rudolph M. Fetal circulation and cardiovascular adjustments after birth. In: *Rudolph's Pediatrics.* 21st ed. New York: McGraw Hill Medical; 2003.

5. Dieckmann R, Pediatric Assessment. In: APLS The Pediatric Emergency Medicine Resource. 4th ed. Sudbury: MA, Jones and Bartlett, 2007.

6. Brown K. The infant with undiagnosed cardiac disease in the emergency department. Clin *Ped Emerg Med.* 2005;6:200-206.

7. Frommelt M, Frommelt P. Cyanosis. In: *Practical Strategies in Pediatric Diagnosis and Therapy.* 2nd ed. Philadelphia: Elsevier; 2004:160-163.

8. Paranon S. Acar P. Ebstein's anomaly of the tricuspid valve: from fetus to adult: congenital heart disease. *Heart.* 2008;94(2):237-243.

9. Celermajer DS, Bull C, Till JA, et al. Ebstein's anomaly: presentation and outcome from fetus to adult. *J Am Coll Cardiol.* 1994;23(1):170-176.

10. Yetman A, Freedom R, McCrindle B. Outcome in cyanotic neonates with Ebstein's anomaly. *Am J Cardiol.* 1998;81:749-754.

11. Yee L. Cardiac emergencies in the first year of life. *Emerg Med Clin N Am.* 2007;25:981-1008.

12. Teitel D. Right-to-left shunts. In: *Rudolph's Pediatrics.* 21st ed. New York: McGraw-Hill Medical; 2003:1814-1832.

13. Nurkalem Z. et al. Total anomalous pulmonary venous return in the fourth decade. *Int J Cardiol.* 2006;113:124-126.

14. Marino B. Diagnosis and management of the newborn with suspected congenital heart disease. *Clin Perinatol.* 2001;28(1):91-136.

15. Rudolph M. Obstructive congenital cardiac lesions. In: *Rudolph's Pediatrics.* 21st ed. New York: McGraw Hill Medical; 2003:1800-1812.

16. Rudolph M. Left to Right shunts. In: *Rudolph's Pediatrics.* 21st ed. New York: McGraw Hill Medical; 2003.

17. Bernstein D. Acyanotic congenital heart disease: The left-to-right shunt lesions. In: *Nelsons Textbook of Pediatrics.* 18th ed. Philadelphia: Saunders; 2003.

18. Inaba A. Congenital heart disease. In: *Pediatric Emergency Medicine.* 1st ed. Philadelphia: Saunders; 2008:277-287.

19. Wessel D, Laussen P. Cardiac intesive care. In: *Pediatric Critical Care.* 3rd ed. Philadelphia: Mosby; 2006:419-460.

20. Caligaro I, Burman C. Pharmacologic considerations in the neonate with congenital heart disease. *Clin Perinatol.* 2001;28(1):209-222.

21. Westlind A. et al. Clinical signs of heart failure are associated with increased levels of natriuretic peptide types B and A in children with congenital heart defects or cardiomyopathy. *Acta Paediatr.* 2004;93:340-345.

22. Braudo M, Rowe RD. Auscultation of the heart-early neonatal period. *Am J Dis Child.* 1961;101:575-586.

23. Frommelt MA. Differential diagnosis and approach to a heart murmur in term infants. *Pediatr Clin N Am.* 2004;51:1023-1032.

24. Tanel RE, Rhodes LA. Fetal and neonatal arrhythmias. *Clin Perinatol.* 2001;28:187-197.

CHAPTER 5

Gastrointestinal Emergencies

Derek Cooney, MD

Richard M. Cantor, MD, FAAP/FACEP

▶ GENERAL CONCEPTS

Feeding patterns vary greatly during the first few weeks of life. Many parents are overly concerned regarding the adequacy of their nutritional efforts. The concept of "food equals love" cannot be overstated because, to the new parent, adequate weight gain and regular intake are often the only measures of their "success" as a parent. That being said, adequate weight gain often rules out most pathologic problems in the young infant.

Variation in times between feedings is the rule in the first few weeks during the establishment of a self-regulated pattern. By the end of first month, more than 90% of infants establish a suitable and reasonably regular schedule.

Most normal newborns lose 5% to 10% of their birth weight over the first week of life. Thereafter, as a general rule, a weight gain of 20 to 30 g per day is considered acceptable. Utilization of standard growth charts will provide guidance in assessing the "problem" feeder.

There are many forms of infant formulas available on the market today. They differ in many aspects, ie, calories, forms of protein, fats, and carbohydrates. These are reviewed in Table 5–1.

▶ CLASSIC COMPLAINTS

It is common for children to present to the emergency department (ED) for evaluation of gastrointestinal (GI) symptoms during the neonatal period. Feeding difficulties, vomiting, diarrhea, constipation, and jaundice are all relatively routine concerns, and each of these are covered in the following. Due to the anxiety that many parents and caregivers experience when their child is suffering from one of these symptoms, it is important to take a detailed history, observe the child and presenting adult(s), perform a thorough examination, and be attentive to the presenting concerns. In addition to details relating

▶ TABLE 5-1. **AVAILABLE INFANT FORMULAS AND COMPOSITION**

Brand Name	Calories per Ounce	Protein Type	Fat Type	Carbohydrate Type	Clinical Indication(s)
Milk-Based Formulas					
Enfamil Low Iron[a] Enfamil with Iron[a] Enfamil Premature Lipil[a] Carnation Good Start[b] Carnation Follow Up[b] Similac[c] Similac with Iron[c]	20 kcal/oz	Milk	Palm, soy, coconut, safflower and sunflower oils	Lactose	Standard formulas
Soy-Based Formulas					
Isomil[c] Enfamil Prosobee[a] Carnation Allsoy[b]	20 kcal/oz	Soy	Soy oil, palm olein, coconut, sunflower and safflower oils	Sucrose, corn syrup solids	Infants with galactosemia or for parents that are strict vegetarians
Formulas for Preterm Infants					
Enfamil EnfaCare Lipil[a] Enfamil Premature[a] Similac Special Care[c]	22-24 kcal/oz	Milk	MCT	Lactose	Premature infants; low birth weight
Predigested Protein Formulas					
Pregestimil[a] Nutramigen[a] Alimentum[c]	20 kcal/oz	Hydrolyzed casein	MCT	Sucrose, corn syrup solids	Infants with digestive problems; cystic fibrosis; cow's milk allergy; fat malabsorption issues
Others					
Similac PM 60/40[c]	20 kcal/oz	Whey protein and sodium Caseinate	High oleic safflower, soy, and coconut oils	Lactose	Infants with inborn errors of metabolism; infants with impaired renal function
BCAD 1 & 2[c]	20 kcal/oz	Amino acids	Soy oil	Corn syrup solids, sucrose, and modified corn starch	Inborn errors of metabolism

(*continued*)

► TABLE 5–1. **(CONTINUED)**

Brand Name	Calories per Ounce	Protein Type	Fat Type	Carbohydrate Type	Clinical Indication(s)
GA[c]	20 kcal/oz	Amino acids	Palm olein oil, coconut oil, soy oil, sunflower oil	Corn syrup solids, sucrose, modified corn starch, maltodextrin	Inborn errors of metabolism

Abbreviation: MCT, medium-chain triglycerides.
[a]Mead Johnson Nutritionals.
[b]Nestle.
[c]Abbott Laboratories.

to the symptomology, other historical details should be gathered. It is important to know basic information about the child's living conditions, feeding schedule, and urine and stool output. Prenatal health of the mother and known complications (preeclampsia, infections, drug use, etc), birth history (prematurity, anoxia, etc), maternal medications during the prenatal and perinatal period, health of siblings, and any congenital conditions of the mother or father should also be reviewed.

► **VOMITING**

Neonatal vomiting is a common complaint. Many times the child is well and experiencing benign episodes of spitting up or reflux. However, it is important to consider that even first-time parents and caregivers may not be overreacting to a minor problem, such as overfeeding. Although seemingly uncommon, the ED practitioner should always consider possible serious causes of vomiting during the evaluation of a neonate.

Historical features of onset, force of emesis, color of vomitus, frequency of episodes, and associated symptoms may help narrow the differential if gathered and considered in the initial phase of evaluation. The association of pain with the episode(s) of vomiting may be an important clue that the cause is pathologic and not a benign.[1] Close attention should be paid to gastric distension, peritonitis, colonic prominence and signs of volume status. When considering serious life-threatening causes of vomiting in the neonate, consultation with a pediatric surgeon and intensive care specialist should be implemented early in the evaluation of the patient.

NONEMERGENT CAUSES

Spitting Up

It is true that many of the neonates and infants presenting for emergent evaluation of vomiting are having episodes of benign regurgitation or spitting up. Spitting up breast milk or formula is common and overfeeding is the primary cause. After a detailed history and physical examination to rule out other causes, parental reassurance and education are all that are needed. It is also wise to take the time to answer any other questions or concerns the parents or caregivers may have, as this may save them unnecessary visits to the ED in the future. Appropriate follow-up with a primary doctor should also be ensured. In this case, it is not appropriate to switch formula type or place the child on non-nutritive substitutes like an electrolyte solution. Simple spitting up from overfeeding should not be confused with gastroesophageal reflux, as this is a different and more complicated entity. Formula allergy can be considered, but changes in formula are usually not indicated on ED evaluation unless significant signs are present. See the section on Formula Intolerance and Cow's Milk Sensitivity later in this chapter.

Gastroesophageal Reflux

Passive regurgitation is common in neonates secondary to the fact that the infant esophagus is relatively short. Coupled with this anatomic disadvantage, infants may also have elements of overfeeding and poor postprandial positioning. Approximately one-half of neonates will exhibit reflux after feeding and this pattern is considered normal.[2] Efforts to educate parents and caregivers about feeding schedules and proper positioning will benefit infant and parents alike.[3] Parental reassurance can be difficult at times, but is crucial. This is especially true for first-time parents in danger of developing a blunted or abnormal bond with their infant. Follow-up with primary care is important. Most cases of reflux are benign; however, symptoms of pathologic reflux, or *gastroesophageal reflux disease (GERD)*, should be recognized and the child referred for additional evaluation.[4] It is sometimes helpful to observe the child feeding in the ED to help differentiate reflux from more serious diagnoses.

Pathologic GERD is more common in children with prematurity and congenital anomalies of the oropharynx, GI tract, chest, lungs, and central nervous system.[5] Failure to thrive, feeding resistance or dysphagia, opisthotonic posturing, irritability, apnea or respiratory distress, and hematemesis are all signs associated with pathologic reflux and should trigger a specific work-up for GERD.[6] There may also be a strong association between reflux and cow milk allergy in up to 50% of infants less that 1 year of age.[7] The evolution of the symptomatology consistent with this condition may be subtle and primary care follow-up is recommended for all children with reflux. Admission may be required if apnea, respiratory symptoms, or significant GI bleeding is noted. If the child appears ill, other causes of vomiting should also be considered.

EMERGENT CAUSES

Necrotizing Enterocolitis

Necrotizing enterocolitis (NEC) is a devastating disease of the newborn that presents in both premature and full-term neonates. NEC represents the most common neonatal GI emergency and is the most common cause of GI perforation in this age group. Mortality for this disorder is 10% to 50%.[8] Low birth weight and prematurity are risk factors; approximately 90% of cases are in premature neonates. The exact cause of NEC is unknown, but is thought to be related to bowel wall injury or hypoxia that leads to inflammation and colonization of the bowel wall by bacterial flora. Some variation in day of onset is possible and seems to be related to gestational age and birth weight. Premature neonates present later than term infants, and this equates to a longer period of vulnerability to the development of this disorder.

Epidemiology

The rate of development of NEC is approximately 0.7 per 1000 births of full-term neonates.[9] Age of presentation is typically 0 to 10 days of life (term neonates day 3 to 4 and premature neonates day 10). Some cases of late presentation include development of NEC as late as 6 months. A number of risk factors have been described including neonatal respiratory distress, maternal preeclampsia, congenital heart disease, hypothyroidism, maternal cocaine abuse, hypotension, and acidosis (Table 5–2). Reports of epidemics in NICU populations may indicate that a specific predisposing pathogen

▶ **TABLE 5-2. RISK FACTORS FOR NEC**

- Premature birth/low birth weight
- Neonatal respiratory distress—hypoxia, perinatal asphyxia, cyanosis
- Maternal preeclampsia
- Congenital heart disease—hypoplastic left heart, coartation of the aorta, patent ductus arteriosis
- Hypothyroidism
- Maternal cocaine abuse
- Hypotension
- Acidosis

also exists. Because most neonates with this condition have other indications for continued hospitalization, it is uncommon to see NEC present to the ED. However, as it becomes more standard practice to plan early discharges for premature neonates, ED presentation may become more common.

History

History may be difficult to obtain from parents of children less than 10 days of age, even when the child has been hospitalized for a short period prior to returning to the ED. One of the earliest symptoms is abdominal distention and should be addressed when commented on by parents of a neonate presenting to the ED. It is important to note that, although common, there may not be a history of abnormal feeding or vomiting. Diarrhea may also be present. Other important features of the clinical history may include irritability, fever, lethargy, and bloody or blood streaked stool.

Clinical Manifestations

Physical examination in the early presentation may be limited to abdominal distension. The child may present with fever, irritability, lethargy, and peritoneal signs. As the course progresses the child will begin to show clinical signs of shock, including hypotension, tachycardia, and tachypnea. Coffee ground or bilious emesis and

guiac positive or grossly bloody stool may also develop at the time of evaluation. Shock indicates late presentation and denotes increased likelihood of intestinal perforation.

Diagnostic Studies

Abdominal radiographs are the diagnostic modality of most importance. Pneumatosis intestinalis, portal vein air, and peritoneal air may all be seen on plain radiographs (Figure 5–1). These are all worrisome signs that should prompt the diagnosis of NEC in this age group. Other radiographic signs that may be present earlier in the course include findings of bowel wall thickening and dilated loops of bowel. Ultrasound evaluation can also reveal portal gas and ascites.[10] Laboratory evaluation is of less diagnostic value, but may show evidence of acidosis and end organ failure denoting septic shock. Blood cultures and baseline labs should be obtained. Blood gas may also be of some value in evaluating disease course.

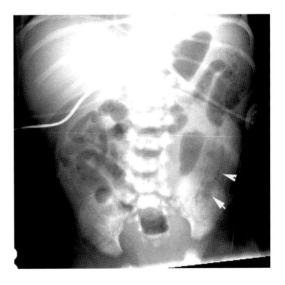

Figure 5–1. An infant with pneumatosis intestinalis in the left lower quadrant *Source:* From Brunicardi CF, Andersen DK, Billiar TR, et al. Schwartz' Principles and Practice of Surgery, 8th ed. New York, NY: McGraw-Hill; 2005.

Management

If the diagnosis is confirmed radiographically, immediate pediatric surgical consultation is required. Fluid resuscitation and broad spectrum antibiotics with coverage for enteric bacteria should be initiated. A nasogastric tube may be placed to decompress the stomach. Because of the severity of this condition, attention should be paid to the patient's response to resuscitation and plans for PICU placement should be initiated. Rapid transport to an appropriate center after initial stabilization is necessary if surgical coverage for neonates is not available. If the diagnosis is in question, admission with serial examinations and radiographs at a center with appropriate surgical coverage is indicated.

Pyloric Stenosis

Hypertrophic pyloric stenosis (PS) is a fairly common cause of nonbilious vomiting in infants between 2 and 8 weeks of age and occurs in 2 to 4 of 1000 births. The diagnosis should be considered in a previously healthy child who develops nonbilious vomiting after the second week and who feeds vigorously after each episode of vomiting. Hypertrophy of the pyloris is thought to occur due to abnormal development of the myenteric plexus of the pyloris. This leads to a lack of response to vasoactive neurotransmitters and a hypertrophy of the pyloris. The resulting gastric outlet obstruction can lead to significant dehydration and metabolic derangements and requires prompt evaluation for surgical correction.

Epidemiology

There is a 2- to 5-fold higher incidence of PS in males versus females.[9] Firstborn males seem to have a higher rate of developing this condition. Caucasian infants are more likely to present with PS and there appears to be a genetic component that is familial in some cases. Preterm infants may present 1 to 2 weeks later than term infants and PS may also present at birth.

History

Infants typically present with a history of worsening reflux that gradually changes to projectile vomiting. It is not unusual for an infant to receive several evaluations for reflux prior to the diagnosis. The child is typically a vigorous feeder and will initially attempt to feed after episodes of emesis. If the infant develops gastritis there may be a history of coffee-ground emesis. A history of loose stool may lead to the misdiagnosis of gastroenteritis. Therefore, the diagnosis must be considered in all infants between 2 to 8 weeks who present with significant nonbilious vomiting.

Clinical Manifestations

Classically a palpable "olive" in the epigastrium has been considered the physical exam finding pathognomic of this disorder. This finding is fairly difficult to appreciate on the average child in the ED. Palpation of the hypertrophic pyloris requires a relaxed infant with an empty stomach. This *may* be appreciated by the astute practitioner after emesis or iatrogenic decompression of the stomach while the infant is sucking on a pacifier or on dextrose solution. Peristaltic waves in the left upper quadrant may also be noted. Other examination findings of note are signs of dehydration and irritability.

Diagnostic Studies

Standard plain radiographs of the abdomen may show a distended stomach with or without peristaltic waves—the so called "caterpillar sign." Typically, gastric outlet obstruction can be deduced, however, this is not specific for PS. Evaluation of the infant with suspected PS should include ultrasound of the pyloris by a trained technician or specially qualified physician. Ultrasound interpretations are subject to institutional variation and can be relative to patient age; however, muscle thickness >3-4 mm, pyloric channel length >14-18 mm, pyloric thickness >10 mm, and a ratio of muscle thickness to pyloric thickness of >0.27

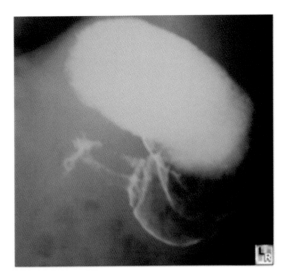

Figure 5-2. The "string sign" in pyloric stenosis.

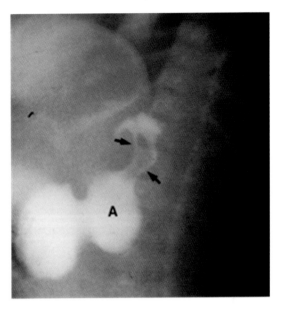

Figure 5-3. The "double track sign" in pyloric stenosis.

are all indicators of a positive test for PS.[11,12] An upper GI series may be obtained if the diagnosis is in question following ultrasound (Figures 5–2 to 5–4). This contrast study is considered positive when a delay of gastric emptying is noted and one of several signs is present. The "shoulder sign" describes the mass impression of the hypertrophic pyloris imposed upon the antrum. A thin linear contrast line passing through the narrowed pyloris creates the "string sign." A double contrast line or "double-track" line may also represent PS. Fluoroscopic evaluation has the potential advantage of being used as a functional study, and may also help make the diagnosis of gastroesophageal reflux as an alternative diagnosis when PS is not present. Unfortunately, fluoroscopy delivers more radiation than a standard radiograph and consideration should be paid to the potential risk to the infant. This test may not be needed if the ultrasound is conclusive.

The classic metabolic finding in an infant with PS is metabolic alkalosis with hypokalemia and hypochloridemia secondary to prolonged vomiting and loss of stomach acid. These findings may be absent if the infant presents early in the course of disease. Laboratory evaluation should include baseline serum studies including CBC, electrolytes, and BUN/creatinine, to evaluate renal function. The child may be jaundiced and liver function tests should be obtained to evaluate for an elevation in unconjugated bilirubin.

Management

Initial fluid resuscitation with normal saline (NS) should be followed by D5 0.45 NS at 1.5 times maintainance to gradually correct the metabolic alkylosis. Potassium replacement with 10 to 20 mEq/L should be given if necessary, but only after urine output has been established. Placement of a nasogastric tube is not required, and may cause an exacerbation of metabolic alkylosis secondary to continued loss of stomach acid. Pediatric surgical consultation should be obtained promptly on identification of the gastric outlet obstruction. If necessary, transfer to an appropriate center should occur after initial stabilization.

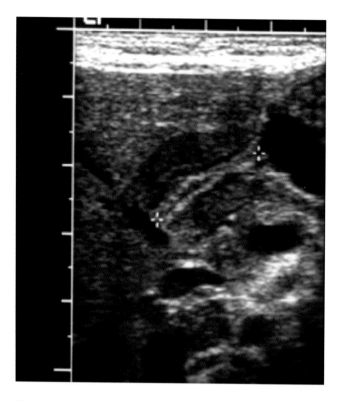

Figure 5–4. Ultrasound findings in pyloric stenosis.

Malrotation/Midgut Volvulus

Malrotation refers to failure of the embryonic gut to rotate 270 degrees around the superior mesenteric vascular axis, resulting in a lack of the usual anatomic arrangement and stability of the small intestine. The distal duodenum does not arrive in the left abdomen and therefore lacks the stability usually provided by the ligament of Treitz. The intestine is then predisposed to twisting around its single mesenteric attachment and obstructs at the distal duodenum or proximal jejunum. This obstruction (or volvulus) may also be associated with vascular compromise secondary to twisting of the superior mesenteric artery and vein.[13] Ladd bands (ie, fibrous attachments arising from the right peritoneal gutter) result from this abnormal development and may lead to intestinal obstructions. Midgut volvulus can cause ischemia and a loss of the entire midgut in a matter of hours and, therefore, represents a surgical emergency.

Epidemiology

Eighty percent of cases of malrotation present during the neonatal period, most within the first 7 to 10 days. There is a 2:1 male to female ratio in incidence.

History

These neonates present with bilious vomiting in 80% to 100% of cases. Bilious vomiting in the neonate should be presumed to be secondary to obstruction, as up to 40% of cases will require surgical intervention. This percentage is lower in the first 72 hours; however, intestinal obstruction should still be considered. In children with midgut volvulus, bilious vomiting may be followed by abdominal distension, irritability, and blood in the child's stool. Bowel necrosis may occur within 2 to 4 hours and shock can ensue quickly.

Clinical Manifestations

Initially the child may appear healthy despite the presence of vomiting. Repeat physical examination is important and may reveal progressive abdominal distension, peritoneal signs, guaiac positive stool, or gross blood and signs of shock as the intestine becomes necrotic.

Diagnostic Studies

Radiographic evaluation of the neonate with bilious emesis is essential. Unfortunately non-contrasted abdominal films may be unremarkable in 20% of cases. Intestinal obstruction and gastric distension are suggestive of midgut volvulus; however, an upper GI is considered the gold standard test and is required to rule out this life-threatening diagnosis (Figures 5–5 & 5–6). Obtaining the upper GI study may also lead to an alternate diagnosis, such as gastroesophageal reflux, pyloric stenosis, hiatal hernia, gastric volvulus, or small bowel atresia. On upper GI of a neonate with volvulus, contrast does not cross over onto the left side of the abdomen and a "corkscrew" sign will be present, representing the twisting of the jejunum.[14] Ultrasound is available in some centers as a screening test. Evaluation of the orientation of the superior mesenteric artery and vein may lead to the diagnosis without need for fluoroscopy and associated radiation.[15] If ultrasound is negative, an upper GI should still be performed to rule out volvulus. CT may also identify malrotation.[16]

Baseline labs should be obtained, including CBC, electrolytes, renal and liver function tests and type and screen. Venous blood gas and coagulation studies should be obtained if the infant appears ill.

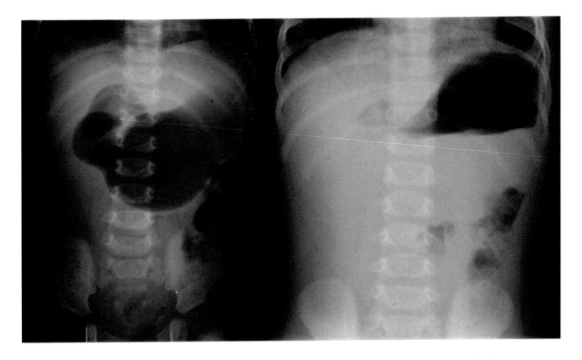

Figure 5–5. Radiographs demonstrating a dilated stomach and duodenal bulb highly suggestive of malrotation with volvulus.

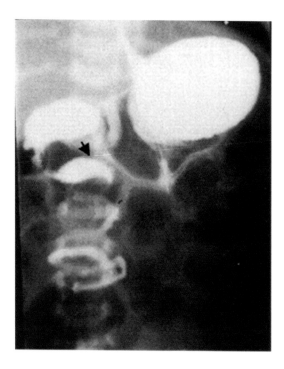

Figure 5–6. Upper GI contrast study in a 1-day-old neonate with bilious vomiting demonstrating malrotation with the duodenum and jejunum descending on the right and the classical "cork screw" appearance of contrast in the duodenum in midgut volvulus.

Management

Early consultation with a pediatric surgeon is essential. Resuscitation with normal saline and broad spectrum antibiotics should be initiated if signs of perforation or shock are present. Due to the severity of this condition, plans for postoperative intensive care should be considered. Rapid transport to an appropriate center after initial stabilization should be initiated if surgical coverage or intensive care for neonates is not available.

Inguinal Hernia

Inguinal hernia in the neonate is usually not considered a significant emergency condition because 90% to 95% can be easily reduced without complication. The child can then undergo outpatient evaluation for surgical repair. Patients are usually brought to the ED for evaluation by a parent that has noticed the inguinal bulging. Infants that present in this way are not symptomatic. If the child is vomiting or appears ill incarceration and possible strangulation should be considered and may require emergent pediatric surgical evaluation.

Indirect inguinal hernia results from incomplete obliteration of the processus vaginalis. Bowel and other peritoneal contents may then enter the inguinal canal and become incarcerated. Strangulation refers to the result of mesenteric vascular supply compromise and can lead to necrosis and perforation. Testes and ovaries may also be involved in the hernia. Special attention should be paid to children with increased intraperitoneal pressures, such as those with abdominal masses or cysts, ascites, or ventriculoperitonel shunting,[17] or neonates undergoing peritoneal dialysis.

Inguinal hernia is the most common abdominal wall defect requiring evaluation in the ED. Major abdominal wall defects are unlikely to present to the ED as they are usually noted in the prenatal or immediate postpartum period. Umbilical hernias are seen frequently in the ED and pediatrician offices. These are unlikely to become incarcerated and rarely require surgical evaluation.

Epidemiology

Inguinal hernia has a prevalence of 0.8% to 4.4%. This is predominately a disorder noted in male children with a ratio of 3:1 to 6:1 male to female. Although less common in female infants, close follow-up and early outpatient surgical evaluation are important as female children have a higher rate of incarceration. Right-sided hernia is more common. In some cases there is a significant family history of inguinal hernia. Incarceration occurs in 6% to 18% of the pediatric population, however, most occur within the first 2 months of life.

▶ **TABLE 5–3. ASSOCIATED RISK FACTORS FOR INGUINAL HERNIA**

Prematurity	Ehlers-Danlos
Undescended teste	syndrome
Ascites	Hunter-Hurler
VP shunt	syndrome
Peritoneal dialysis	Marfan syndrome
Intraabdominal mass	Mucopolysaccharidosis
Abdominal wall	Family history
defects	Hypospadia
	Testicular feminization

Associated congenital anomalies should also be considered and connective tissue disorders have also been described as risk factors for developing inguinal hernia (Table 5–3).

History

Details of time of onset, location of bulge or swelling, variations during sleep verses wakefulness, and recent increased size or firmness are all usual aspects of the inguinal hernia history. In addition to parental description of the groin bulging or scrotal swelling, other historical features are important and should be gathered by the examining clinician. Symptoms related to bowel obstruction and ischemia should be reviewed with the parents to ensure there is no clinical suspicion of incarceration. Irritability may be the first and only historical feature; however, as time passes, the infant may suffer vomiting, abdominal distension, and obstipation. Lethargy and bloody stools are ominous signs of strangulation and possible necrosis and perforation.

Clinical Manifestations

Although the examination of a neonate for presence of indirect inguinal hernia is not difficult, attention should be paid to several points. First, male infants should be carefully examined for presence of both testes in the scrotum, as an undescended teste may be mistaken for a hernia. The hernia bulge should be in the expected location and should not

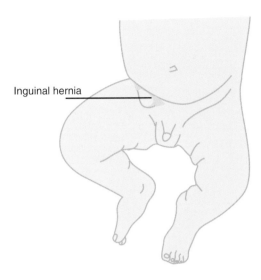

Inguinal hernia

Figure 5–7. Drawing of an inguinal hernia.

appear fluctuant (Figure 5–7). Tumors and abscesses can sometimes be mistaken for hernia as well. If the hernia bulge is noted to be intensely tender or discoloration is noted, care should be taken not to attempt reduction. Similarly, necrotic bowel from strangulation should not be reduced in the ED. An indirect inguinal hernia that cannot be reduced in the usual fashion should be evaluated for possible incarceration. Examination findings of abdominal distension, vomiting, blood per rectum, and signs of shock should all be considered consistent with incarceration with strangulation until proven otherwise.

Diagnostic Studies

Radiographic evaluation with plain x-ray will reveal air-fluid levels when partial or complete intestinal obstruction is present (Figure 5–8). Small bowel dilation is also a prominent feature of obstruction from incarcerated hernia; however, midgut volvulus should also be considered when small bowel obstruction is identified in the neonate. Free air may be present if strangulation has led to perforation. Ultrasound may be used to differentiate hernia bulge from

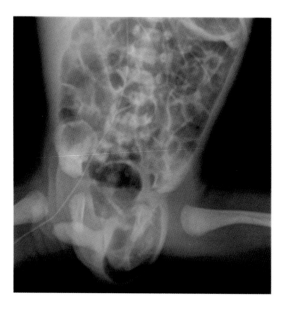

Figure 5-8. Inguinal hernia with accompanying bowel obstruction.

abscess and tumor mass. Evaluation for hydrocele and testicular pathology is also possible during ultrasound evaluation. Baseline blood labs are of little value unless the infant appears ill or strangulation is suspected.

Management

In cases of uncomplicated indirect inguinal hernia, reduction in the ED can lead to discharge with parental instructions and close follow-up for surgical evaluation and repair. If the hernia cannot be easily reduced without significant discomfort to the infant, then analgesics and possible sedation should be given to facilitate relaxation of the abdomen. If the hernia is initially thought to be incarcerated but can eventually be reduced in the ED, the child should be seen by surgery and considered for admission, as recurrence and complications are of a greater concern in these patients.

Before the initial attempt at bimanual reduction, the child should be placed in a Trendelenburg position and comforted in a way to encourage relaxation. If the hernia

reduces then the child is unlikely to incur complications as an outpatient referral to surgery and can be discharged. If the hernia sac fails to reduce, bimanual reduction using gentle, steady compression of the distal sack should be initiated in an effort to evacuate the contents of the bowel from the herniated portion. Gentle proximal support should be employed to guide the sac back through the external inguinal ring as the distal hand is used to apply slightly more pressure in support of reducing the sac. If reduction does not occur within 5 minutes of applying pressure, efforts should be suspended and sedation may be required. A cold pack may also be applied to the groin. Appropriate procedure sedation should take place only after discussion with the parent and consent is obtained. Bimanual reduction should be attempted again after the child falls asleep.

If the neonate is found to have an incarcerated inguinal hernia, pediatric surgical evaluation is necessary. In cases where signs of obstruction, strangulation, or shock are present, immediate surgical consultation is required. In the presence of strangulation with potential necrosis of the bowel, bimanual hernia reduction should not be performed in the ED, but rather by the surgeon. Intravenous resuscitation with normal saline and broad spectrum antibiotics, along with other supportive measures, should be initiated in anticipation of surgical treatment and appropriate intensive care unit placement. A nasogastric tube can be placed to alleviate gastric distension in patients with bowel obstruction.

Small Bowel Atresias

Small bowel atresia affects as many as 1 in 1500 to 4000 births.[18] There appears to be a higher rate in children of low birth weight. Duodenal atresia is commonly associated with chromosomal abnormality,[19,20,21] whereas jejunal and ileal are general not. Small bowel atresia can also be found in conjunction with atresias of the stomach and colon in some families of French-Canadian descent. When atresia is severe the child will often be diagnosed by prenatal ultrasound along with maternal polyhydramnios or with small bowel obstruction in the immediate postpartum period. Due to the variability in luminal narrowing, presentations may be more subtle and therefore diagnosis may be delayed.

Duodenal Atresia

Abnormal embryonic GI development can lead to duodenal webs, stenosis, and atresia. This condition may present at any time in the neonatal period, or even later. Variability in the degree of narrowing of the duodenum makes the clinical presentation of this entity more variable. Although narrowing may be secondary to annular pancreas, Ladd bands, and volvulus, duodenal atresia should also be considered in severe cases of proximal small bowel obstruction. The etiology of this condition is not clear; however, the prevailing theory appears to be a lack of complete recanalization of the duodenum during early development.[22] Severe cases are likely to be detected in the prenatal and immediate postpartum period, and are therefore less likely to present primarily to the ED. Because of this fact, midgut volvulus must be the diagnosis of primary consideration in the neonate with bilious (or bile streaked) vomiting in the ED.

Epidemiology

Duodenal obstruction has in incidence of about 1 in 10,000 live births.[23] Many times this condition is associated with other abnormalities and is seen with some frequency in children with trisomy 21 (Down syndrome) and Feingold syndrome.[24] Cardiac and renal anomalies are also fairly common. A number of other GI malformations are associated with this condition and should also be considered (Table 5–4).[25]

▶ **TABLE 5-4. GI ABNORMALITIES ASSOCIATED WITH DUODENAL ATRESIA**

Annular pancreas (most common)	Anomalous bile duct communication
Malrotation	Pancreatic duct atresia
Biliary atresia	Esophageal atresia
Preduodenal portal vein	Imperforate anus
Choledochal cyst	

History

Vomiting is typically bilious or bile streaked in nature. This is due to the fact that 85% of cases are associated with obstruction distal to the ampulla of Vater. The other 15% may not have bile in their emesis and may appear to vomit clear fluid or a recent feeding. If the narrowing is of a lesser degree, the infant may have a delayed diagnosis. Historical features may then also include constipation and a failure to gain weight.

Clinical Manifestations

Abdominal distension and vomiting are usually noted at the time of evaluation. The infant may also present with tachycardia signs of dehydration. When comparison to birth weight is made, the child will likely not have made appropriate weight gain.[26]

Diagnostic Studies

Plain radiography of the abdomen will usually reveal a distended stomach and proximal small bowel (Figure 5–9). This is the classic "double bubble" sign. The absence of gas beyond the proximal small bowel is very suggestive of duodenal obstruction, but does not exclude malrotation as the cause. Therefore, even when the "double bubble" sign is noted in the absence of distal bowel gas, an upper GI and/or ultrasound should be performed to exclude the diagnosis of midgut volvulus. In cases where clinical features are less severe, it may also be appropriate to obtain a CT to further delineate the duodenal

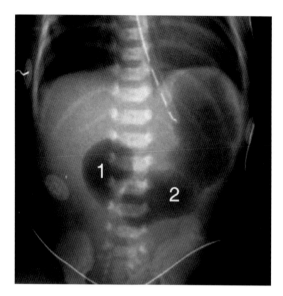

Figure 5–9. The "double bubble" sign in duodenal atresia. *Source:* From Brunicardi CF, Andersen DK, Billiar TR, et al. Schwartz's Principles and Practice of Surgery, 8th ed. New York, NY: McGraw-Hill; 2005.

pathology.[27] CT scanning should only be done in consultation with a pediatric surgeon and is not considered a standard diagnostic modality for the diagnosis of duodenal atresia.

Management

Supportive measures, including resuscitation with normal saline, should be initiated in response to signs of dehydration. If a proximal small bowel obstruction is identified, a nasogastric tube for decompression may be indicated. Pediatric surgical consultation and admission are necessary as operative management is almost always indicated.

Jejunal Atresia

Jejunal atresia is also a cause of bilious vomiting in the neonate. Presentation is fairly variable, however, and infants may present with nonbilious emesis. Jejunal atresia, in contrast to duodenal atresia, is not commonly associated with chromosomal abnormalities or with congenital

malformations in cardiac or renal systems. However, there may be a familial component.[28]

Epidemiology

Jejunal atresia is more common than duodenal atresia and may present in as many as 1 in 1500 neonates. Maternal polyhydramnios, prematurity, and low birth weight have all be associated with this condition.

History & Clinical Manifestations

The infant will have some history of feeding difficulty. Vomiting may or may not be bilious in nature. In some cases the neonate will fail to pass meconium. Parents who bring their newborn to the ED may report abdominal distension and constipation in addition to vomiting. Severe atresia usually results in significant bilious vomiting.

Diagnostic Studies & Management

Abdominal plain films will reveal multiple loops of distended small bowel and air fluid levels. Management is similar to that of duodenal atresia and should involve pediatric surgical evaluation and consideration of other causes of small bowel obstruction.[29]

Other GI Causes

There are a number of other GI disorders of the neonate that may cause vomiting as the primary presenting symptom. These conditions are almost always diagnosed in the immediate postpartum period and the neonate is not likely to present to the ED unless the mother had minimal (or no) prenatal care and an out-of-hospital delivery. It is worthwhile to mention several of them here as out-of-hospital delivery may be common with respect to geographic, socioeconomic, and cultural considerations.

Tracheoesophageal fistula and *esophageal atresia* usually present with the first feeding and is rarely missed, later to present to the ED. The neonate will attempt to feed, but will experience spitting, coughing, choking, and sometimes cyanosis. Inability to pass a nasogastric tube is usually considered diagnostic in this situation. Upper GI is not recommended due to the risk of aspiration. Immediate pediatric surgical consultation is needed.[30] *Pyloric atresia* differs from pyloric stenosis in that the defect is structural rather than functional and will therefore present at or shortly after birth. A single gas bubble, representing the distended stomach, will be present with a complete absence of intestinal gas. Gastric perforation may occur. Nasogastric tube and resuscitation are initiated while awaiting pediatric surgical consultation. *Intussusception* is extremely uncommon in neonates and infants under 3 months. Presentation is usually between 3 months and 6 years and abdominal mass, rectal bleeding, vomiting and intermittent abdominal pain are classically described.[9] Air or contrast enema is typically used to diagnose the condition, however, ultrasound may also be employed.[11,12] Immediate surgical consultation is required. Infants may sometimes present with only lethargy.

Extragastrointestinal Causes

When evaluating the neonate presenting with vomiting it is important to consider causes outside of the alimentary tract. A number of important conditions involving other systems of the body may be overlooked due to a readiness to evaluate only the GI causes of vomiting. The emergency physician must consider conditions related to increases in intracranial pressure, metabolic derangements,[31,32,33] and infections.

Proper attention to these causes of vomiting will avoid unnecessary delay in diagnosis and potential mismanagement (Table 5–5).

▶ DIARRHEA

Despite the fact that diarrhea in the neonate is usually caused by a self-limited process it can be a life-threatening condition. Aggressive management is sometimes needed to avoid dehydration with its potential complications. Diarrhea is caused by a lack of normal function of the bowel mucosa and is usually caused by enteritis of some type. Inflammation of the bowel wall can be caused by atopy, infection, and even ischemia.[34] Other causes of diarrhea include congenital atrophy of the villi and short gut syndrome (following loss of intestine to some other condition).[35,36] A complete history and physical examination is important. Basic information that must be reviewed includes amount of oral intake, urinary output, number and character of stools (whether they are bloody or nonbloody, and their color and consistency), change in behavior, irritability, and fever or other signs of infection. Exposure to sick contacts (especially those with diarrheal illness), presence of other children in the home, and child care history should also be reviewed.

NONEMERGENT CAUSES

Normal Stool Changes

Neonates typically have loose stool after the passage of meconium is complete. During

▶ TABLE 5-5. **VOMITING FROM CAUSES OTHER THAN THE GI SYSTEM**

Neurologic	Metabolic	Infections	Other
• Intracranial mass • Intracranial bleeding • Hydrocephalus • Closed-head trauma	• Inborn errors of metabolism • Hypothyroidism • Congenital adrenal hyperplasia	• Meningitis • Sepsis • Urinary tract infection • Otitis media	• Narcotic withdrawal

the first 5 days the character of the stool will change from the thick dark meconium to a more liquid greenish-brown. The stool is commonly yellow in color and seedy in consistency by the fifth day of life. Normal healthy infants may have a stool after every feeding. This is especially common in breastfed neonates. First-time parents and caregivers may be alarmed by this initial change in stool consistency and may present for evaluation of diarrhea. If the child appears healthy and is gaining weight parental assurance and education may be all that is required.

Overfeeding

Neonates and infants that are fed excessively may present with very frequent stooling. This is commonly a problem when the infant is fed in response to every cry or other sign of discomfort. A careful feeding history may lead to this conclusion in an otherwise normal healthy infant. Education concerning comforting and coping techniques is essential especially for first-time parents and caregivers. These children may also suffer from excessive spitting up, reflux, and colic.

EMERGENT CAUSES

Infectious Enteritis

Pathogens causing injury to the proximal small intestine lead to inflammation and dysfunction of the mucosa, producing watery diarrhea and sometimes vomiting usually associated with viral pathogens. Bacterial pathogens usually affect the colon and blood may also be present in the stool. Parasitic infections causing diarrhea are rare in the neonate.

Epidemiology & History

Rotavirus is the most common viral pathogen causing diarrhea and is most commonly seen in the winter. Rotavirus has been known to be associated with electrolyte abnormalities (including hypocalcemia), seizures, development of necrotizing enterocolitis, and increased frequency of both apnea and bradycardia. Dehydration can be significant and IV rehydration was the standard therapy for many years. Despite the usual history of vomiting, recent literature has shown that oral rehydration therapy is appropriate in most cases of mild to moderate dehydration. Rotavirus can be found in asymptomatic carriers and outbreaks in newborn nurseries are not uncommon. *Adenovirus, enteroviruses,* and *Norwalk agent,* among other viral pathogens, also cause a similar presentation.

Escherichia coli has a number of forms and may have a variable presentation dependent of the strain of pathogen responsible for the infection. Enteroinvasive and enterohemorrhagic strains of *E. coli* present with bloody diarrhea, whereas other strains typically present with green watery diarrhea without blood or mucus. As with viral pathogens, the primary concern is with regard to dehydration and electrolyte disturbances. Other pathogens responsible for bloody diarrhea include *Shigella, Campylobacter, Yersinia,* and *Aeromonas.*

Clinical Manifestations

A thorough physical examination is warranted to determine if there are any other sources of infection. Temperature and pulse are important indicators of infection and dehydration. A rectal examination is important for obtaining a stool sample but also for checking for anal fissures as possible etiology of bloody diarrhea. The patient should be weighed unclothed for an accurate weight. Close attention to respirations, detection of sunken fontanel, skin elasticity, whether patient makes tears, mucous membranes, urinary output, and capillary refill will help determine the degree of dehydration.

Diagnostic Studies

In cases of significant dehydration it may be helpful to obtain labs to evaluate electrolytes and renal function. Bloody diarrhea may prompt the clinician to consider a diagnostic evaluation for GI bleeding. Sending stool cultures and smear may be helpful in the overall management of the neonate, but does not affect the initial management of the patient. Results of stool cultures may lead to antibiotic therapy in select cases.

Management

Any neonate with diarrhea and any evidence of dehydration deserves admission for further evaluation and care. Mild dehydration (3% to 5%) should be treated with oral rehydration therapy if possible. If dehydration is moderate (6% to 9%) or severe (>10%), then generally IV fluid rehydration is needed. Antimotility agents such as loperamide, opium, and diphenoxylate should not be used. In addition, antibiotics should not be given unless culture results yield a specific bacterial agent, and the pathogen and the patient's clinical condition correspond to warrant antimicrobial therapy.

Noninvasive strains of *E. coli* can be treated with oral neomycin or colistin sulfate. Neomycin therapy may eradicate the bacteria and shorten the course of illness. An absorbable antibiotic, such as ampicillin or trimethoprim-sulfamethoxazole, may be indicated for enteroinvasive bacteria causing diarrhea. *Salmonella* infection in the neonate can be treated with ampicillin, amoxicillin, bactrim, cefotaxime, or ceftriaxone. In cases of neonates with confirmed bacterial enteritis, it may be appropriate to obtain a consultation with a pediatric infectious disease specialist.

Formula Intolerance/ Cow's Milk Sensitivity

Sensitivity to protein in formula derived from cow's milk and/or soy can cause significant difficulty for the neonate. Immunologic reaction to these proteins causes an inflammation of the small and large bowel and can therefore present as diarrhea and/or vomiting. Symptoms are typically evident within a few days to weeks after initial ingestion of the cow's milk protein. Diagnostic testing to determine sensitivity may not be necessary if symptoms cease after withdrawing the cow's milk or soy based formula.

Epidemiology

Around 3% of infants will have a sensitivity to cow's milk protein.[7] Soy protein sensitivity is less common and is found in about 1%. Some infants will be sensitive to both.[37] Most children will overcome this sensitivity by age 3.

History

Children usually present with significant diarrhea and vomiting that usually occurs within 2 hours of ingestion. Infants presenting with this disorder may have been previously hospitalized for a septic workup due to a previous presentation with lethargy.

Clinical Manifestations

In addition to vigorous vomiting and diarrhea, infants commonly present with heme positive (or grossly bloody) stool and may also have a tender abdomen. Irritability and lethargy may also be present. The child may even present in apparent shock. Avoidance of the offending protein leads to resolution of symptoms.

Diagnostic Studies

Stool studies and baseline CBC, electrolytes, and renal function should be obtained. Ill-appearing neonates should be considered septic until proven otherwise, and a full septic workup may be indicated in relation to this important differential. Fecal leukocytes with eosinophils are usually seen. Serum studies may reveal an increase in polymorphonuclear leukocyte count. If deemed appropriate by an allergy/immunology specialist, a protein challenge may be performed. This should not be done in the ED or while the infant is still symptomatic.

Management

Supportive care and avoidance of the offending food protein(s) is the mainstay of care for these patients. Immediate care includes resuscitation and possible administration of steroids. Admission should be considered in any neonate with significant diarrhea and/or GI bleeding. Consultation with an allergy/immunology specialist is indicated. Follow-up at regular intervals is appropriate. Infants with confirmed, or suspected, food protein sensitivity should be placed on hydrolyzed formula or amino acid-based formula. Switching from cow's milk formula to soy-based formula may not be effective, as some infants may be sensitive to both.

Other Causes

Systemic infection, autoimmune enteropathy, congenital microvillus atrophy, and congenital nutrient malabsorption are all rare causes of neonatal diarrhea. The clinician should also consider causes of partial bowel obstruction or chronic constipation that may lead to diarrhea. Unfortunately, diarrhea in the infant is also a presentation of Munchausen syndrome by proxy and this entity must also be considered.

▶ CONSTIPATION

A lack of significant bowel output is a common concern for parents and caregivers. After passage of meconium, it is common for neonates to have small amounts of stool 1 to 2 times daily. This can be especially true when children are breastfed. Children presenting for constipation within the first 5 days should have a review of their diaper count and consideration for pathologic causes of inadequate bowel output. During the first 2 days of life, the neonate is expected to pass meconium 1 or more times per day. On days 3 to 5 the bowel output should consist of 2 or more brownish-green stools followed by a change to a more yellow color after 5 days. A neonate with less than 2 stools per day should be evaluated for dehydration and potential nutritional

deficiency. If there are any signs of abdominal distension or vomiting other pathologic causes should be investigated.

NONEMERGENT CAUSES

Some parents and caregivers have been instructed to expect a stool after each feeding or may have had a previous child with a similar pattern of bowel output. Although this is common for neonates and infants, it is not absolutely necessary for successful weight gain. As long as the child appears healthy and has passed meconium and at least 2 to 4 stools per day for the first week, there may be no need for concern.

Breastfed neonates usually have more bowel output than formula-fed children. In contrast to the 2-6 stools expected in the formula-fed neonate, it is common for breastfed neonates to have a stool following every feeding. A low number of stools in this group may be of more concern because underfeeding can occur and the neonate may become dehydrated because their intake is not as easily quantified. If there is any question as to the nutritional status of the child, weight gain should be closely monitored by their primary physician. Dehydrated neonates, or those with jaundice or inadequate bowel output, should be admitted for further evaluation and care. In some cases of lactation failure the neonate may develop hypernatremic dehydration, a serious condition requiring aggressive resuscitation with isotonic fluids, followed by correction of water losses and electrolyte abnormalities.

EMERGENT CAUSES

Hirschsprung Disease

Hirschsprung disease (HD) is a congenital absence of ganglion cells in part or all of the colon, and rarely the small bowel, that leads to an inability for the effected region to relax. This effectively causes a functional colonic obstruction to develop. Due to the fact that migration of embryonic ganglion cells is cephalocaudal, the aganglionic region will be without gaps and will involve the distal colon. HD (also known as congenital megacolon) is an important cause of constipation, as it can lead to significant complications in the neonatal period and requires surgical consultation. Presentation varies and in some cases the disorder may go unrecognized until later childhood when the diagnosis is made as the result of evaluation for chronic constipation.

Epidemiology

HD is not uncommon and is found in 1 in 5000 live births.[38] The development of this disease is thought to be multifactorial. There is a family history in 10% of cases.[39] Male infants are more commonly affected with a 4:1 male to female ratio. Infants are usually the product of an uneventful pregnancy with a normal delivery history and are usually of adequate birth weight. HD is more common in children with trisomy 21 (Down syndrome) and Waardenburg syndrome. The rectosigmoid colon is involved in 75% of cases. However, the entire colon can be effected in up to 10% of patients. In severe cases (<1%), the entire intestine may be involved.

History

Early diagnosis can be attributed to careful attention to bowel history. Ninety to 95% of cases will have a failure to pass meconium within the first 24 to 48 hours of life. The infant is usually otherwise healthy and appears normal. Postpartum discharge within 24-48 hours is now common and the diagnosis can therefore be missed. Parents may report a lack of stool over a number of days and may have even reported this at the time of newborn follow-up, only to be told that the child appears normal. In some cases, the infant may manifest only chronic constipation and the diagnosis will be delayed into infancy and even childhood or adulthood. A history of delayed passage of meconium or retention of the meconium plug requiring evacuation should lead to an evaluation for aganglionic colon. Some infants will present with a history of constipation with infrequent, voluminous, and sometimes explosive bowel movements. Parents may also comment on a foul odor to the stool.

Neonates with more severe obstructive pathology will present earlier with additional symptoms of obstipation, abdominal distension, and vomiting. Vomiting may be bilious or even feculent in nature. Patients who develop megacolon can manifest Hirschsprung enterocolitis and present with a history of fever, lethargy and obtundation.

Clinical Manifestations

Depending on the severity of the condition and the time of presentation the child will frequently appear well. Some abdominal distension may be present with hyperactive bowel sounds. Rectal examination often reveals a vacant ampulla. The examiner may witness a rapid evacuation of gas and stool after completion of the rectal examination. Infants with enterocolitis may present with fever, lethargy, tachycardia, and signs of shock. Peritoneal signs should be considered consistent with perforation.

Diagnostic Studies

Initial evaluation should include a plain abdominal radiograph. Large bowel obstruction is expected to be seen (Figure 5–10). In addition, this film should be closely evaluated for the presence of free air. Barium enema reveals a "saw-tooth" pattern of contrast in the aganglionic colon with a proximal area of significant dilation. Barium enema has been reported with various levels of sensitivity and a negative result does not rule out the diagnosis in all cases. If clinical suspicion is significant, a surgical consultation for anorectal manometry and to evaluate for rectal biopsy should be obtained.[40]

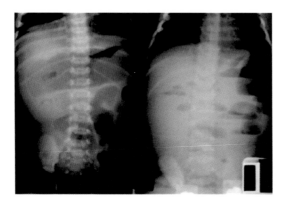

Figure 5-10. Plain radiographs demonstrating air-fluid levels in the intestine and no gas in the rectum, suggestive for Hirschsprung disease.

Management

Supportive measures and pediatric surgical consultation are the mainstay of therapy. Infants presenting with sepsis and/or perforation will require fluid resuscitation and broad spectrum antibiotics. These patients should be initially stabilized and transferred to a center with pediatric surgical services and appropriate intensive care if such resources are not available at the presenting facility.

Meconium Ileus

Meconium can create an intestinal obstruction in neonates deficient in pancreatic enzymes. The blockage is usually located at the terminal ileum and, as such, causes a clinical picture consistent with distal small bowel obstruction. Ten to 15% of infants with cystic fibrosis will develop meconium ileus. When meconium fails to pass within 24 to 48 hours in a full-term infant, other conditions should also be considered (Table 5–6).

Epidemiology

Meconium ileus is found in 1 in 2800 live births. Essentially a complication of cystic fibrosis, 90% to 95% of neonates with meconium ileus have a positive sweat chloride

▶ TABLE 5-6. **FAILURE TO PASS MECONIUM**

Muconium ileus	Small left colon syndrome
Muconium plug syndrome	Hypogangliosis
Hirschsprung disease	Neuronal intestinal dysplasia
Anorectal stenosis/ lack of patency	Megacystis-microcolon-intestinal hypoperi stalsis syndrome

test. Other GI manifestations of cystic fibrosis include constipation, distal intestinal obstructive syndrome, aquired megacolon, rectal prolapse, and pancreatits.

History

Meconium ileus is usually diagnosed prior to postpartum discharge when the child does not pass meconium in the first 24 to 48 hours of life. Bilious vomiting and abdominal distension usually follow. The child may return to the ED after having had treatment to relieve the obstruction, as infants with cystic fibrosis are prone to recurrence of intestinal obstruction.

Clinical Manifestations

The abdomen will appear distended and tender. Loops of distended bowel may be palpable. In cases of associated volvulus or meconium peritonitis (secondary to perforation) the infant may be tachycardic and exhibit signs of shock.

Diagnostic Studies

Despite the fact that meconium ileus represents a functional distal small bowel obstruction, plain abdominal radiographs are expected to show specific characteristic signs (Figure 5–11).[41] The meconium is usually visualized in the right lower quadrant and is described as having a "soap bubble" or "ground glass" appearance as it is mixed with gas.[42] Multiple distended loops of small bowel are notable; however, the expected air fluid

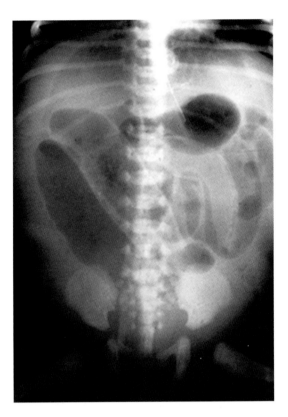

Figure 5–11. A 3 day old with multiple dilated loops of gut and a supine pneumoperitoneum. Perforation of a meconium ileus was found at surgery.

levels of a typical small bowel obstruction are absent. When contrast enema is obtained, the colon appears narrow. This is known as "microcolon" and is because the colon has not been used. Free air and the presence of calcifications are consistent with perforation and should be cause for emergent surgical consultation. Baseline labs and a sweat chloride test should also be obtained.

Management

Fortunately, response to therapy is usually good. Enemas are largely effective, and contrast medium may serve a therapeutic and diagnostic role in this regard. If obstruction cannot be alleviated after multiple enemas, or

if signs of perforation develop, surgical exploration is necessary.[43] After relief from obstruction, recurrence should be prevented by proper treatment of the underlying cause. Intestinal malabsorption is typically treated with pancreatic enzyme preparation in order to prevent further GI complications.

Meconium Plug Syndrome

Meconium plug syndrome (MPS) refers to colonic obstruction by meconium. Despite the fact that MPS is seemingly not related to cystic fibrosis or Hirschsprung disease, both of these more serious conditions should be considered at the time of presentation. Mostly a benign cause of colonic obstruction, MPS is usually present in children with a predisposition to poor bowel motility.

Epidemiology

MPS has an incidence of 1 in 500 to 1000 neonates.[44] Neonates of low birth weight or immaturity are at risk for this condition. Other associated risks are maternal diabetes and hypothyroidism. An iatrogenic cause of MPS is the administration of magnesium sulfate to the mother in the peripartum period.

History

Symptoms of obstruction may present several days after birth. Bilious vomiting, abdominal distension, and failure to pass meconium may be reported by the parents.

Clinical Manifestations

The abdomen is usually not tender on examination. Rectal examination may result in dislodgment of the meconium plug, relieving the colonic obstruction and confirming the diagnosis.

Diagnostic Studies

Plain radiographic evaluation of the abdomen will reveal signs of distal small bowel or large bowel obstruction.

Management

Water enema will usually dislodge the meconium plug and serve as diagnostic and therapeutic. Close follow-up is important, as 10% to 15% of patients thought to have this condition will ultimately be diagnosed as actually having Hirschsprung disease.

Anorectal Malformations

Failure of the completion of the usual embryonic development of the urologic structures and rectum lead to a variety of anorectal malformations. *Anal stenosis* and *anal atresia* (low type) may be overlooked at the time of delivery and subsequently present to the ED. It is common for anorectal malformations to be detected during the newborn examination and therefore diagnosis is usually made prior to discharge from hospital.[45]

Anal atresia refers to the lack of the usual anus as an opening to the outside of the body. Developmentally speaking, this has a high and low type and leads to the development of different fistulas to allow for the passage of stool from the body. *Anal stenosis* represents around 20% of anorectal malformations and is essentially a very tight anus. This may be strictly a small opening, or may be secondary to the presence of anal web.

Epidemiology

One in 5000 infants will be born with an anorectal malformation.[10] About half of these children will also have one or more associated conditions. These may include duodenal atresia, esophageal atresia, tracheoesophageal fistula, cloacal extrophy in females, cardiac and urologic malformations, vertebral and upper limb abnormalities, and Down syndrome. Males are slightly more likely to present with anorectal malformations, but are much more likely to present with high type anal atresia when compared with females.

History

If the child has been discharged home after passing meconium, the child may present with a history of thin, stringy, or ribbon-like stools that are passed with apparent difficulty. If an associated urologic malformation is present, the child may present with fever or other signs of urinary tract infection. Parents may report cloudy or dark urine. Female children may have a history of stool coming from the vagina.

Clinical Manifestations

Anal atresia that presents as a classic imperforate anus is not likely to be missed at the time of the newborn examination shortly after delivery. If a child is the product of an out-of-hospital birth, however, the examiner may find just that. The presence of an apparent anus is more likely in children who were born in-hospital and initially missed. A close inspection of the perineum may reveal a tight-appearing anus that lies slightly anterior to the expected location of the anus. This may represent the perineal fistula in males and the anocutaneous or rectofourchette fistula in females.[10]

Diagnostic Studies & Management

Diagnostic studies are usually not indicated. Once the abnormality is discovered or suspected, pediatric surgical consultation should be obtained. Children suffering from urologic abnormalities should be tested for renal function and urinary tract infection.

Other Causes

Other, rarer causes of apparent constipation exist but are unlikely to present to the ED. *Colonic atresia* and *colonic stenosis* are commonly associated with other abnormalities of the GI system, abdominal wall, and urologic structures. When presenting as an isolated malformation, clinical presentation will include constipation (or failure to pass meconium), abdominal distension, and bilious vomiting. Plain radiographs will show an obstructive picture. The diagnosis is confirmed by contrast enema that reveals a blind end to a microcolon. *Duplications* of the GI system may occur anywhere along the alimentary tract and may contain heterotopic tissues, such as gastric mucosa or pancreatic tissue. The duplications may be tubular, cystic, or fusiform. Presentation is variable, creating some diagnostic difficulty. However, these abnormalities are often identified in utero by prenatal ultrasound.

▶ JAUNDICE

Sixty percent of normal newborns and 80% of preterm infants become clinically jaundiced during the first week of life.[46,47] Normal neonates produce bilirubin at around 2 to 3 times the rate an average adult. Details concerning the initial time of presentation and duration of the jaundice are key to determining the etiology. Neonates are rarely jaundiced at the time of delivery and presentation within the first 24 hours is considered pathologic until proven otherwise.

Indirect or *unconjugated*, bilirubin is predominately present in the body as a breakdown product of hemoglobin, but also represents a byproduct of precursor cell breakdown and, in some cases, inefficient hemoglobin synthesis. Neonates have larger red cells with greater hematocrit and a shorter life span of around 90 days. *Direct* bilirubin refers to the *conjugated* form that is normally excreted into the bowel and transported out of the body with feces. This mechanism can be derailed by obstruction of the biliary system or of the small or large bowel.

Bilirubin encephalopathy or *kernicterus* is a serious neurologic condition related to the deposition of unconjugated bilirubin in the brain. This lipid soluble form of bilirubin may cross the blood brain barrier and results in disruption of brain cell metabolism, especially in the basal ganglia.[48] For the development of this condition, levels greater than 20 mg/dL are usually required in healthy term newborns. Severe infection, hypoxia, hemolysis, and specific drug exposures may lead to neurologic damage in patients with levels below 20 mg/dL. Preterm neonates are also at increased risk. Presentation or jaundice with fever, bulging fontonel, lethargy, irritability, poor feeding, tremor, seizure, or other neurologic signs should raise immediate concern for *bilirubin encephalopathy*.

Nonemergent Causes

Physiologic jaundice typically becomes apparent on days 2 or 3 and peaks between the days 2 or 4 of like. Resolution should be seen by the day 7. Breast milk jaundice typically presents after the day 7 of life, peaks around week 2 to 3, and resolves from week 3 to 10.

Physiologic Jaundice

Physiologic jaundice is the result of increased bilirubin production from the breakdown of fetal red blood cells in addition to the limitation of the conjugation of bilirubin by the immature neonatal liver. In more detail, the increased bilirubin load on liver cells may be secondary to an increased erythrocyte volume, decreased erythrocyte survival, increased early-labeled bilirubin, or an increased enterohepatic circulation of bilirubin. A decreased hepatic uptake of bilirubin from plasma may occur. The most common reason is secondary to a decrease in ligandin, which is the bilirubin-binding protein in liver cells. Phenobarbital has been shown to increase the ligandin levels. A decrease in bilirubin conjugation is caused by uridine diphosphoglucuronosyl transferase. The purpose of this enzyme is to convert insoluble unconjugated bilirubin to bilirubin glucuronide, the water-soluble conjugated bilirubin, allowing for excretion. And lastly, defective bilirubin excretion impairs bilirubin excretion.

Breast Milk Jaundice

Breast milk jaundice is associated with increased enterohepatic circulation of bilirubin. Decreased caloric intake may lead to decreased stool production. Breastfed infants produce stool that contains less bilirubin compared with formula-fed infants. Unconjugated bilirubin is associated with unabsorbed fat in the intestine. In the breastfed infant there is an increase in intestinal fat absorption, thereby increasing the amount of unconjugated bilirubin. Moreover, breast milk slows the formation of urobilin in the intestine, which increases the reabsorption of bilirubin. An increased activity of beta-glucuronidase in breast milk produces unconjugated bilirubin, which can be reabsorbed in the gut. And lastly, mutations of the Igene (Gilbert sydrome) prolong breast milk jaundice.[49]

Epidemiology

Elevations in bilirubin may be related to familial, ethnic, and other genetic predisposing factors. Hispanics tend to have a higher incidence of elevated total serum bilirubin (TSB) levels. Black infants, on the other hand, tend to have lower TSB. Siblings of children with a history of elevated TSB also tend to have higher TSBs. Also of note, *physiologic jaundice* may be more prominent in infants of Asian and Greek descent. Asian and Native American infants may have a higher rate of *breast milk jaundice*.

History

The complex differential causes of jaundice in the neonate make it imperative to obtain a detailed history including family, pregnancy and delivery, and postnatal history. Physiologic jaundice, and breast milk jaundice to a lesser degree, should be a diagnosis of exclusion.

Family history of Gilbert syndrome, hemolytic disorders, maternal illness, delayed cord-clamping, birth trauma, breastfeeding history, loss of stool color, and parental nutrition are some of the important details of the history sometimes necessary to determine the cause of jaundice. A pharmacologic history is also important as some drugs alter the bilirubin-albumin binding affinity. Anticonvulsants, diuretics, antibiotics, and sedatives may all be causative agents.

Physiologic jaundice usually becomes noticeable on the day 3 of life in term infants and by day 5 in preterm children. *Breast milk jaundice* presents later, around days 7 to 14. The child may have a history of difficulty initiating feeding or the mother may note a slow onset of milk production. Both types can be more prominent in neonates with a history of inadequate oral intake or dehydration.

Other Causes of Jaundice in the Young Infant

There are many additional causes of hyperbilirubinemia in the young infant.[50] These are broken down by types of hyperbilirubinemia and presented in Table 5–7.

▶ **TABLE 5–7. CAUSES OF HYPERBILIRUBINEMIA BY BILIRUBIN SUBGROUP**

Unconjugated Predominance	Conjugated Predominance
Physiologic jaundice	Urinary tract infection
Breast milk jaundice	Congenital viral
Birth trauma	infection (CMV)
(cephalohematoma)	Biliary atresia
Polycythemia (delayed	Dubin-Johnson
cord clamping)	syndrome
Hemolysis (ABO	Rotor syndrome
incompatability RBC	
defects)	
Intestinal obstruction	
Hypothyroidism	

► TABLE 5–8. **ETIOLOGY OF HYPERBILIRUBINEMIA BY LABORATORY PROFILE**

Coombs Testing	Anemia	Most Likely Diagnosis
Positive	Present	Blood group incompatability
Negative	Present	RBC defect
Negative	Absent	Breast milk jaundice

Diagnostic Studies & Management

In general, almost all causes of conjugated hyperbilirubinemia mandate consultation and probable admission. In contrast, most causes of unconjugated hyperbilirubinemia are self limited and benign (with the exception of blood group incompatibilities).[51] In this regard, diagnostic studies should include a CBC with peripheral smear (to look for hemolysis), bilirubin fractionization, blood typing, and Coombs testing. Some general characteristics of laboratory findings are listed in Table 5–8.

Most jaundiced infants may be safely discharged from the ED as long as adequate follow-up is arranged. General guidelines for phototherapy are provided in Table 5–9.

► GI BLEEDING

Gastrointestinal bleeding in the neonate requires investigation due to the fact that it may herald serious life-threatening conditions that require emergent surgical or medical intervention. This being stated, a common cause for upper and lower GI blood is simply the swallowing of maternal blood at the time of birth or even from cracked nipples of the breastfeeding mother. Historical details and a careful physical examination are crucial when evaluating the neonate with apparent GI bleeding. In cases of significant GI bleeding, diagnostic evaluation with baseline labs, radiographs, and appropriate consultation are required to ensure timely diagnosis and treatment.

Upper GI Bleeding

Hematemesis within the first several days of life may represent swallowing of maternal blood during delivery. The neonate will usually appear well otherwise, and an Apt test would be expected to be negative. If the Apt test is positive, this benign process is ruled out and causes of GI bleeding should be considered. More serious causes of upper GI bleeding in the neonate include milk protein sensitivity, esophagitis, stress gastritis, or ulcer and vascular malformations.[52] Neonates

► TABLE 5–9. **MANAGEMENT OF HYPERBILIRUBINEMIA IN THE HEALTHY TERM INFANT WITH NO RISK FACTORS**

	25-48 h	49-72 h	>72 h (3 days)
Consider phototherapy	12-15mg/dL	15-18 mg/dL	18-20 mg/dL
Phototherapy	>15 mg/dL	>18 mg/dL	>20 mg/dL
Consider exchange transfusion	19-22 mg/dL	22-24 mg/dL	24-25 mg/dL
Exchange transfusion	>22 mg/dL	>24 md/dL	>25 mg/dL

Note: (1) Infants with jaundice in the first 24 h are not considered healthy infants. (2) TSB of 25 mg/dL or higher is a medical emergency and the child should be admitted immediately.

Source: Adapted from 1994 AAP Practice Guideline.

born in the out-of-hospital setting may present with hematemesis as a presenting sign of hemorrhagic disease of the newborn secondary to vitamin K deficiency. Ill neonates may present with disseminated intravascular coagulation (DIC) or liver failure and may be septic. Surgical emergencies such as necrotizing enterocolitis and midgut volvulus must also be considered.[38]

Lower GI Bleeding

Anal fissure is the most common cause of rectal bleeding in the neonate. If identified in the otherwise healthy-appearing infant, no other diagnostic evaluation may be needed. Other causes to be considered are allergic enterocolitis, infectious enterocolitis, necrotizing enterocolitis, midgut volvulus, and Hirschsprung disease.[53] Vitamin K deficiency, DIC, and liver failure may also present as lower GI bleeding.

Diagnostic Studies

Neonates with significant GI bleeding in the first several days of life should have the blood tested for source (maternal vs neonate). This can be done with the Apt test. If negative, and the child appears well, observation only may be appropriate. If the Apt test is positive or cannot be completed in a timely manner, additional diagnostic evaluation is appropriate. All ill neonates with GI bleeding should have further diagnostics.[54] This evaluation should include CBC, coagulation tests, liver function tests, BUN and creatinine, and plain films for obstruction. Other diagnostic testing and consultation should be guided by the differential diagnosis established by patient history and examination.

Management

If the child is not septic, no surgical emergency can be identified, and coagulation testing is normal, admission to the pediatrics service or gastroenterology unit is still appropriate in cases where Apt testing is positive

and no rectal fissure or other benign explanation can be identified. The neonate may require endoscopy and both gastroenterology and pediatric surgery may be required at the institution where the child is to be admitted.

REFERENCES

1. Reyna TM, Reyna PA. Gastroduodenal disorders associated with emesis in infants. *Semin Pediatr Surg.* 1995;4(3):190-197.
2. Hyman PE, Milla PJ, Benninga MA, Davidson GP, Fleisher DF, Taminiau J. Childhood functional gastrointestinal disorders: neonate/toddler. *Gastroenterology.* 2006;130(5):1519-1526.
3. Gremse DA. Gastroesophageal reflux: life-threatening disease or laundry problem? *Clin Pediatr (Phila).* 2002;41(6):369-372.
4. Naik-Mathuria B, Olutoye OO. Foregut abnormalities. *Surg Clin North Am.* 2006;86(2):261-284, viii.
5. Poets CF. Gastroesophageal reflux: a critical review of its role in preterm infants. *Pediatrics.* 2004;113(2):e128-e132.
6. Rasquin-Weber A, Hyman PE, Cucchiara S, et al. Childhood functional gastrointestinal disorders. *Gut.* 1999;45(Suppl 2):II60-II68.
7. Salvatore S, Vandenplas Y. Gastroesophageal reflux and cow milk allergy: is there a link? *Pediatrics.* 2002;110(5):972-984.
8. Hostetler MA, Schulman M. Necrotizing enterocolitis presenting in the Emergency Department: case report and review of differential considerations for vomiting in the neonate. *J Emerg Med.* 2001;21(2):165-170.
9. Louie JP. Essential diagnosis of abdominal emergencies in the first year of life. *Emerg Med Clin North Am.* 2007;25(4):1009-1040, vi.
10. Rao P. Neonatal gastrointestinal imaging. *Eur J Radiol.* 2006;60(2):171-186.
11. Maclennan AC. Investigation in vomiting children. *Semin Pediatr Surg.* 2003;12(4):220-228.
12. Vasavada P. Ultrasound evaluation of acute abdominal emergencies in infants and children. *Radiol Clin North Am.* 2004;42(2):445-456.
13. Green P, Swischuk LE, Hernandez JA. Delayed presentation of malrotation and midgut

volvulus: imaging findings. *Emerg Radiol*. 2007; 14(6):379-382.

14. Hajivassiliou CA. Intestinal obstruction in neonatal/pediatric surgery. *Semin Pediatr Surg*. 2003;12(4):241-253.

15. Blumer SL, Zucconi WB, Cohen HL, Scriven RJ, Lee TK. The vomiting neonate: a review of the ACR appropriateness criteria and ultrasound's role in the workup of such patients. *Ultrasound Q*. 2004;20(3):79-89.

16. Zissin R, Osadchy A, Gayer G, Shapiro-Feinberg M. Pictorial CT of duodenal pathology. *Br J Radiol*. 2002;75(889):78-84.

17. Duong M, Dinoulos JG, Gupta A, et al. Index of suspicion. *Pediatr Rev*. 2005;26(1):23-33.

18. Prasad TR, Bajpai M. Intestinal atresia. *Indian J Pediatr*. 2000;67(9):671-678.

19. Al-Salem AH, Qaissaruddin S, Karthikeya Varma K. Pyloric atresia associated with intestinal atresia. *J Pediatr Surg*. 1997;32(8):1262-1263.

20. Celli J, van Bokhoven H, Brunner HG. Feingold syndrome: clinical review and genetic mapping. *Am J Med Genet A*. 2003;122(4):294-300.

21. Pameijer CR, Hubbard AM, Coleman B, Flake AW. Combined pure esophageal atresia, duodenal atresia, biliary atresia, and pancreatic ductal atresia: prenatal diagnostic features and review of the literature. *J Pediatr Surg*. 2000;35(5):745-747.

22. Berrocal T, Torres I, Gutiérrez J, Prieto C, del Hoyo ML, Lamas M. Congenital anomalies of the upper gastrointestinal tract. *Radiographics*. 1999;19(4):855-872.

23. Escobar MA, Ladd AP, Grosfeld JL, et al. Duodenal atresia and stenosis: long-term follow-up over 30 years. *J Pediatr Surg*. 2004;39(6):867-871; discussion 867-871.

24. Sajja SB, Middlesworth W, Niazi M, Schein M, Gerst PH. Duodenal atresia associated with proximal jejunal perforations: a case report and review of the literature. *J Pediatr Surg*. 2003;38(9):1396-1398.

25. Kelly DA, Davenport M. Current management of biliary atresia. *Arch Dis Child*. 2007;92(12):1132-1135.

26. Nixon HH. Duodenal atresia. *Br J Hosp Med*. 1989;41(2):134, 138, 140.

27. Jayaraman MV, Mayo-Smith WW, Movson JS, Dupuy DE, Wallach MT. CT of the duodenum: an overlooked segment gets its due. *Radiographics*. 2001;21 Spec No:S147-S160.

28. Shorter NA, Georges A, Perenyi A, Garrow E. A proposed classification system for familial intestinal atresia and its relevance to the understanding of the etiology of jejunoileal atresia. *J Pediatr Surg*. 2006;41(11):1822-1825.

29. Kays DW. Surgical conditions of the neonatal intestinal tract. *Clin Perinatol*. 1996;23(2):353-375.

30. Stark Z, Patel N, Clarnette T, Moody A. Triad of tracheoesophageal fistula-esophageal atresia, pulmonary hypoplasia, and duodenal atresia. *J Pediatr Surg*. 2007;42(6):1146-1148.

31. Burton BK. Inborn errors of metabolism in infancy: a guide to diagnosis. *Pediatrics*. 1998;102(6):E69.

32. Cappellini MD, Fiorelli G. Glucose-6-phosphate dehydrogenase deficiency. *Lancet*. 2008; 371(9606):64-74.

33. Kwon KT, Tsai VW. Metabolic emergencies. *Emerg Med Clin North Am*. 2007;25(4):1041-1060, vi.

34. Armon K, Stephenson T, MacFaul R, Eccleston P, Werneke U. An evidence and consensus based guideline for acute diarrhoea management. *Arch Dis Child*. 2001;85(2):132-142.

35. Galea MH, Holliday H, Carachi R, Kapila L. Short-bowel syndrome: a collective. *J Pediatr Surg*. 1992;27(5):592-596.

36. Sigalet DL. Short bowel syndrome in infants and children: an overview. *Semin Pediatr Surg*. 2001;10(2):49-55.

37. Sicherer SH. Food protein-induced enterocolitis syndrome: clinical perspectives. *J Pediatr Gastroenterol Nutr*. 2000;30(Suppl):S45-S49.

38. Kessmann J. Hirschsprung's disease: diagnosis and management. *Am Fam Physician*. 2006;74(8):1319-1322.

39. Pearl RH, Irish MS, Caty MG, Glick PL. The approach to common abdominal diagnoses in infants and children. Part II. *Pediatr Clin North Am*. 1998;45(6):1287-1326, vii.

40. Lewis NA, Levitt MA, Zallen GS, et al. Diagnosing Hirschsprung's disease: increasing the odds of a positive rectal biopsy result. *J Pediatr Surg*. 2003;38(3):412-416; discussion 412-416.

41. McAlister WH, Kronemer KA. Emergency gastrointestinal radiology of the newborn. *Radiol Clin North Am*. 1996;34(4):819-844.

42. Gupta AK, Guglani B. Imaging of congenital anomalies of the gastrointestinal tract. *Indian J Pediatr.* 2005;72(5):403-414.

43. Rescorla FJ, Grosfeld JL. Contemporary management of meconium ileus. *World J Surg.* 1993;17(3):318-325.

44. Loening-Baucke V, Kimura K. Failure to pass meconium: diagnosing neonatal intestinal obstruction. *Am Fam Physician.* 1999;60(7):2043-2050.

45. Peña A, Hong A. Advances in the management of anorectal malformations. *Am J Surg.* 2000;180(5):370-376.

46. Maisels MJ, McDonagh AF. Phototherapy for neonatal jaundice. *N Engl J Med.* 2008;358(9):920-928.

47. Maisels MJ, Watchko JF. Treatment of jaundice in low birthweight infants. *Arch Dis Child Fetal Neonatal Ed.* 2003;88(6):F459-F463.

48. Wennberg RP, Ahlfors CE, Bhutani VK, Johnson LH, Shapiro SM. Toward understanding kernicterus: a challenge to improve the management of jaundiced newborns. *Pediatrics.* 2006;117(2):474-485. Erratum in: *Pediatrics.* 2006;117(4):1467.

49. Gartner LM, Herschel M. Jaundice and breastfeeding. *Pediatr Clin North Am.* 2001;48(2):389-399.

50. Ip S, Chung M, Kulig J, et al. An evidence-based review of important issues concerning neonatal hyperbilirubinemia. *Pediatrics.* 2004;114(1):e130-e153.

51. Dennery PA, Seidman DS, Stevenson DK. Neonatal hyperbilirubinemia. *N Engl J Med.* 2001;344(8):581-590.

52. Chawla S, Seth D, Mahajan P, Kamat D. Upper gastrointestinal bleeding in children. *Clin Pediatr (Phila).* 2007;46(1):16-21.

53. Leung AK, Wong AL. Lower gastrointestinal bleeding in children. *Pediatr Emerg Care.* 2002;18(4):319-323.

54. Raine PA. Investigation of rectal bleeding. *Arch Dis Child.* 1991;66(3):279-280.

CHAPTER 6

Neonatal Genitourinary Emergencies

Brian Stout, MD

Congenital genitourinary abnormalities often present during the neonatal period. As such, a firm understanding of these problems is necessary for any emergency physician. This chapter serves to elucidate the most common of these conditions and includes a discussion of renal abnormalities, collecting system abnormalities, bladder abnormalities, penile and urethral abnormalities, scrotal abnormalities, various gynecologic abnormalities, and urinary tract infections.

▶ RENAL ABNORMALITIES

Renal abnormalities invariably include some form of renal dysgenesis due to abnormal development of the kidney in utero. These abnormalities are often identified prenatally, however some patients will present in the neonatal period.

Embryologically, the kidney originates from the ureteral bud and the metanephric blastema. During week 5 of gestation, the ureteral bud develops from the Wolffian duct and penetrates the metanephric blastema. This ureteral bud undergoes multiple divisions and by week 20 of gestation forms the entire collecting system including the ureters, renal pelvis, calyces, papillary ducts, and the collecting tubules. Nephron differentiation begins during week 7 of gestation and over 30% of nephrons are present by week 20 of gestation.[1] At any point during renal development dysgenesis can occur. Dysgenesis refers to multiple forms of abnormal renal development including aplasia, dysplasia, hypoplasia, and cystic disease.

UNILATERAL RENAL AGENESIS

Epidemiology

Unilateral renal agenesis is a relatively common condition with an incidence of 1 in 450

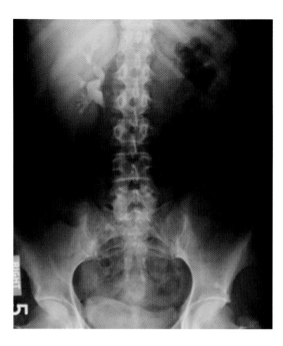

Figure 6–1. Renal agenesis.

to 1000 live births and is found with increased frequency in the neonate with a single umbilical artery (Figure 6–1).[1]

Clinical Presentation

This condition is often found while evaluating a neonate for urinary tract symptomatology. True renal agenesis is defined by no ureter or hemitrigone, as well as no kidney on the same side. Often, the contralateral kidney undergoes compensatory hypertrophy that can be palpated during the neonatal abdominal examination. Fifteen percent of patients with unilateral renal agenesis have vesicoureteral reflux.[1] Males have an absent ipsilateral vas deferens while females can have Mullerian duct abnormalities.

Diagnostic Testing

Renal ultrasound as well as renal function testing and urinalysis should be obtained.

Management

Referral to a pediatric nephrologist is appropriate and any issues with renal function should be addressed in an inpatient admission.

RENAL DYSPLASIA

Pathophysiology

Renal dysplasia refers to persistence of primitive ducts in the kidney derived from abnormal metanephric differentiation. This entity can affect all or a portion of the kidney. The pathophysiology leading to this disease is due to ureteral bud development in an abnormal location that causes inappropriate penetration and induction of the metanephric blastema.[1]

Clinical Presentation

Renal dysplasia can also be associated with posterior urethral valves and an absent portion of the ureter. If cysts are present, the disease process is termed cystic dysplasia. If the entire kidney is affected with many cysts, the disease is termed a multicystic dysplastic kidney. Multicystic kidney disease is the most common cause of an abdominal mass in a neonate and is present in approximately 1 of 2000 live births.[1] These kidneys often have little or no function. Contralateral vesicoureteral reflux is present in 15% of patients. Five to 10% of patients will have contralateral hydronephrosis.[1]

Diagnostic Testing

Ultrasound of the kidney will demonstrate a kidney replaced by cysts of various sizes with no communication. No renal parenchyma is present (Figure 6–2).

Management

Management of the patients in the emergency department (ED) would include an ultrasound, renal function profile, urinalysis, and consultation

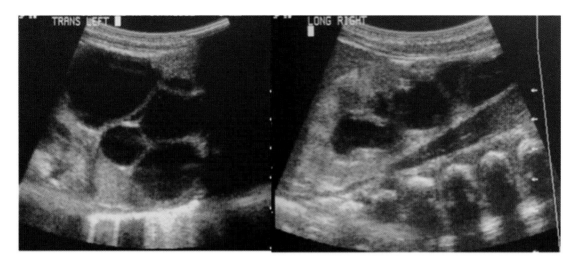

Figure 6–2. Multicystic kidneys.

with a pediatric nephrologist. A confirming renal scan should be performed along with a VCUG looking for reflux. These can be accomplished on an outpatient basis if no abnormalities are present on the renal panel. Later complications include rennin-mediated hypertension and Wilms tumor. These patients require annual follow-up with a pediatric nephrologist.

RENAL HYPOPLASIA

Pathophysiology

Renal hypoplasia refers to a kidney that is structurally normal but small in size. The kidney is small due to a less than normal number of nephrons and calyces. Like many renal conditions identified in the neonatal period, this entity is often found while evaluating a patient for other urinary problems. Because of the reduced number of nephrons and calyces, these kidneys usually do not have normal function. If renal hypoplasia is present bilaterally, chronic renal failure can ensue.

Clinical Presentation

Symptoms include polyuria and polydipsia.

Management

If found on ultrasound, these patients should undergo a renal function profile, urinalysis, and pediatric nephrology consultation. Any abnormalities in renal function should be addressed with an inpatient admission.

Abnormalities in shape and position of the kidneys are a relatively common finding in neonates and may be found in the evaluation of a neonate in the ED. In normal development, the kidneys ascend from the pelvis to a position behind the ribs. If this process is incomplete, renal ectopic or nonrotation can develop, leading to an abnormal position or shape of the kidney.

RENAL ECTOPIA & FUSION ABNORMALITIES

Pathophysiology

Renal ectopia refers to an abnormal location of the kidney with an incidence estimated at 1 of 900 live births.[1] Pelvic, iliac, thoracic, or contralateral placement of the kidney has been described. Ninety percent of patients with a contralateral kidney have fusion of 2 kidneys.[1]

Fusion abnormalities, leading to an abnormality in shape, are even more common than ectopia alone. Horseshoe kidney is the most common fusion abnormality, occurring in 1 of 500 live births.[1]

Clinical Presentation & Diagnostic Testing

The large, fused kidney is often palpable in the neonatal patient and can be diagnosed on ultrasound. The risk of Wilms tumor is fourfold in patients with a horseshoe kidney.[1] There is an increased incidence of multicystic dysplastic kidney usually affecting one side of the kidney. Crossed-fused ectopia is another common fusion abnormality involving the fusion of the parenchyma of the 2 kidneys. Most commonly, the left kidney crosses the midline to fuse with the lower pole of the right kidney.

Management

A renal function panel should assess renal function initially and any abnormalities should be addressed with an inpatient admission. If all results are normal, further workup can be arranged as an outpatient.

► COLLECTING SYSTEM & BLADDER ANOMALIES

The renal collecting system is made up of calyces, ureters, bladder, and urethra. Problems can develop in any of these areas that lead to specific disease processes (Figure 6–3).

VESICOURETERAL REFLUX

Epidemiology & Pathophysiology

Vesicoureteral reflux (VUR) is one of the most common collecting system problems found in

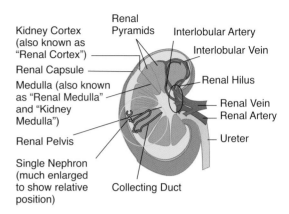

Figure 6–3. Normal renal architecture.

neonatal patients and is defined by the retrograde flow of urine from the bladder to the ureter or renal pelvis. This entity occurs as the result of an abnormal attachment of the ureter to the bladder. Normally the attachment is oblique, forming a flap-like valve (Figure 6–4).

If this tunnel into the bladder is short or absent, reflux develops (Figure 6–5). This is considered a birth defect and is found in approximately 1% of children.[2] VUR is an important issue due to the increased risk of recurrent urinary tract infection in patients

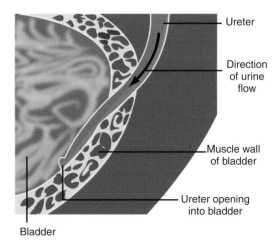

Figure 6–4. Normal ureter entering bladder.

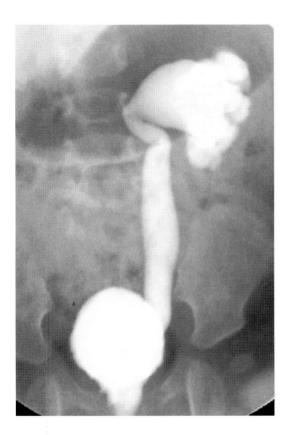

Figure 6–5. Vesicoureteral reflux. *Source: From Brunicardi FC, Andersen DK, Billiar TF. Schwartz's Principles of Surgery, 8th ed. New York, NY: McGraw-Hill; 2005.*

with this abnormality. Prior to the wide-spread knowledge regarding this entity, VUR accounted for 15% to 20% of end stage renal disease in children and young adults.[2]

Grading of vesicoureteral reflux has been established on a scale from I to V; grade V represents the most severe form. VUR can be primary or secondary depending upon the cause.

Duplication anomalies are one of the most common causes for vesicoureteral reflux and occur in approximately 1 of 125 children.[2] In this condition, 2 ureters drain 1 kidney. At least 1 of the ureters is in an abnormal position on the bladder. Reflux occurs in approximately 50% of patients with duplication anomalies.[2] If the ureter drains outside the bladder, it is considered an ectopic ureter. If the ureter drains into the bladder neck, vesicoureteral reflux is almost universally present. Duplication anomalies are also associated with ureteral diverticulae and ureterocele.

Neuropathic bladder and posterior urethral valves are also associated with vesicoureteral reflux with an occurrence rate of 25% and 50%, respectively.[2] Fifteen percent of patients with vesicoureteral reflux also have renal agenesis, multicystic dysplastic kidney, or ureteropelvic junction obstruction.[2]

As stated previously there is a genetic link to VUR. Approximately 35% of siblings have reflux that is often asymptomatic.[2] In these siblings, 12% will have evidence of renal scarring.[2] Fifty percent of children of mothers with reflux will also have reflux.[2]

Clinical Presentation

From a clinical standpoint, many patients with reflux will be asymptomatic and the disease will be found in the evaluation for a urinary tract infection (UTI). Typically, these patients are diagnosed by a VCUG and ultrasound. Any neonate found to have a UTI should be admitted for antibiotic treatment but should undergo ultrasound and voiding cystourethrogram, usually done during the inpatient admission.

Management

Treatment usually involves medical management because most reflux tends to improve over time. Typically, antibiotic prophylaxis with Bactrim or nitrofurantoin is used. Surgical therapy is resolved for more severe cases that are unlikely to resolve.

The prognosis is good for most patients, in that reflux tends to improve over time except in the most severe cases. Reflux without infection does not lead to renal scarring.

URINARY TRACT OBSTRUCTION

Pathophysiology

Obstruction to urine flow can occur anywhere along the urinary tract from the urethral meatus to the calyces. These obstructions can be due to a variety of causes, including congenital causes, trauma, neoplasia, calculi, inflammation, or surgery. Early fetal obstruction leads to renal dysplasia, whereas late fetal obstruction causes dilatation of the collecting system and renal parenchymal damage.

Clinical Presentation

Clinically, neonatal patients with urinary obstruction will present with abdominal pain or flank pain secondary to the collecting system dilatation and hydronephrosis. This can be difficult to identify in the neonatal patient and the initial presentation may be only irritability. Also, failure to thrive may be a significant component in their history.

Diagnosis can prove to be difficult in these patients as many of will be asymptomatic. If a palpable abdominal mass is present, this typically indicates a dysplastic kidney. If the bladder is palpable in a male patient, this may indicate an intravesicular obstruction. A patent urachus is also indicative of a urinary obstruction. Abdominal ascites is a common finding in patients with posterior urethral valves. UTI may also be present.

Diagnostic Testing

Numerous imaging modalities may be required to evaluate neonates with presumed urinary obstruction; these include renal ultrasound, VCUG, and radioisotope studies to evaluate renal function.

Differential Diagnosis & Management

Hydrocalycosis refers to dilatation of the calyx secondary to infundibular stenosis. This entity can result from a developmental or infectious process. It is often discovered during evaluation for pain or urinary tract infection.

Ureteral pelvic junction (UPJ) obstruction is the most common form of obstruction found in childhood and can present in the neonatal period.[3] Typically, this is an intrinsic form of stenosis. UPJ obstruction can present in a number of ways including fetal hydronephrosis found on ultrasound; palpable abdominal mass found on a neonate or infant; abdominal, flank, or back pain; febrile urinary tract infection; or hematuria after minimal trauma. Sixty percent of patients have obstruction on the left side and 10% will have bilateral obstruction.[3] There is a male to female preponderance of 2 to 1.[3] Renal function may be impaired secondary to elevated pressures. In these cases, surgery is required for definitive treatment. Primary evaluation of UPJ obstruction should include a renal function panel, renal ultrasound, a CT scan of the abdomen and pelvis in some cases (Figure 6–6), and VCUG. Inpatient admission is usually indicated in the neonatal patient.

Midureteral obstruction is a rare congenital condition that can be identified in the

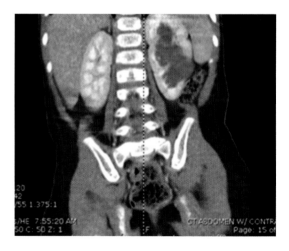

Figure 6–6. Ureteral pelvic junction obstruction.

neonatal patient. Similar to other obstructive lesions, this can present as a palpable abdominal mass due to hydronephrosis of the ipsilateral kidney. Often, this is due to a retrocaval ureter. Treatment universally involves surgery and, as such, pediatric urology should be involved immediately upon diagnosis.

Ectopic ureter defines a condition where a ureter is abnormally placed in the bladder wall or drains outside of the bladder. This entity is 3 times more common in females than males.[3] In females, 35% of patients have a ureter entering the bladder neck, 35% have a ureter entering the urethrovaginal septum, and 25% have a ureter entering the vagina.[3] Other locations include the cervix, uterus, and Gartner duct. Urinary incontinence occurs with ectopic placement of the ureter except when the ureter is implanted in the bladder neck.

In males, the ectopic ureter is implanted in a variety of locations. Forty-seven percent of patients have a ureter entering in the posterior urethra, 33% have a ureter entering in the seminal vesicle, 10% have an entrance in the prostatic utricle, 5% in the ejaculatory duct, and 5% in the vas deferens.[3] Unlike females, males do not have any incontinence, though the abnormality can be associated with a UTI or epididymitis.

Diagnosis is usually established by an ultrasound obtained for a palpable mass found on physical examination. A hydronephrotic kidney is invariably present on the side of the ectopic ureter. A VCUG needs to be obtained along with a urologic consult.

Surgical repair may involve ureteral reimplantation or nephrectomy.

Ureterocele is defined as a cystic dilatation of the terminal ureter. These lesions are obstructive due to a pinpoint orifice. Similar to an ectopic ureter, there is a female preponderance over males. These lesions are almost always associated with ureteral duplication.

The first type of ureterocele is the simple ureterocele. The simple ureterocele is a simple cystic dilatation of the ureter with a normal insertion location on the bladder. There is no duplication associated with the simple ureterocele. Often, this lesion is found during an evaluation of a patient for a UTI. Treatment involves drainage though the lesion itself and may cause reflux, in which case surgical reimplantation is required. In small lesions, no treatment may be required at all.

In more complicated cases of ureterocele involving ureteral duplication and abnormal insertion, treatment almost universally involves surgery. Typically, this involves excision of the affected pole of the kidney and the ectopic ureter. If the ureterocele is small, drainage alone is sometimes successful. In a septic infant, immediate urologic consultation is required with drainage of the ureterocele.

Megaureter defines a ureter that is dilated through its entire length. There are numerous causes including many nonobstructive causes. Diagnosis is established through an ultrasound or VCUG, during or after an evaluation for a UTI (Figure 6–7).

Typical symptoms include abdominal pain and hematuria. Nonobstructive management is conservative while obstructive lesions usually require surgery.

Prune-belly syndrome, also known as Eagle-Barrett or triad syndrome, is a rare condition occurring in approximately 1 of 40,000 live births and causes massive dilatation of the ureter and upper tracts of the collecting system.[3] Ninety-five percent of affected patients are males.[3]

The clinical findings in prune-belly syndrome typically include a large, distended bladder and can include a patent urachus or urachal diverticulum. Vesicoureteral reflux is typically present. The prostatic urethra is dilated while the prostate itself is hypoplastic. The kidneys are usually dysplastic and in males, posterior urethral valves may be present.

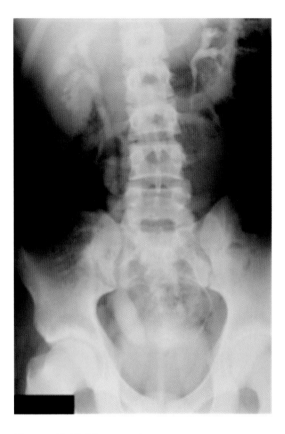

Figure 6–7. Megaureter.

All patients with this entity should receive prophylactic antibiotics. If no obstruction is present, this is all the treatment required at the time. If obstruction is present, vesicostomy is required. Thirty percent of patients will go on to have end-stage renal disease.[3]

Bladder neck obstruction is usually a secondary form of collecting system obstruction caused by an ectopic ureterocele, bladder calculi, or tumor of the prostate. Typical symptoms include difficulty voiding, urinary retention, and urinary tract infection. Bladder distension is universal, often with overflow incontinence.

Posterior urethral valves are the most common cause of severe renal and urologic disease. This entity only affects males and has an incidence of 1 in 8000 live births.[3] This congenital abnormality with the presence of valves in the urethra obstructs the flow of urine, leading to dilatation of the prostatic urethra to bladder muscle hypertrophy. Vesicoureteral reflux will develop in 50% of patients if untreated.[3] Renal changes ranging from hydronephrosis to dysplasia can occur. Without effective treatment, 30% of patients will go on to end stage renal disease or chronic renal insufficiency.[3]

The diagnosis can often be established prenatally, however some patients will be missed. The diagnosis should be suspected in any male neonate with a palpable, distended bladder or a weak urine stream. Initial workup should include a renal ultrasound, and, if posterior urethral valves are suspected, a voiding cystourethrogram should be obtained. A renal function panel should be obtained to evaluate renal function. Pediatric urologic consultation should be sought immediately.

Treatment involving antibiotic prophylaxis is required in all patients and definitive treatment is accomplished by valve ablation. Postoperative incontinence is common and some patients will also have polyuria lasting for weeks. Some patients may have residual hydronephrosis of the kidneys.

Urethral atresia is an obstructive condition that is often diagnosed in utero and will present in the first days of life due to absent urine production. Due to obstruction, the bladder distends, ultimately causing bilateral hydroureteronephrosis. Emergent urinary diversion using a vesicostomy is required.

Urethral hypoplasia is an obstructive condition in which the urethral lumen is small. This is a rare condition that, similar to urethral atresia, causes a distended bladder and bilateral hydronephrosis. Renal dysplasia can develop causing end stage renal disease. Treatment involves a vesicostomy, followed by urethral reconstruction, dilatation, or diversion.

Urethral stricture is a condition in which a portion of the urethra is significantly narrowed causing an obstruction. This condition is much more common in males than females. The most common cause for this condition is

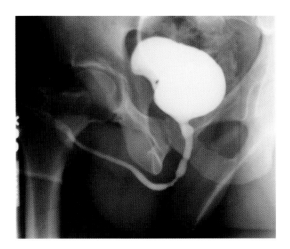

Figure 6-8. Urethral stricture.

urethral trauma. Symptoms develop gradually, as does the lesion, and includes bladder instability, hematuria, and dysuria. Diagnosis is accomplished by IV urography or retrograde urethrography and ultrasound (Figure 6–8). Treatment is accomplished by dilatation or urethroplasty.

Anterior urethral valves are another rare obstructive condition. This can be associated with a diverticulum in the penile urethra. This expands and can lead to a palpable mass on the ventral surface of the penis. Other physical examination findings are consistent with those for posterior urethral valves. The urinary stream is typically weak. Diagnosis is established by VCUG and treatment involves excision of the valves and diverticula.

Bladder abnormalities can also cause urinary obstruction. These conditions include bladder diverticula, urachal abnormalities including urachal cyst, and patent urachus.

Neurogenic bladder usually results congenitally from spinal abnormalities, such as spina bifida. Symptoms include urinary incontinence, UTI, and upper tract deterioration. Ten to 15% of patients have hydronephrosis and 25% have vesicoureteral reflux.[3]

Diagnosis involves ultrasound, postvoid bladder residuals, and VCUG.

▶ **PENILE & URETHRAL ABNORMALITIES**

HYPOSPADIAS

Epidemiology & Pathophysiology

Hypospadias is a common, congenital condition present in 1 of 250 live births where the urethral opening is abnormally located on the ventral surface of the penis.[4] In most infants, hypospadias is an isolated abnormality. Associated abnormalities include incomplete development of the prepuce, chordee, absent foreskin ventrally, and inguinal hernia. A bifid scrotum can also be present. Ten percent of patients have undescended testes.[5] The etiology of this congenital malformation is unclear. There is an increased incidence of hypospadias in infants where the mother received antiandrogenic or estrogenic compounds.

Classification of the condition is based upon the location of the urethral opening. Sixty percent of patients will have a distal hypospadias, 25% subcoronal or midpenile, and 15% proximal.[5] Less common locations include glanular, coronal, subcoronal, midpenile, penoscrotal, scrotal, and perineal (Figure 6–9).

Clinical Presentation

The abnormal location of the urethral opening leads to several complications including deformity of the urinary stream, sexual dysfunction secondary to curvature of the penis, infertility, and meatal stenosis.

Management

Surgical treatment represents the definitive therapy and is usually performed at 6 to 12 months of age. Circumcision should never be performed in the infant with hypospadias until the repair is complete.

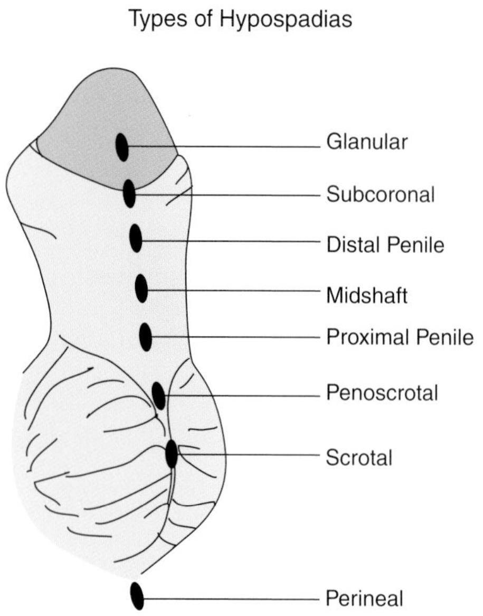

Types of Hypospadias

- Glanular
- Subcoronal
- Distal Penile
- Midshaft
- Proximal Penile
- Penoscrotal
- Scrotal
- Perineal

Figure 6–9. Hypospadias.

CHORDEE

Chordee refers to a ventral curvature of the penis due to tight bands in the penis. Usually there is incomplete development of the foreskin; in the neonate there is a dorsal hood similar to that seen in hypospadias. If this condition is identified in the evaluation of a neonate, it is important to refer the patient to a pediatric urologist for surgical repair

PHIMOSIS

Phimosis is a penile condition in which there is an inability to retract the prepuce. It is important to note that at birth there is physiologic phimosis that normally resolves by year 3 of life.

COMPLICATIONS OF CIRCUMCISION

Circumcision is the most common elective surgical procedure performed on newborn boys in the United States and 0.2% to 3% of boys who underwent circumcision require a subsequent operative procedure.[5]

Clinical Presentation

Many neonates are brought to the ED following this procedure with concerns regarding bleeding or the appearance of the circumcision site. After circumcision, the penis normally demonstrates an erythematous glans with a white healing eschar. This appearance often may cause concern, particularly to new parents. After a thorough physical examination, the concerns of the parents should be addressed and reassurance given. The most common complications of a circumcision include bleeding, wound infection, meatal stenosis, secondary phimosis, removal of insufficient foreskin, and penile adhesions.

Management

For bleeding complications postcircumcision, direct pressure is always the first line of treatment and usually the only treatment needed. Topical treatments include topical thrombin as well as silver nitrate cauterization. If bleeding continues despite these local treatments, urologic consultation should be obtained. Rare, serious complications include sepsis, amputation of the distal part of the glans, removal of an excessive amount of foreskin, and development of a urethrocutaneous fistula.

PENILE TORSION

Penile torsion is a condition that may present to the ED due to parental concern about the appearance of the penis. The condition involves a rotation deformity of the shaft of the penis, usually counterclockwise. This condition is invariably cosmetic in nature and the parents can be reassured and referred to pediatric urology for outpatient treatment.

INCONSPICUOUS PENIS

Another penile issue that may present to the ED is the inconspicuous penis. This essentially refers to a penis that is small, at least in appearance. There are a variety of different subtypes of inconspicuous penis. A webbed penis refers to a penis that has the scrotum extending onto the anterior ventral penis. The penis itself is not small but appears to be small due to concealment of the penile shaft by the scrotum. If circumcision is performed, the penis can retract into the scrotum and secondary phimosis can develop.

A second type of inconspicuous penis is the concealed penis. In this condition, the penis is hidden by suprapubic fat. The cause can be congenital or iatrogenic after circumcision. Again, it is important to note that the penis itself is not small in this case.

A third type of inconspicuous penis is the trapped penis, which is acquired after circumcision. In this case, the penis is literally embedded in the suprapubic fat. UTIs and urinary retention can develop and patients presenting with this condition should be evaluated for these complications. Again, the penis itself is normal size.

The fourth type of inconspicuous penis is the micropenis, which is a true small penis. Micropenis is defined by a penile size that is 2.5 standard deviations below the mean, which equates to penile length less than 1.9 cm in the stretched position.[5] The etiology of micropenis is usually related to a congenital hormone problem in the infant. These patients need no emergent treatment but referrals to a pediatric urologist and an endocrinologist should be made.

MEATAL STENOSIS

Meatal stenosis refers to stenosis of the urethral meatus. This is most commonly seen after circumcision and it is due to severe inflammation postcircumcision. Typically, due to the pinpoint orifice, parents will describe a forceful, fine stream of urine possibly with a dorsal deflection. Referral to a pediatric urologist should be made for definitive treatment by meatoplasty.

▶ URINARY TRACT INFECTION

EPIDEMIOLOGY & PATHOPHYSIOLOGY

Urinary tract infection can be a serious and potentially life-threatening problem in neonates and must be considered in any neonate presenting with a fever. The infection can be present in the urinary bladder or the kidney itself. The overall prevalence of a febrile infant having a UTI is approximately 5%; however, the prevalence of UTI in the neonatal population is most likely higher.[4] Congenital abnormalities including vesicoureteral reflux and posterior urethral valves place the affected infant at increased risk for infection.

CLINICAL PRESENTATION

Clinically, the neonate with a UTI can present with a variety of symptoms and severity. Some neonates may appear quite well with minimal symptoms such as vomiting and poor feeding while others can appear septic with high fevers.

DIAGNOSTIC TESTING

A thorough history and physical examination should be performed along with a urinalysis, urine Gram stain, and urine culture if a UTI is suspected. It is important to obtain a sterile specimen by catheterization to avoid skin contamination commonly seen when bagged specimens are collected. The gold standard for diagnosis is the urine culture; however, most culture results will not be available for at least 24 hours. As such, the diagnosis is based upon the urinalysis and/or Gram stain. A white blood cell count in the urine of 5 or greater per high power field would be consistent with a UTI. However, given the age of the patient, any abnormality on the urinalysis indicating infection, such as a positive nitrite or leukocyte esterase, should be given strong weight and prompt treatment. Also, bacteremia from the UTI can be a problem for patients in this age range. In a study looking at the utility of blood cultures in febrile children with UTIs, Pitetti and Choi found that the prevalence of bacteremia was 22.7% in children younger than 2 months in this setting.[6] Given this fact, a complete blood count and blood cultures and lumbar puncture should be obtained in febrile neonates who may have UTIs.

MANAGEMENT

Initial treatment of UTI in neonates involves broad-spectrum antibiotics, usually ampicillin and cefotaxime or gentamycin. Admission is required until the 48-hour culture results return. A renal ultrasound is usually indicated and a VCUG should be obtained once the infection has resolved. *E. coli* is the most common pathogen responsible for UTI in the neonate.

▶ SCROTAL ABNORMALITIES

UNDESCENDED TESTES

Epidemiology & Pathophysiology

Scrotal abnormalities encompass a wide variety of conditions that include abnormalities of the scrotum itself as well as abnormalities involving the scrotal contents. In many of these conditions, the primary cause of the observed defects is due to an abnormality in the descent of the testes to their intrascrotal location.

The testes originate in the retroperitoneal area and, during gestation, descend to the level of the internal inguinal ring. They do not complete their descent until shortly before or soon after birth. If an abnormality develops where both or one of the testes does not complete its descent, it is referred to as an undescended testis.

Clinical Presentation

An undescended testis is a common disorder with an incidence that is approximately 30% in premature boys compared to 3% in term boys.[4] If the testis is going to descend on its own, it usually does so by about 3 months of age. If there is no descent by 6 months of age, the testis likely will not complete its descent. Bilateral cryptorchidism occurs in about 10% to 20% of patients.[7] Undescended testes are usually located in the inguinal canal though they can be ectopic in location as well, including intra-abdominal locations. In 15% of patients, the missing testis will be nonpalpable and in those, only 50% will actually have a testis present.[7] If both testes are nonpalpable, strong consideration should be given to the diagnosis of a virilized female with congenital adrenal hyperplasia.

Problems associated with this condition include infertility, malignancy, hernia, torsion of the undescended testis, and psychological issues later in life. Fertility is often a significant concern of parents and it is important to note that 85% of boys with a unilateral undescended testis are fertile and that 50% to 65% of boys with bilateral undescended testes are fertile after repair.[7]

Diagnosis

This diagnosis is made after a thorough physical examination. If the testis is palpated in the inguinal canal of the neonate and cannot be milked down into the scrotum, the parents should be reassured and the patient monitored by the pediatrician for descent of the testis. If no testis can be palpated, the patient should undergo an abdominal ultrasound to look for the undescended testis.. This does not need to be done on an emergent basis but should be discussed with the parents; the patient should be referred to a pediatric urologist for further evaluation and management.

Management

Treatment is accomplished through orchiopexy at age 9 to 15 months. If the testis is not found on ultrasound, laparoscopy is usually performed due to the risk of malignancy developing in an undescended testis.

ENLARGED SCROTUM & SCROTAL SWELLING

Scrotal swelling is a common complaint in many neonates presenting to the ED. There are a variety of conditions that can be the cause of scrotal swelling. It is important on history to note if the swelling is acute or chronic and whether it is painful or painless.

Diagnosis & Management

Hydrocele is one of the most common causes of scrotal swelling in the neonate. It occurs in approximately 1% to 2% of males.[7] The hydrocele may communicate with the abdominal cavity or may be noncommunicating. Communicating hydroceles will typically be small in the morning and will enlarge by the evening. They will disappear with compression on physical examination. Noncommunicating hydroceles will not vary in size. They are typically smooth and not tender on physical examination. Most noncommunicating hydroceles will disappear by age 1 year. If they do not or are large they will require surgical intervention, usually after 2 years of age.[8]

Neonatal testicular tumors are rare. Typically, a mass can be palpated off the testicle or the testicle itself may be enlarged. Most of these tumors will not transilluminate as they are solid masses. Gonadal stromal tumors are the most common; yolk sac tumors and mature teratomas are next most common.[4] If a mass is palpated, an ultrasound should be obtained to delineate the mass. Tumor markers such as alpha-fetoprotein and beta-human chorionic gonadotropin along with screening labs such as a complete blood count, comprehensive metabolic profile, and urinalysis should be obtained. Finally, immediate urologic consultation in conjunction with pediatric oncology consultation should be obtained to determine the need for surgical intervention.

Neonatal or extravaginal torsion may present as acute scrotal swelling in early life. Testicular torsion presents as the acute unilateral swelling of the scrotum usually with an ipsilateral swollen, and possibly tender scrotum. The scrotum itself may be red and inflamed. Typically, the mass does not transilluminate. When diagnosing this condition, a urinalysis should be obtained as well as an ultrasound to examine the mass and blood flow to the testicle. Urologic consultation should be obtained although salvage of the testicle is unlikely as often, the testicle has undergone torsion during its descent from the abdominal cavity in utero. Surgery for this condition is usually performed for fixation of the contralateral testicle.

Scrotal hematoma is another neonatal condition that may present as acute scrotal swelling with a scrotal mass. This lesion can present secondary to a tumor or torsion. Typically, this mass will be solid and will not transilluminate. Similar to torsion, an ultrasound to determine if the testicle is intact and urinalysis should be obtained, in addition to a coagulation profile and complete blood count. If a tumor is suspected or found, tumor markers should be obtained as well. Immediate urologic consultation should be obtained as well.

Inguinal hernias can present as a scrotal mass in the neonatal period. Typically, parents will notice a bulge in the inguinal canal or scrotum that may or may not remit. This is usually the inciting event for presentation to the ED. If the hernia is incarcerated, feeding issues may be present along with vomiting. On physical examination, a palpable bulge may be felt in the scrotum extending up to and into the inguinal canal. The scrotum may be swollen and inflamed. The mass may or may not transilluminate. If the mass is compressible, reduction can be attempted with traction and gentle but firm pressure trying to push the hernia through the inguinal ring. If it is reducible, surgery should be consulted for possible surgical correction. If vomiting has been present, a basic metabolic profile along with fingerstick blood sugar should be obtained early on. If the hernia is not reducible, an ultrasound should be obtained along with immediate surgical consultation because most likely the hernia is incarcerated and will require surgical intervention.

► AMBIGUOUS GENITALIA

CLINICAL PRESENTATION

Most patients with ambiguous genitalia have been thoroughly evaluated prior to any presentation to the ED. However, surgical therapy for these patients may not be performed until later in life. For this reason, emergency medicine physicians must be familiar with these patients and their comorbid conditions.

The most common physical examination findings in these patients include clitoral enlargement with palpable labial/scrotal masses or microphallus with varying degrees of hypospadias and clitoromegaly with labial fusion.

DIAGNOSIS & MANAGEMENT

Salt wasting may be a comorbid condition when the cause of ambiguous genitalia is 21-hydroxylase deficiency. In the most severe cases, these patients have a deficiency of both aldosterone and cortisol ultimately leading to an adrenal crisis. Unless patients are diagnosed prenatally or soon after birth and treatment is initiated, they will present in crisis, appearing septic, at about 2 weeks of age. Signs and symptoms typically include weight loss, anorexia, vomiting, dehydration, weakness, hypotension, hypoglycemia, hyponatremia, and hypokalemia. An appropriate history should be obtained with careful attention to fever, vomiting, diarrhea, and urine output. A careful physical examination should be performed as well. Appropriate laboratory evaluation includes a full septic workup with a basic metabolic profile and fingerstick blood sugar. Treatment in the ED involves IV fluids, antibiotics, and corticosteroids.

Inguinal hernia is also associated with ambiguous genitalia. Diagnosis and treatment is identical to that discussed earlier.

► GYNECOLOGIC ABNORMALITIES

Gynecologic abnormalities in the neonate are relatively uncommon but emergency medicine physicians should be familiar with the most common conditions that could present to the ED.

MASTITIS

Clinical Presentation

Mastitis typically presents as an inflamed, tender, and swollen breast bud. Due to maternal estrogen, often the breasts of a neonate (male or female) may be swollen and draining so-called "witch's milk." Breast bud tissue may be palpable. To distinguish this normal condition from mastitis, in mastitis the nipple and surrounding tissue will be red, swollen, and tender. Often, discharge of purulent material from the nipple may be present. Staphylococcal and streptococcal bacteria are common causes. Fever may be present as well.

Diagnostic Testing

Diagnosis is based upon the clinical presentation; however, given the likelihood of a bacterial cause and the age of the patient, a full septic workup should be performed including urinalysis, urine Gram stain, urine culture, complete blood count and differential, blood culture, and lumbar puncture.

Management

Treatment should be initiated with broad-spectrum antibiotics such as ampicillin and cefotaxime or gentamycin once blood cultures have been obtained. If drainage is present, it should be cultured as well and if there is any concern for an abscess, immediate surgical consultation should be obtained.

IMPERFORATE HYMEN

Clinical Presentation

Imperforate hymen is another condition that may present in a neonate. Typically, the female neonate will present with a vaginal and possibly a palpable suprapubic mass. Depending upon the size and time course, obstructive symptoms may be present due to hydronephrosis and renal failure. On physical examination, a large vaginal mass that is grayish-white to blue in color is typically present. The urethral meatus should appear normal.

Diagnostic Testing

An ultrasound should be obtained as it can determine if the vagina is fluid-filled or if there is a solid mass present. If urinary obstruction is being considered, a renal ultrasound should be obtained as well. Immediate urologic consultation should be obtained, plus

a urinalysis, urine Gram stain, urine culture, and basic metabolic profile to assess renal function.

GYNECOLOGIC MASSES

Gynecologic masses are exceedingly rare in the neonatal population. Typically, these present as vaginal masses that protrude out between the labia. A Gartner duct cyst is one of the most likely masses to be encountered. This typically presents as a smooth, translucent mass protruding out of the vaginal introitus. The urethral meatus is usually normal. These masses often drain spontaneously, though some might require surgical intervention.[8]

The other mass most likely to be encountered in the neonatal female patient is sarcoma botryoides, which is a rhabdomyosarcoma of the vagina. This mass resembles a "cluster of grapes" protruding from the vaginal introitus. Similar to the Gartner duct cyst, the urethral meatus is usually normal. Basic screening labs should be obtained on any patient with a vaginal mass and urologic or gynecologic consultation should be obtained immediately.

REFERENCES

1. Elder JS. Congenital anomalies and dysgenesis of the kidneys. In: Kliegman RM, et al., eds. *Nelson Textbook of Pediatrics*. 18th ed. Philadelphia, PA: Saunders Elsevier; 2007:2221-2223.
2. Elder JS. Vesicoureteral reflux. In: Kliegman RM, et al., eds. *Nelson Textbook of Pediatrics*. 18th ed. Philadelphia, PA: Saunders Elsevier; 2007:2228-2234.
3. Elder JS. Obstruction of the urinary tract. In: Kliegman RM, et al., eds. *Nelson Textbook of Pediatrics*. 18th ed. Philadelphia, PA: Saunders Elsevier; 2007: 2234-2243.
4. Mesrobian HO, Balcom AH, Durkee CT. Urologic problems of the neonate. *Pediatr Clin North Am.* 2004;(51):1051-1062.

5. Elder JS. Anomalies of the penis and urethra. In: Kliegman RM, et al., eds. *Nelson Textbook of Pediatrics.* 18th ed. Philadelphia, PA: Saunders Elsevier; 2007:2253-2260.

6. Pitetti RD, et al. Utility of blood cultures in febrile children with UTI. *Am J Emerg Med.* 2002;(20):271-274.

7. Elder JS. Disorders and anomalies of the scrotal contents. In: Kliegman RM, et al., eds. *Nelson Textbook of Pediatrics.* 18th ed. Philadelphia, PA: Saunders Elsevier; 2007:2260-2265.

8. Leslie JA, Cain MP. Pediatric urologic emergencies and urgencies. *Pediatr Clin North Am.* 2006;(53):513-527.

CHAPTER 7

Orthopedic Emergencies in the Neonate

P. David Sadowitz, MD

Lisa Keough, MD

Norma Cooney, MD

Despite improvements in obstetrical care, birth injuries represent a significant cause of neonatal morbidity. Many of these entities may not be readily apparent at birth and thus are "discovered" during visits to the primary care physician and emergency medicine physician. This chapter reviews and summarizes these entities. Congenital orthopedic problems, the neonatal septic hip and osteomyelitis, and nonaccidental trauma (NAT) will also be discussed.

► NONACCIDENTAL TRAUMA

Unrecognized fractures, intracranial bleeding, and internal organ injury are entities to consider in the irritable or crying infant. It is imperative to get a complete history including the time of the injury if known and the mechanism of reported injury. In addition, it is important to document the reliability of the historian, ie, is the history believable and is the person telling the story consistent in the details. Fractures represent the second most common presentation of NAT. Eighty percent of fractures occurring in infants less than 1 year of age have been attributed to abuse.[1] The entire body should be carefully examined and palpated looking for deformities, crepitus, tenderness, and decreased range of motion. If a fracture is suspected then radiologic images should be obtained and, in most cases, an infant skeletal survey if there is any suspicion of NAT. Fractures with a high specificity for NAT include fractures present in the absence of trauma, metaphyseal fractures, midshaft extremity fractures, posterior rib fractures, spinous process fractures, and sternal fractures.[2,3] A CBC with differential and platelet count, PT-PTT-TT, bone scan, dilated retinal examination, and CT-MRI of the brain should be obtained as a part of the workup if NAT is suspected. Social work and child protective services should be consulted in the setting of suspected NAT.

▶ FRACTURES

CLAVICLE FRACTURE

Pathophysiology & Epidemiology

The most common neonatal fracture is a fractured clavicle that occurs during the birthing process and is present in 1% to 3% of newborns.[4,5] This is particularly the case during difficult delivery of the shoulder in vertex presentations and the extended arms in breech presentations.

Clinical Presentation

The majority of fractures are found shortly after birth during the newborn's examination. However, 40% of fractures are not discovered until the infant is home.[6] Parents may notice that the infant is not moving one arm or a deformity or tenderness in the clavicle area.

Diagnosis

The clinician can usually diagnose a clavicle fracture clinically or with radiologic imaging (Figure 7–1).

During the clinical examination the clinician may notice a deformity in the clavicle area with crepitus and/or pain to palpation. In addition, an absent Moro reflex may be observed on the affected side.

Management

Most clavicle fractures have an excellent prognosis and will heal without treatment.[4] If the infant appears to be uncomfortable, the affected arm may be immobilized against the abdomen to help decrease movement and thus decrease pain. Acetaminophen may also be used to decrease the infant's discomfort.

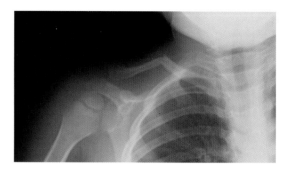

Figure 7–1. Clavicular fracture.

LONG BONE FACTURES

Pathophysiology & Epidemiology

Long bone fractures represent an uncommon birth injury. Humeral fractures occur in 0.05 of 1000 live births and femoral fractures are found in 0.13 of 1000.[7,8] Low birth weight, breech presentation, and caesarian section are the most common settings for these injuries.[9]

Clinical Presentation

The initial clinical presentations include decreased movement and swelling of the affected extremity, pain with movement of the extremity, and crepitance at the fracture site. On occasion, these fractures are not detected on the initial physical examination.

Diagnosis

The diagnosis of an extremity fracture is confirmed by radiographic studies. Ultrasound examination may be useful for the diagnosis of fractures occurring at the epiphyseal region, as this portion of the bone is not ossified at birth.[10]

Management

Splinting and immobilization are the most common treatment options. Proximal femur fractures may require a Pavlik harness or spica cast. Long-term sequelae from long bone fractures are rarely seen.[8]

▶ BRACHIAL PLEXUS INJURIES

PATHOPHYSIOLOGY & EPIDEMIOLOGY

Brachial plexus injuries occur in 0.1% to 0.2% of live births.[11] The significant risk factors for this injury include fetal malpresentation, forceps delivery, shoulder dystocia, and macrosomia.[11] Brachial plexus injuries are characterized by decreased mobility of the affected extremity and are generally discovered shortly after birth but may not be discovered until after the child has been discharged from the hospital. Bilateral injuries are seen in 4% of cases. When parents discover this entity

at home they usually seek immediate evaluation to determine the cause.

Brachial plexus injuries are primarily caused by trauma during delivery and are the result of a stretching injury from lateral flexion of the head with slow prolonged traction or shoulder dystocia deliveries. There are 4 types of associated neuronal injury. Type 1 injuries are characterized by a temporary conduction block (neuropraxia). Type 2 injuries occur when the axon is severed but the surrounding neurologic elements are intact (axonotmesis). In type 3 injuries there is complete postganglionic nerve disruption (neurotmesis). Type 4 brachial plexus injury is characterized by an avulsion of the brachial plexus with complete preganglionic separation from the spinal cord (Figure 7–2).

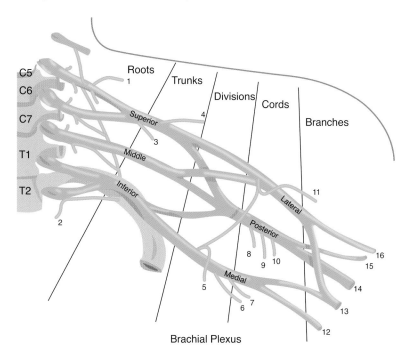

1) Dorsal scapular
2) Long Thoracic
3) To subclavius
4) Suprascapular
5) Medical pectoral
6) Medial cutaneous nerve of arm
7) Medial cutaneous nerve of forearm
8) Upper subscapular
9) Lower subscapular
10) Lateral pectoral
12) Ulnar
13) Median
14) Radial
15) Axillary
16) Musculocutaneous

Figure 7–2. Normal brachial plexus.

CLINICAL PRESENTATION

The child with a brachial plexus injury typically presents with a limp arm held against the trunk. Deep tendon reflexes may be absent. If there is involvement of the entire arm, a careful examination for Horner syndrome (ptosis, meiosis, anhydrosis) should be performed. Intrinsic hand weakness suggests a stellate ganglion injury. Any impairment of respiratory status should suggest the possibility of phrenic nerve injury. Erb palsy is the most common type of brachial plexus injury (90% of cases) in the neonatal period.[12] This injury involves the C5 and C6 nerve roots with resultant inability to abduct the shoulder, externally rotate the arm, and supinate the forearm. The arm hangs limply at the shoulder and is adducted and internally rotated, the elbow is extended and forearm pronated (waiter's tip position) (Figure 7–3).

The hand and wrist are spared and there is a normal grip. The bicep reflex is absent. The Moro reflex will be asymmetric. Rarely, the nerve fibers supplying the diaphragm are involved and there may be a paralysis of the diaphragm on the ipsilateral side. Klumpke paralysis (1% of brachial plexus injuries) involves C8-T1 nerves.[13] Affected infants will have weakness of the hand muscles and impaired flexion of the wrist and fingers. If the sympathetic fibers from T1 are involved, the infant may have an ipsilateral ptosis and meiosis (Horner syndrome). This type of neurologic injury is much less common than Erb palsy and more likely to result in permanent impairment. Ten percent of infants with brachial plexus injury have disruption of the entire plexus, producing a totally flaccid extremity with absent reflexes.

DIAGNOSIS

There are multiple studies that can be used to delineate the source and extent of injury.

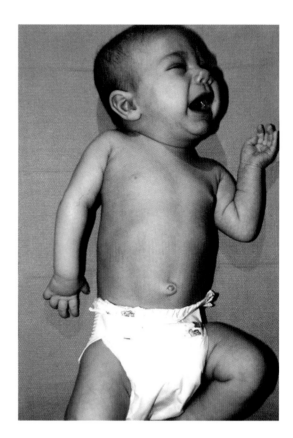

Figure 7–3. Erb palsy.

Initially shoulder films are obtained to rule out bony injury to the clavicle and shoulder. A chest x-ray is often obtained in any situation where phrenic nerve injury and hemidiaphragm paralysis is suspected. High resolution MRI of the cervical spine may delineate complete avulsion of the nerve root and is the best imaging study for diagnosing and evaluating nerve. The differential diagnosis of brachial plexus injury includes fractured clavicle, fractured humerus, congenital malformation, spinal cord lesions, and brain lesions.

MANAGEMENT

In general treatment consists of immobilizing the arm across the abdomen for the first week to decrease pain. After the first week it is best to start physical therapy that should involve passive range of motion at the shoulder, elbow, wrist, and hand. Ultimately, active range of motion and strengthening exercises are important to minimize bony deformities and contractures.[14] Surgical intervention remains controversial and there is a lack of consensus regarding to the timing of surgical intervention.[15] The majority of neonates with brachial plexus injuries will recover completely; however, 3% to 10% will have permanent impairment of arm and hand movement.[16,17] If no improvement is seen in the week 1 of life then complete recovery is unlikely. Rare causes of brachia plexus injury include neoplasms and hemangiomas that may cause compression injury to the brachial plexus.

▶ MUSCULAR TORTICOLLIS

PATHOPHYSIOLOGY & EPIDEMIOLOGY

Congenital muscular torticollis is characterized by a palpable mass or tightness in the sternomastoid muscle with the head tilted toward the abnormal sternocleidomastoid muscle and the chin rotated away from the abnormal muscle. This entity is present in 0.4% to 2% of live births.[18] The cause of this developmental abnormality remains unclear. Many investigators believe that intrauterine trauma occurs, causing muscle fiber tears in the sternomastoid muscle with formation of a hematoma and subsequent fibrosis in the muscle. A second theory is that fetal positioning may cause muscle inflammation and edema leading to compartment syndrome, muscle necrosis, and fibrosis. Histologic examination of the sternomastoid region reveals fibrosis and muscle atrophy. In support of these theories is the observation of an increased incidence of torticollis

in infants delivered with forceps or in breech deliveries.

CLINICAL PRESENTATION

There are 3 types of congenital torticollis described: postural torticollis (torticollis with no evidence of a muscle mass or tightness), muscular torticollis (muscle tightness with no mass), and sternomastoid tumor (mass present in the muscle). The diagnosis of torticollis is typically made between days 7 and 28 of age. The characteristic clinical presentation is a child with a palpable mass or tight sternomastoid muscle with the head tilted toward the lesion and the chin turned away from the lesion.[19] Children with congenital torticollis often have associated musculoskeletal abnormalities including hip dysplasia (7%), C1-C2 subluxation, metatarsus adductus, talipes equinovarus, and plagiocephaly.[19-21]

DIAGNOSIS

Cervical spine abnormalities involving the muscles, nerves, or bone can cause torticollis. Craniosynostosis occurring in unilateral fashion can lead to plagiocephaly and torticollis.[22,23] Klippel-Feil syndrome is a disorder characterized by congenital fusion of cervical vertebrae with associated torticollis. Additional abnormalities include Sprengel deformity (elevation of the scapula), scoliosis, congenital heart disease, renal anomalies, and deafness.[24] Pterygium colli is a congenital condition marked by a web of skin extending from the acromial process to the mastoid, limiting neck motion.[25] This entity is seen in Turner syndrome, Noonan syndrome and trisomy 18. Brachial plexus palsy is also associated with torticollis.

The diagnosis of congenital muscular torticollis is usually made on careful physical examination with palpation of a mass within the sternocleidomastoid muscle and the characteristic head tilt toward the abnormal muscle with the chin turned away from the lesion. Cervical spine films should be obtained to rule out congenital cervical spine abnormalities. Ultrasound has been used in some centers as a means to confirm the diagnosis.

MANAGEMENT

Congenital muscular torticollis may resolve spontaneously; however, in many cases significant craniofacial deformity will develop without treatment. The principle therapy for this lesion is frequent passive and active stretching of the abnormal muscle. All infants with a range of motion limited by 10 degrees or less had an excellent outcome with stretching of the abnormal sternomastoid muscle. More than 90% of infants with torticollis were effectively treated with manual stretching of the sternomastoid muscle if the initial passive motion was limited no more than 10 degrees. In contrast, infants at 6 months of age with persistent head tilt and a restriction of range of motion of 15% or greater will require surgery.[26,27] If the lesion remains uncorrected, the patient can develop plagiocephaly and permanent head tilt. Parents can enhance movement and stretching of the affected muscle by positioning the child to rotate the chin toward the affected muscle during feeding. Toys can be positioned so that the child must rotate the chin toward the affected muscle in order for the child to visualize the toy. Parents are taught to gently rotate the chin to touch the shoulder of the affected muscle and to tilt the head away from the affected muscle until the ear touches the shoulder of the unaffected side.

Surgical intervention may be required if there is significant limitation of motion, plagiocephaly, or facial asymmetry after 6 to 12 months of conservative therapy.[28]

► DEVELOPMENTAL HIP DYSPLASIA

The term developmental dysplasia of the hip (DDH) has replaced the term congenital hip dislocation to cover the spectrum of abnormalities that can occur in the development of the shape and position of the femoral head with respect to the acetabulum.[29,30] Specific entities are outlined in Table 7–1.

EPIDEMIOLOGY

Many infants have ligamentous laxity in conjunction with immature development of the acetabulum in the first few weeks of life that resolves over the first 1 to 2 months of life with no need for intervention.[31] True dislocation of the hip is present in 1% to 2% of live births, is 4 times more common in females, and may be bilateral in 20% of cases, but may not be detected on the

► **TABLE 7–1. DEVELOPMENTAL DYSPLASIA OF THE HIP: SPECIFIC ENTITIES**

Dislocation	The femoral head is completely outside the acetabulum
Subluxation	The femoral head is partially outside the acetabulum
Dislocatable	At rest the hip is within the acetabulum but can be dislocated during physical exam maneuvers
Subluxatable	The hip is within the acetabulum at rest and can be partially dislocated during physical exam maneuvers
Reducible	The hip is dislocated at reset but can be reduced with manipulation
Dysplasia	Abnormal developmental of the acetabulum or femoral head

initial newborn examination.[31-33] Hip dysplasia occurs more commonly in first-born infants and in breech presentations. The etiology of hip dysplasia is multifactorial and is believed to result from abnormal positioning in the uterus in conjunction with ligamentous laxity.[33,34] This entity is often seen in association with torticollis and metatarsus adductus (Figure 7–4).[35,36]

FACTORS

Conditions that limit fetal mobility pose an increased risk of DDH and include oligohydramnios, congenital abnormalities (torticollis, plagiocephaly), multiple gestations, and breech presentation. In breech presentations, 12% of female infants and 2.6% of male infants have DDH.[33]

PATHOPHYSIOLOGY

The etiology of hip dysplasia is multifactorial and is believed to result from a combination of ligamentous laxity and abnormal pressure on the developing femoral head.[34] The resultant pressure on the femoral head

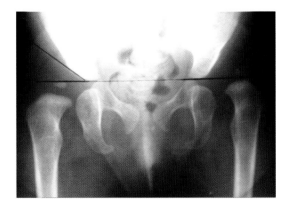

Figure 7–4. Developmental dysplasia of the hip.

directs the head out the acetabulum, preventing the normal growth and deepening of the acetabular socket and development of the labrum.

CLINICAL PRESENTATION & DIAGNOSIS

The diagnosis of DDH is made by careful physical examination, the Ortalani test, and the Barlow maneuver (Figure 7–5).

RISK

The Ortolani test demonstrates a click with abduction of the hip and medial pressure on he thigh in the supine infant. Barlow maneuver is performed by pushing the femur posteriorly with the hip flexed and the knee flexed 90 degrees. The test is positive if the hip dislocates. The Galeazzi sign may be present in the affected infant. The knee on the affected side will appear lower when the hips and knees are flexed at 90 degrees. The diagnosis is made by the classic physical examination findings. X-rays in the first few months of life may demonstrate abnormalities of the femoral head and acetabulum but cannot be used to establish the diagnosis in all cases of DDH. Ultrasound can be very useful in diagnosis and can aid in reduction of the true hip dislocation.

MANAGEMENT

Orthopedic consultation should be obtained. Generally a Pavlik harness is used to keep the femoral head positioned correctly. Open, surgical reduction is reserved for patients who do not respond to the above noted measure.

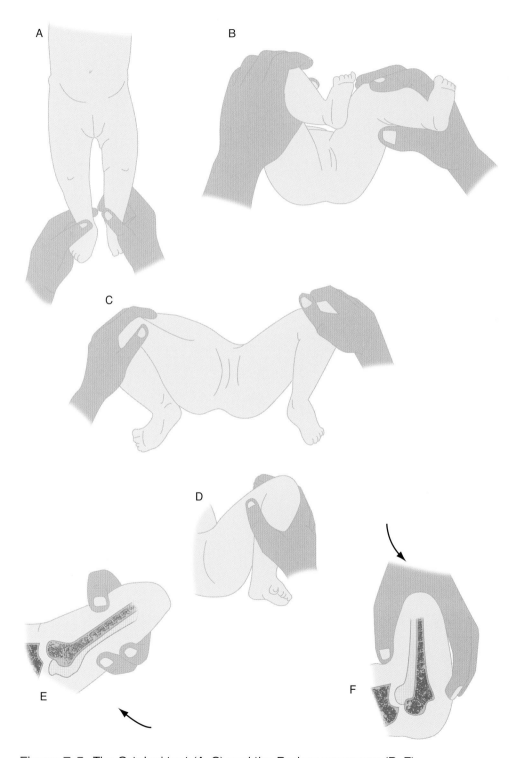

Figure 7–5. The Ortalani test (A–C) and the Barlow maneuver (D–F).

► SEPTIC ARTHRITIS AND OSTEOMYELITIS

EPIDEMIOLOGY & PATHOPHYSIOLOGY

Septic arthritis and osteomyelitis are uncommon diseases in the neonate. The failure to rapidly diagnose and treat these entities can lead to complete destruction of the articular cartilage, destruction of the growth plate, and dislocation of the affected joint causing permanent disability. In most cases there is no one precipitating event that causes septic arthritis. Septic arthritis and osteomyelitis have been reported following a variety of interventions in the neonate including heel punctures, umbilical artery catheterization, urinary catheterization, and femoral vein puncture.[37] Hematologic dissemination of a bacterial infection to the bone or joint represents the most common source of bacteria causing bone and joint infections in the neonate.

The pathogenesis of osteomyelitis differs in the neonate in comparison to the older child and adult. During the neonatal period there are blood vessels that cross the growth plate, linking vessels in the metaphysis to vessels in the epiphysis. The blood flow in these transphyseal vessels is sluggish at best and may predispose to sequestration of bacteria, which can then rapidly proliferate within the epiphysis and rupture into the joint space.[38] As the result of an immature immune system, neonates may present with multiple foci of infection (multifocal osteomyelitis) along with contiguous joint infection. The most common sites of septic arthritis in the neonate are the hip and shoulder, which may be secondary to their anatomic structure. The synovial membrane in the shoulder and hip inserts into the epiphysis, which is located within the joint allowing for a natural bridge for infection.[38]

MICROBIOLOGY

In a review of 92 cases, the pathogens included *Staphylococcus* species (62%), *Candida* species (17%), enteric gram-negative species (13%), and *Streptococcus* species and *Haemophilus influenzae* (4%).[39,40]

CLINICAL PRESENTATION

The initial presentation of the infant with septic arthritis or osteomyelitis may be a difficult challenge as the typical signs of infection such as fever, redness, or swelling may be absent. The initial findings may be fever and irritability that are common to many neonatal infections. A careful physical examination is needed to document pain or irritability on movement of the affected extremity or joint. There may be decreased movement of the affected arm or leg. A neonate with the classic presentation for a septic hip will maintain the affected leg with hip flexion and external rotation of the leg. Internal and external rotation may be limited. On examination, the hip will be in a position of flexion and external rotation. In addition, there may be localized redness and swelling over the affected area as well as tenderness to the sacroiliac joint. As noted earlier it is imperative to recall that erythema and swelling are late findings; the absence of these findings does not exclude the diagnosis of a septic joint. Given the often subtle findings on physical examination, a detailed history and physical examination in conjunction with appropriate laboratory studies and imaging are needed to make an accurate diagnosis of a septic joint.

DIAGNOSIS

Laboratory Studies

Laboratory studies that are useful to establish the diagnosis of osteomyelitis and septic joints include include a complete blood count, erythrocyte sedimentation rate (ESR), C-reactive protein, and aspiration of the affected bone or synovial fluid for analysis to include Gram stain, culture, cell count, and glucose. The peripheral white blood cell count in a neonate with a septic joint is typically >12,000/μL. The ESR is also usually greater than 40 mm/h and the C-reactive protein is also typically elevated. A minimal amount of synovial fluid is required for analysis—only a few drops are needed for Gram stain and culture. A WBC count in the synovial fluid >50,0000/μL (range 50,000-200,000/μL) with 75% neutrophils is very suggestive of septic arthritis.[41] The effusion in infected joints typically exhibits a low glucose. Appropriate cultures of the affected join or bone are crucial in appropriately treating septic arthritis and osteomyelitis especially in this era where the incidence of methicillin resistant staphylococcal infection is increased.

Radiographic Studies

Early diagnosis of septic arthritis is essential to avoid debilitating sequelae. Radiographic imaging early in course of the disease may show evidence of soft tissue swelling or joint capsular distension (widening of the joint space or even subluxation). Ultrasound examination of the affected joint is very useful in determining the presence and extent of joint effusion and in guiding the aspiration of fluid from the joint (Figure 7–6).

Skeletal scintigraphy using technetium-labeled isotopes (bone scan) is another modality of evaluation for osteomyelitis. The MRI represents the gold standard for skeletal and muscle imaging and to evaluate for the presence of fluid in the joint space (Figure 7–7).[42] However the MRI is limited by the need for sedation in order to obtain the scan.

MANAGEMENT

Once septic arthritis is suspected, immediate orthopedic consultation is required for surgical drainage and washout of the hip. Initiation of antibiotics in a timely manner is exceedingly important. It is ideal to obtain cultures of the joint aspirate prior to antibiotic therapy so that bacteria-specific antibiotics may be used based on culture results; however, if there is any delay in expected time to surgical drainage, kefzol 20 mg/kg IV q12 in the first 7 days of life, then 20 mg/kg IV q8h after day 7, zosyn 75 mg/kg IV q6h, or Cefotaxime 50 mg/kg/IV every 8 hours are acceptable antibiotic choices pending culture results. Vancomycin

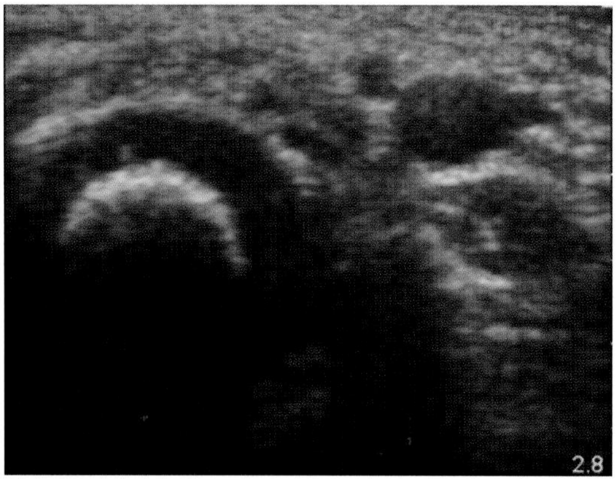

Figure 7–6. Joint effusion on ultrasound.

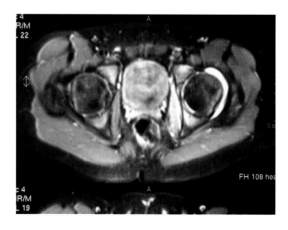

Figure 7–7. MRI demonstrating hip effusion.

15 mg/kg IV every 8 hours should be given if methicillin resistant staphylococcal infection is suspected.

COMPLICATIONS

There are many complications of septic arthritis. Specific to the hip, complications include aseptic necrosis of the femoral head. The injury to the femoral head can lead to failure of acetabular development and dislocation of the femoral head.

REFERENCES

1. Pierce MH, Bertocci G. Fractures resulting from inflicted trauma: assessing injury and history compatibility. *Clin Pediatr Emerg Med.* 2006;7:143.

2. Leventhal JM, Thomas SA, Rosenfield NS, et al. Distinguishing child abuse from unintentional injuries. *AMJ Dis Child.* 1993;147(1):87.

3. Kleinman PK. *Diagnostic Imaging of Child Abuse.* 2nd ed. St. Louis, MO: Mosby; 1998:9.

4. Hsu TY, Hung FC, Lu YJ, et al. Neonatal clavicle fracture: clinical analysis of incidence, predisposing factors, diagnosis and outcome. *Am J Perinatol.* 2002;19(1):17.

5. Many A, Brenner SH, Yaron Y, et al. Prospective study of incidence and predisposing factors for clavicle fracture in the newborn. *Acta Obstet Gynecol Scand.* 1996;75(4):378.

6. Joseph PR, Rosenfeld W. Clavicle fractures in neonates. *Am J Dis Child.* 1990;144(2):165.

7. Erkaya S, Tuncer RA, Kutlar I, et al. Outcome of 1040 consecutive breech deliveries: clinical experience of a maternity hospital in Turkey. *Int J Gynaecol.* 1997;59(2):115.

8. Morris S, Cassidy N, Stephens M, et al. Birth-associated femoral fractures: incidence and outcome. *J Pediatr Orthop.* 2002;22(1):22.

9. Nadas S, Gudenchet F, Capasso P, et al. Predisposing factors in obstetrical fractures. *Skeletal Radio.* 1993;22(3):195.

10. Fisher NA, Newman B, Lloyd J, Mimouni. Ultrasonographic evaluation of birth injury to the shoulder. *J Perinatol.* 1995;22(3):398.

11. Perlow JH, Wigton T, Hart J, et al. Birth trauma. A five year review of incidence and associated perinatal factors. *J Reprod Med.* 1996;41(10):754.

12. Eng GD, Binder H, Getson P, O'Donall R. Obstetrical brachial plexus injury (OBPI) outcome with conservative management. *Muscle Nerve.* 1996;19(7):884.

13. al-Qattan MM, Clarke HM, Curtis CG. Klumpke's birth palsy. Does it really exist? *J Hand Surg Br.* 1995;20(1):19.

14. Shenaq SM, Berzin E, Lee T, et al. Brachial plexus birth injuries and current management. *Clin Plast Surg.* 1998;25(4):527.

15. McNeely PD, Drake JM. A systematic review of brachial plexus surgery for birth-related brachial plexus injury. *Pediatr Neurosurg.* 2003;38(2):57.

16. Greenwald AG, Schute PC, Shiveley JL. Brachial plexus birth palsy: a 10 year report on the incidence and prognosis. *J Pediatr Orthop.* 1984;4(6):689.

17. Michelow BJ, Clarke HM, Curtis CG, et al. The natural history of brachial plexus palsy. *Plast Reconstr Surg.* 1995;93(4):675.

18. Cheng JC, Au AW. Infantile torticollis: a review of 624 cases. *J Pediatr Orthop.* 1994;14:802.

19. Tunnessen, WW. Torticollis. In: Tunnessen WW, Roberts KB, eds. *Signs and Symptoms in Pediatrics.* 3rd ed. Philadelphia: Lippincott, Williams, & Wilkins; 1999:353.

20. Hollier L, Kim J, Grayson BH, et al. Congenital muscular torticollis and the associated craniofacial changes. *Plast Reconstr Surg.* 2000;105:827.

21. Cheng JC, Kun A, Chen TM, et al. The clinical presentation and outcome of treatment of congenital muscular torticollis in infants—study of 1086 cases. *J Pediatr Surg.* 2000;35:1091.

22. Slate RK, Posnick JC, Armstrong DC, et al. Cervical spine subluxation associated with congenital muscular torticollis and craniofacial asymmetry. *Plast Reconstr Surg.* 1993;91:1187.

23. Raco A, Raimondi AJ, De Ponte FS, et al. Congenital torticollis in association with Craniosynostosis. *Childs Nerv Syst.* 1999;15:163.

24. Staheli LT. Spin and neck. In: Staheli LT, ed. *Fundamentals of Pediatric Orthopedics.* 2nd ed. Philadelphia: Lippincott Raven; 1998:73.

25. Green M. The neck. In: Green M, ed. *Pediatric Diagnosis: Interpretation of Symptoms and*

Signs in Children and Adolescents. 6th ed. Philadelphia: WB Saunders; 1998:63.

26. Cheng JC, Wong MW, Tang SP, et al. Clinical determinants of the outcome of manuel stretching in the treatment of congenital muscular torticollis in infants. A prospectice study of eight hundred and twenty-one cases. *J Bone Joint Surg Am.* 2001;83-A:679.

27. Emery C. The determinants of treatment duration for congenital muscular torticollis: results of conservative management with long-term followup in 85 cases. *Arch Phys Med Rehabil.* 1987;68:222.

28. Stassen LF, Kerawala CJ. New surgical technique for the correction of congenital muscular torticollis (wry neck). *Br J Oral Maxillofac Surg.* 2000;38:142.

29. American Academy of Orthopaedic Surgeons Advisory Statement. *"CDH" should be "DDH."* Park Ridge, IL: American Academy of Orthopaedic Surgeons; 1991.

30. Ilfield FW, Westin GW, Makin M. Missed or developmental dislocation of the hip. *Clin Orthop.* 1986;203:276.

31. von Rosen S. Diagnosis and treatment of congenital dislocation of the hip joint in the newborn. *J Bone Joint Surg Br.* 1962;44B:284.

32. BIalik V, Bialik GM, Blazer S, et al. Developmental dysplasia of the hip: a new approach to incidence. *Pediatrics.* 1999;103:93.

33. Clinical practice guideline: early detection of developmental dysplasia of the hip. Committee on Quality Improvement, Subcommittee on Developmental Dysplasia of the Hip. American Academy of Pediatrics. *Pediatrics.* 2000;105:896.

34. Massie WK, Howorth MB. Congenital dislocation of the hip. III. Pathogenesis. *J Bone Joint Surg Am.* 1951;33:190.

35. Tien YC, Su JY, Lin GT, et al. Ultrasonographic study of the coexistence of muscular torticollis and dysplasia of the hip. *J Pediatr Orthop.* 2001;21:343.

36. Kumar SJ, Macewen GD. The incidence of hip dysplasia with metatarsus adductus. *Clin Orthop.* 1982;2(3):234.

37. Knudson CJ, Hoffman EB. Neonatal osteomyelitis. *J Bone Joint Surg.* 1990;72(6):846.

38. Ogden JA. Pediatric osteomyelitis and septic arthritis: the pathology of neonatal disease. *Yale J Biol Med.* 1979;52:543.

39. Deshpande SS, Taral N, Modi N, Singrakhia M. Changing epidemiology of neonatal septic arthritis. *J Orthop Surg (Hong Kong).* 200412(1):10.

40. Dan M. Septic arthritis in young infants: clinical and microbiological correlation and therapeutic implications. *Rev Infect Dis.* 1984;6:147.

41. Swan A, Amer H, Dieppe P. The value of synovial fluid assays in the diagnosis of joint disease: a literature review. *Ann Rheum Dis.* 2002;61:493.

42. Morrison WB, Schweitzer ME, Bock GW, et al. Diagnosis of osteomyelitis: Utility of fat-suppressed-contrast-enchanced MR imaging. *Radiology.* 1993;189:251.

CHAPTER 8

Dermatologic Disorders in the First 30 Days of Life

James D'Agostino, MD

Skin lesions occurring in the neonatal period often prompt the parents to present the infant for evaluation. Thorough knowledge of neonatal skin physiology and benign vs pathologic conditions are parental expectations of professionals providing neonatal care. This chapter assists those professionals, providing an understanding of the common, benign, pathologic, worrisome, and rare dermatologic disorders that can present in the first 30 days of life.

▶ SKIN ANATOMY

Skin is divided into 3 layers: epidermis, dermis, and the subcutaneous tissue. The skin is thicker on the dorsal and extensor surfaces with the exception of the palms and soles. The thickness of the epidermis (stratified squamous epithelium) ranges from 0.05 mm on the eyelids to 1.5 mm on the palms and soles. The dermis (papillary outer layer and reticular lower layer) varies in thickness from 0.3 mm on the eyelids to 3.0 mm on the back.

The skin of the newborn differs from the adult skin in several ways. Although the epidermal thickness is similar, the newborn skin is less hairy, has less sweat and sebaceous gland secretions, has decreased collagen and elastic fibers in the dermis, a thinner dermis with fewer intercellular attachments, and fewer melanosomes. The preterm (less than 32 weeks of gestation) infant's epidermis and dermis are thinner and the differences detailed above are significantly magnified compared to a full-term newborn. The significance of these differences is that the newborn has increased transepidermal water loss, increased permeability to topical agents, and increased tendency for the skin to blister. With the decreased collagen and elastic fibers the newborn skin is less elastic. The newborn is less equipped to tolerate thermal stress or excess sunlight and is more likely to develop blisters or erosions in response to heat, chemical irritants, mechanical trauma, and inflammatory skin conditions.

▶ EXAMINATION

The newborn infant should have a thorough physical examination, including the skin, within 24 hours of birth to identify anomalies, birth injuries, jaundice, or cardiopulmonary disorders.[1] The normal newborn's skin varies from light to dark pink. A ruddy, plethoric neonate may have polycythemia. A polycythemic neonate may appear cyanotic despite normal oxygenation due to the high content of unsaturated hemoglobin. Pallor may indicate anemia in the neonate. The hands, feet, and perioral areas may reveal acrocyanosis, which is normal due to vasoconstriction. Dark, musky coloration of the tongue and mucous membranes, however, suggests cyanosis from hypoxemia.

The skin should be inspected for abnormalities that may suggest an underlying systemic disorder. Yellow appearance of the skin often suggests jaundice and is best seen in natural light. Jaundice that occurs within the first 24 hours of birth is always pathologic and requires an extensive investigation. Prolonged exposure to intrauterine meconium may cause the newborn skin to appear green. If there are grunting respirations, meconium aspiration is a possibility. Look for abnormal pigmentation, congenital nevi, macular vascular stains (particularly in the first branch of the trigeminal nerve or forehead region), hemangiomas, and other unusual lesions and document these in the patient's record.

BIRTHMARKS

Birthmarks or nevi are circumscribed malformations of the skin that may be predominantly epidermal, adnexal, melanocytic, or vascular, or a compound overgrowth of these tissues. Nevi can be divided into 3 groups: pigmented, vascular, and those resulting from abnormal development.

Pigmented Birthmarks

Congenital nevi (Figure 8–1) are present at birth and may vary from a few millimeters to several centimeters. They may contain hair and if so it is usually course. Most are flat at

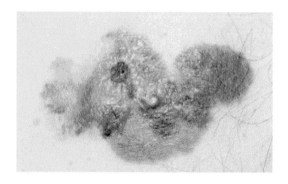

Figure 8–1. Congenital nevus. *Source: Wolff K, Johnson RA, Suurmond D. Fitzpatrick's Color Atlas and Synopsis of Clinical Dermatology,* 5th ed. New York, NY: McGraw-Hill; 2005.

birth but become thicker during childhood. Congenital melanocytic nevi occur in up to 0.2% to 2.1% of infants at birth.[2] The risk of developing melanoma in very large nevi is significant.[3] Congenital melanocytic nevi are thought to arise from disrupted migration of melanocyte precursors in the neural crest. Colors range from brown to black. Melanoma developed in 0.5% to 0.7% of patients with mostly large lesions.[2,4] The mean age at diagnosis for melanoma was 15.5 years.[2] Management of these lesions can be challenging for the family and physician. Large, thick lesions should be removed as soon as possible.[5] There is a great risk of melanoma in patients with nevi covering greater than 5% of body surface area.[5] The risk for malignant degeneration for smaller congenital nevi is unknown. A dermatologist should check all congenital nevi or moles. If the congenital nevus is not surgically removed, it should be examined on a regular basis. Unfortunately, nevi invariably change as the child grows, making evaluation challenging. Because of the possibility of malignant degeneration of congenital nevi, some experts recommend that all congenital nevi be considered for prophylactic excision.[6] Nevertheless, any nevus that changes color, shape, or thickness warrants further evaluation to rule out

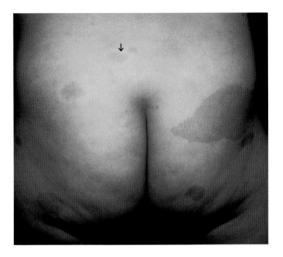

Figure 8–2. Café-au-lait spot. *Source:* From Wolff K, Goldsmith LA, Katz SI, et al. *Fitzpatrick's Dermatology in General Medicine*, 7th ed. New York, NY: McGraw-Hill; 2008.

melanoma. Patients should be followed regularly, even after the congenital melanocytic nevus has been removed, because of recurrence at the original site and because one-third of melanomas arise in different sites from the original nevus.[2,7]

Café-au-lait spots (Figure 8–2) are pale, brown macular lesions that may be present at birth and vary in size from 0.5 to 20 cm; they are estimated to be present in 10% to 20% of normal children and increase in number and size with age. Six or more spots greater than 1.5 cm in diameter are presumptive evidence for neurofibromatosis in children over age 5 years. Café-au-lait macules have smooth, regular borders, the shape of which has been compared to the coast of California and are present in 90% to 100% of patients with neurofibromatosis. Similar look-a-like lesions having irregular borders are seen in polyostotic fibrous dysplasia (Albright syndrome), the shape of which has been compared to the coast of Maine.[8]

Dermal melanosis or *"Mongolian spots"* (Figure 8–3) is another type of birthmark. These flat, bluish-gray or brown lesions arise

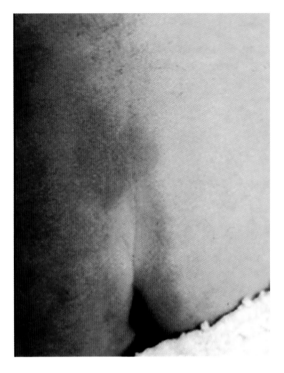

Figure 8–3. Mongolian spot.

when the melanocytes are trapped deep in the skin. These lesions most commonly arise on the lower back and buttocks. They are easily mistaken for bruises. These lesions should be well documented on the patient's record because their appearance at later visits in some settings may raise the suspicion of child abuse. These lesions are more common in African American, Native American, Asian, and Hispanic populations.[9] Most lesions fade by 2 years of life and do not need treatment.[10]

Vascular Birthmarks

Congenital vascular lesions are easily grouped into 2 major categories: hemangiomas and vascular malformations. Hemangiomas, a collection of dilated arterial vessels in the dermis surrounded by masses of proliferating endothelial cells, are present at birth 40% of the time and the remainder appear during the first year of life. This is in contrast to vascular malformations, 99% of which are present at birth. Hemangiomas occur in 1.1% to 2.6% of newborns[11] and are present in 10% of infants by the age of 1 year.

Hemangiomas

At birth hemangiomas may be unapparent or marked by a pale patch of skin. Congenital and infantile hemangiomas are referred to as strawberry hemangiomas. The lesions begin as nodular masses or flat, telangiectatic macules that may be mistaken for bruises. Look-a-like lesions are other forms of nodules (ie, melanoma). Perform the "pressure test" on the suspected nodule: After pressing firmly on the nodule for 30 sec, near total involution is characteristic of hemangiomas. The proliferating endothelial cells are responsible for the unique growth characteristics of hemangiomas as the lesions age. The strawberry hemangiomas, therefore, grow rapidly in the first few months of life. They are bright red lesions with well-defined borders forming nodular, protuberant, and compressible masses. Fifty percent resolve by 5 years of age, 70% by 7 years of age, and 90% by 10 years of age.[12,13] Regression of the lesions is followed by normal-appearing skin in 70% of patients or by atrophy, scarring, telangiectasia, pigmentation changes, and deformity.

Lesions that are small with an indolent growth pattern should be left untouched to involute spontaneously. There is a potential for bleeding or ulceration, which can be managed with cool, wet compresses. Hemangiomas that compress the eye (Figure 8–4A & B), auditory canal, airway (particularly found in the subglottic area), or vital organs require immediate referral. Although uncommon, brain imaging studies are recommended on all asymptomatic infants with large facial hemangiomas to assess for the presence of hydrocephalus and fourth ventricle anomalies. Multiple cutaneous hemangiomas should alert physicians to the possibility of hemangiomas in the liver, gastrointestinal tract, and subglottic area; the former 2 could cause obstruction or bleeding

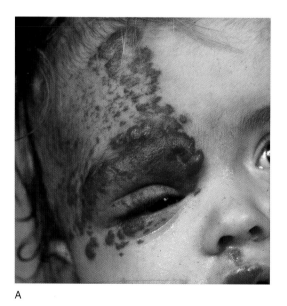

A

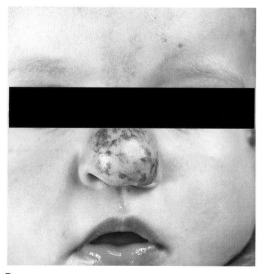

B

Figure 8–4A & B. Hemangioma. *Source:* Wolff K, Johnson RA, Suurmond D. *Fitzpatrick's Color Atlas and Synopsis of Clinical Dermatology*, 5th ed. New York, NY: McGraw-Hill; 2005.

and the latter eventual upper airway stridor with growth or upper airway infection as in croup. Management of these lesions have been successful using prednisone 3 mg/kg daily for 6 to 12 weeks[14] or 2 to 4 mg/kg/day given in divided doses twice a day.[15] Periorbital hemangiomas have been associated with strabismus and amblyopia. Ophthalmologists frequently use intralesional steroids when these lesions do not respond to oral steroids.

Cavernous hemangiomas (Figure 8–5) are collections of dilated arterial vessels deep in the dermis and subcutaneous tissue and are present at birth. They appear as large, pale masses that are skin-, red-, or blue-colored, ill-defined, and rounded. Like their strawberry counterparts, they grow rapidly at first followed by an involution phase. They can limit the range of motion of a limb if present near or over a joint. Orthopedic referral is advised. Otherwise, cavernous hemangiomas are treated in a similar manner as strawberry hemangiomas. Giant hemangiomas can consume large quantities of platelets and clotting factors. A variant of disseminated intravascular coagulation (DIC) can

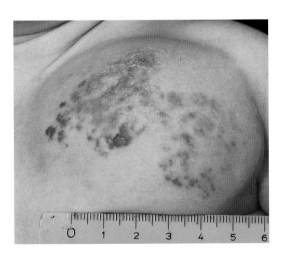

Figure 8–5. Cavernous hemangioma. *Source:* Wolff K, Johnson RA, Suurmond D. *Fitzpatrick's Color Atlas and Synopsis of Clinical Dermatology*, 5th ed. New York, NY: McGraw-Hill; 2005.

occur known as Kasabach-Merritt syndrome. It is not exactly known why DIC occurs. The static blood in the venous sinusoids may encourage an environment for platelets and clotting factors to be activated by contact with abnormal endothelium. Thrombocytopenia, microangiopathic hemolytic anemia, and an acute or chronic consumptive coagulopathy may be seen in association with an enlarging hemangiomas.[16] Kasabach-Merritt syndrome occurs most often in infants during the first few weeks of life. The majority of lesions is huge and occurs on the limbs or trunk. Prednisone 2 to 4 mg/kg/day is indicated when the hemangiomas rapidly enlarge and the platelet count drops.

Vascular Malformations

Congenital vascular malformations are poorly circumscribed lesions present at birth 99% of the time. Unlike hemangiomas that have a rapid neonatal growth with slow involution. Vascular malformations have no change in size and grow only in proportion to the growth of the child. There is no involution stage. Vascular malformations are predominantly venous, but any combination of capillary, arterial, and lymphatic components can occur.

Nevus flammeus or *port-wine stains* (Figure 8–6) are vascular malformations that occur in up to 0.3% of newborns.[9] At birth these lesions are flat, usually unilateral, irregular, dark, red to purple in color which does not fade. With time the lesions become papular and simulate a cobblestone surface. They may be a few millimeters in size or cover an entire limb. They may develop varicosities, nodules, or granulomas and do not require treatment. The entire depth of the dermis contains numerous dilated capillaries. These lesions tend to darken with age and present a significant cosmetic concern since they frequently occur on the face. Pulsed dye laser therapy can be used to lighten lesions. Optimal timing of treatment is before 1 year of age and 5 sessions of pulsed dye laser therapy reduces lesion size by 63%.[17]

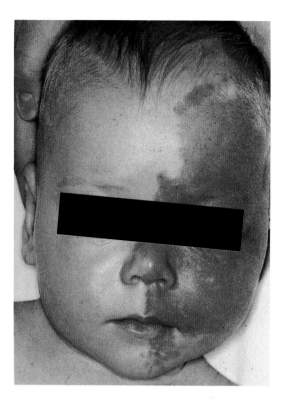

Figure 8–6. Port-wine stain.

Port-wine stains involving the first branch of the trigeminal nerve (forehead) are associated with ipsilateral glaucoma. Therefore, infants with port-wine stains near the eye should be referred to an ophthalmologist for glaucoma testing.[18] Port-wine stains of the eyelids, bilateral distribution of the birthmark, and unilateral lesions involving all 3 branches of the trigeminal nerve are associated with a significant likelihood of having eye and CNS complications known as Sturge-Weber syndrome. Patients with this syndrome are at increased risk for mental retardation and hemiplegia.[19] The classic triad of glaucoma, seizures and port-wine stains is associated with angiomas of the brain and meninges, and these patients therefore should be studied for glaucoma and CNS lesions.[20]

Nevus simplex or *salmon patches* (Figure 8–7) are vascular birthmarks that occur in

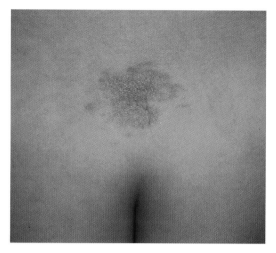

Figure 8–7. Salmon patch. *Source:* From Knoop KJ, Stack LB, Storrow MD. *Atlas of Emergency Medicine*, 2nd ed. New York, NY: McGraw-Hill; 2002.

33% to 70% of newborns.[9] They are variants of nevus flammeus that are flat, salmon-colored, irregular macular patches caused by telangiectasias or dilation of dermal capillaries. They are most common on the nape of the neck where the lesion is referred to as a "stork bite." Unlike the port-wine stains, salmon patches on the face commonly occur bilaterally in a symmetric pattern. Patches that occur on the glabella and upper eyelids are at times mistaken for birth trauma or forceps clamp marks; 40% resolve in the neonatal period while most resolve by 18 months of age. Patches on the nape of the neck may persist for life. Salmon patches are benign lesions of no clinical significance.[9]

Supernumerary nipples or *extra mammary glands* that arise during embryogenesis may be unilateral or bilateral. They may include an areola, nipple, or both and because of their pigmentation, they are occasionally mistaken for congenital melanocytic nevi. In children presenting for routine well-child care, 5.6% exhibited 1 or more supernumerary nipple. These lesions are considered benign, although there is conflicting evidence suggesting an association with renal or urogenital anomalies.[21] There is insufficient evidence to warrant imaging studies or removal of the lesions in the absence of clinical concern.

Midline lumbosacral skin lesions, such as lipomas, dimples, dermal sinuses, tails, hemangiomas, and hypertrichosis (growth of hair in excess of normal), are potential cutaneous markers for occult spinal dysraphism (incomplete fusion of the midline elements of the spine).[22] A review of 200 patients with occult spinal dysraphism found that 102 had a cutaneous sign.[23] Patients with high risk (any one of dermal sinus, lipomas, or tail) or intermediate risk (any one of aplasia cutis congenita, atypical dimple, or deviation of the gluteal furrow) lumbosacral lesions should undergo imaging studies (MRI, ultrasonography) as should those with 2 or more lesions of any type, which is the strongest predicter for occult spinal dysraphism.[24] A tethered cord is a potential consequence of occult spinal dysraphism and failure to detect and surgically release a tethered cord can lead to excessive traction on the cord and neurologic compromise.[22] Those at low risk for occult spinal dysraphism (any one of hemangioma, hypertrichosis, Mongolian spot, nevus simplex, port-wine stain, and simple dimple) require no evaluation in most cases.[24]

Transient Vascular Phenomenon

In the first 4 weeks of life, a newborn's immature skin vascular physiology may result in several transient vascular conditions that concern parents or mimic other more serious conditions. Acrocyanosis, cutis marmorata, and harlequin color change are three transient vascular conditions that result from vascular changes to a decrease in the ambient temperature. Acrocyanosis of the hands and feet is a common occurrence in the neonate. The exaggerated vasoconstriction that occurs in these areas to cold stress causes the skin

to appear cyanotic without edema or skin lesions. The condition resolves with warming of the hands and feet. The dark, musky coloration of the tongue and mucous membranes, however, suggest central cyanosis from hypoxemia, which occurs in association with pulmonary or cardiac disease. Rewarming of the infant will not affect the color of central cyanosis. Acrocyanosis usually resolves in 2 to 4 weeks of life.

Cutis marmorata (Figure 8–8) is a reticulated mottling of the skin that occurs in a symmetrical pattern over the trunk and extremities. The reticulated pattern is red to cyanotic in color giving the skin a marbled (veined or mottling) appearance. Like acrocyanosis, rewarming of the infant's skin resolves the combination of vascular constriction and dilatation brought on by cold stress. No treatment is required. Physicians may confuse this condition with the mottling of dehydration or septic conditions. Hypothermia or hyperthermia of the neonate, with or without skin manifestations, is a serious concern and requires

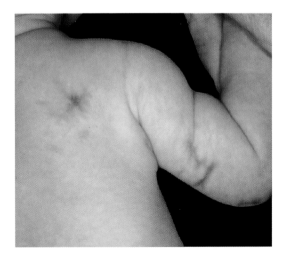

Figure 8–8. Cutis marmarata. *Source:* From Wolff K, Goldsmith LA, Katz SI, et al. *Fitzpatrick's Dermatology in General Medicine*, 7th ed. New York, NY: McGraw-Hill; 2008.

immediate investigation. Cutis marmorata is a transient condition that usually resolves within 4 weeks of life. Mottling may persist for several weeks or months, or sometimes into early childhood.[25] Conditions that persist beyond 6 months of age may be a sign of hypothyroidism, trisomy 18, Down syndrome, Cornelia de Lange syndrome, or other causes of CNS-induced neurovascular dysfunction. A look-a-like mottling condition is cutis marmorata telangiectatica congenita. The mottling persists in localized patches on the trunk or extremities. Rewarming does not resolve the condition, which may be associated with reticulated cutaneous atrophy or musculoskeletal or vascular abnormalities.[26] Another look-a-like condition is livedo reticularis seen with collagen vascular diseases such as neonatal lupus erythematosus. As in cutis marmorata telangiectatica congenita, this condition does not resolve with rewarming.

Harlequin color change (Figure 8–9) is an interesting vascular flushing of the neonate's skin when the infant is placed horizontally. The dependent portions of the neonate, particularly premature infants, become flushed red with blood leaving the nondependent areas pale. The condition usually occurs suddenly, persists for 30 sec to 20 min, and resolves with increased muscle activity, crying, or returning the infant to a supine position. This phenomenon occurs in up to 10% of full-term infants and often goes unnoticed due to infant bundling. The condition commonly occurs during the first week of life and recurs up to 3 to 4 weeks of age. This condition is not associated with serious underlying disease and although the underlying cause is not exactly known, some have suggested that it is caused by immaturity of the hypothalamic center that controls the dilation of peripheral blood vessels.[27]

Transient Skin Eruptions of the Neonate

Skin disorders in this category are erythema toxicum neonatorum, transient neonatal pustular melanosis, acne neonatorum, milia, miliaria, and seborrheic dermatitis. These benign, innocent pustular eruptions must be differentiated from potentially serious infectious dermatoses. Erythema toxicum neonatorum (Figure 8–10) is the most common pustular eruption in newborns. It is estimated to occur in 40% to 70% of newborns,[28] particularly in term infants weighing more than 2500 grams (5.5 lb).[29] This condition may present at birth but most commonly presents on the day 2 or 3 of life; it has been reported to have an onset up to 2 to 3 weeks of age. The lesions typically begin as erythematous, 2- to 3-mm macules and papules that eventually evolve into pustules[30] within several hours. A large, blotchy erythematous base giving the infant a "flea bitten" appearance surrounds each pustule. Lesions commonly occur on the face, trunk, and proximal extremities. The palms and soles are not involved. The lesions typically fade away in 5 to 7 days and recurrences may occur for several weeks. In healthy infants the diagnosis of erythema toxicum neonatorum is made clinically. If done, a Gram or Wright stain of a pustule reveals sheets of eosinophils and occasional neutrophils. Peripheral eosinophilia may also be present.[31] Infants who appear ill or have atypical rashes should be

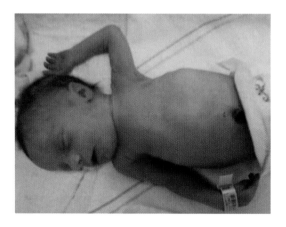

Figure 8–9. Harlequin infant.

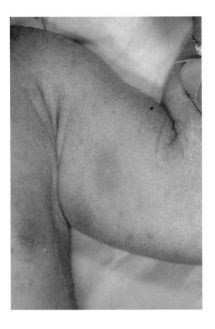

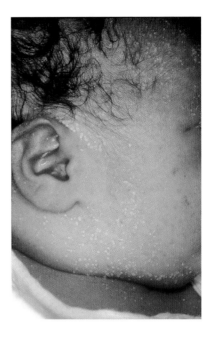

Figure 8–10. Erythema toxicum neonatorum. *Source:* From Wolff K, Goldsmith LA, Katz SI, et al. *Fitzpatrick's Dermatology in General Medicine*, 7th ed. New York, NY: McGraw-Hill; 2008.

Figure 8–11. Transient neonatal pustulosis. *Source:* From Wolff K, Goldsmith LA, Katz SI, et al. *Fitzpatrick's Dermatology in General Medicine*, 7th ed. New York, NY: McGraw-Hill; 2008.

tested for several infections that may present with vesicopustular lesions in the neonatal period such as herpes simplex, *Candida*, and *Staphylococcus* infections.[32]

Transient neonatal pustular melanosis (Figure 8–11) is a vesiculopustular rash that occurs in up to 5% of African American newborns and less than 1% of Caucasian newborns.[30] In contrast to erythema toxicum neonatorum, the lesions of transient neonatal pustular melanosis more commonly are present at birth and lack surrounding erythema. Characteristic lesions of transient neonatal pustular melanosis are 2- to 5-mm diameter pustules on a nonerythematous base involving all areas of the body including the palms and soles. Over several days the lesions either rupture or form central crusts that desquamate, leaving behind hyperpigmented macules and a collarette of scales that fade over 3 to 4 weeks. Light complexioned infants may have little to no hyperpigmentation remnants. Often the only manifestation of transient neonatal pustular melanosis is the presence of brown macules with a rim of scale at birth; the lesions may appear at different stages of development simultaneously. The pigmented macules within the vesiculopustules of transient neonatal pustular melanosis are unique to this condition. Physicians who clinically recognize this condition may avoid unnecessary diagnostic testing and treatment for infectious disorders because these pigmented macules do not occur in any of the infectious rashes.[33] Gram stain of a pustule will reveal polymorphic neutrophils and occasionally eosinophils.

Acne neonatorum (Figure 8–12) consists of closed comedones (a plug of sebaceous material causing whiteheads) on the forehead,

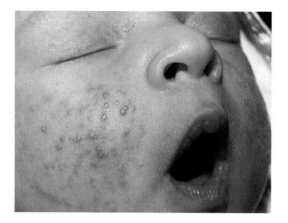

Figure 8–12. Neonatal acne. *Source:* From Wolff K, Goldsmith LA, Katz SI, et al. *Fitzpatrick's Dermatology in General Medicine*, 7th ed. New York, NY: McGraw-Hill; 2008.

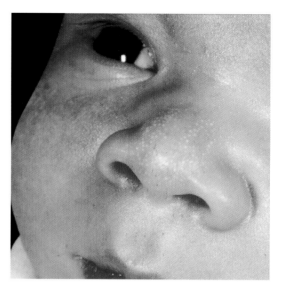

Figure 8–13. Milia. *Source:* From Wolff K, Goldsmith LA, Katz SI, et al. *Fitzpatrick's Dermatology in General Medicine*, 7th ed. New York, NY: McGraw-Hill; 2008.

nose, and cheeks that are present in 20% of newborns,[34] more commonly at 2 to 4 weeks of life. Open comedones (blackheads), inflammatory papules, and pustules may also develop. The large sebaceous glands on the face of newborns are stimulated by maternal or endogenous androgens, thus causing an increased activity of the pilosebaceous unit. With this activity the sebaceous cells mature, die, fragment, and then extrude into the sebaceous duct where they combine with desquamating cells to finally arrive at the surface of the pilosebaceous unit as sebum. Sebum is the pathogenic factor in acne and it is irritating and comedogenic. Sebaceous glands are located throughout the body except the palms, soles, dorsa of the feet, and the lower lip. These glands are large in newborn infants but regress shortly after birth; therefore, the lesions clear without treatment within 4 months without scarring since the large sebaceous glands that had been stimulated by androgens become smaller and less active. Severe, unrelenting neonatal acne, especially accompanied by other signs of hyperandrogenism, should prompt an investigation for adrenal cortical hyperplasia, virilizing tumors, or underlying endocrinopathies.[34]

Milia (Figure 8–13), another transient neonatal condition, are 1- to 2-mm, pearly white or yellow papules that occur in up to 50% of newborns.[35] They are caused by retention of keratin (protein material present in the epidermis) within the upper dermal layer. Milia occur most commonly on the forehead, cheeks, nose, and chin. Other areas may include the upper trunk, extremities, penis, or mucous membranes. When milia are present in the mouth they are referred to as Epstein pearls and approximately 60% of newborns will have these lesions on their palates.[36] Milia have a benign, self-limited course as the cystic spheres rupture onto the skin surface and exfoliate their contents, usually resolving within the first month of life, although they may persist into the second or third month of life.[35] Large numbers of lesions or persistence beyond 3 months of age may suggest the possibility of the oral-facial-digital syndrome or hereditary trichodysplasia. Look-alike lesions are those of molluscum contagiosum, an acquired viral

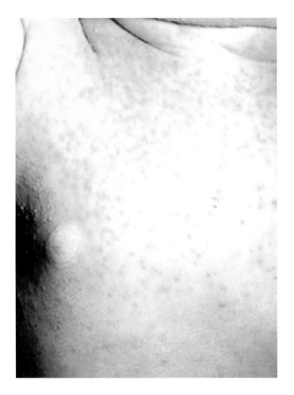

Figure 8–14. Miliaria. *Source:* Courtesy of Peter Lio, MD.

infection, which usually do not appear in the immediate neonatal period.

Miliaria or heat rash (Figure 8–14) affects up to 40% of infants during the first month of life.[37] The rash commonly occurs in warm climates, while the neonate is warmed in an incubator, during a fever, or from wearing occlusive dressings or warm clothing. Eccrine sweat-duct occlusion is the initial event. The duct ruptures, leaks fluid into the surrounding tissue, and an inflammatory response occurs. Occlusion of the eccrine sweat-duct system occurs at 2 different levels resulting in 2 clinically distinguishable subtypes: miliaria crystallina and miliaria rubra.

In miliaria crystallina, superficial eccrine duct closure occurs at the skin surface resulting in accumulation of sweat under the stratum corneum. The lesions consist of 1- to 2-mm vesicles without surrounding erythema,

giving the appearance of clear dewdrops. The lesions are most common on the head, neck, and trunk and, as each vesicle evolves, rupture is followed by desquamation, which may persist for hours to days.

A deeper, intraepidermal level of eccrine duct gland obstruction causes miliaria rubra, classically referred to as heat rash. Here papules and vesicles form, surrounded by a red halo or diffuse erythema as the inflammatory response develops. Both miliaria crystallina and miliaria rubra are benign, self-limited conditions; however, avoidance of overheating, removal of excess clothing, cool water compresses or cool baths, and proper ventilation, especially air conditioning, are recommended for the management and prevention of these disorders.[30]

Sucking blisters are most commonly solitary oval bullae or erosions on noninflamed skin in the newborn.[38] The lesions are found on the newborn's radial forearm, wrist, hand, dorsal thumb, and index finger. The lesions result from vigorous sucking by the infant on effected areas. Herpetic lesions should be easily differentiated from sucking blisters in that the former are grouped vesicles on an erythematous base. Likewise bullous impetigo lesions occur on an erythematous base. These 2 conditions will be discussed further under infectious conditions of the neonate.

Seborrheic dermatitis (Figure 8–15) is a common rash that develops within the first month of life. Erythema and greasy scales characterize it and most parents are familiar with this rash as "cradle cap" since the scalp is a common location. Other affected areas include the face, ears, and neck; the rash may spread to the diaper area and it is therefore important to consider this condition in the evaluation of diaper dermatitis.[39] Erythema has a tendency to occur in the flexural folds and intertriginous areas, whereas scaling predominates on the scalp.[40] Seborrheic dermatitis may be difficult to clinically distinguish from atopic dermatitis. While the onset of the former is within the first month of life, the age

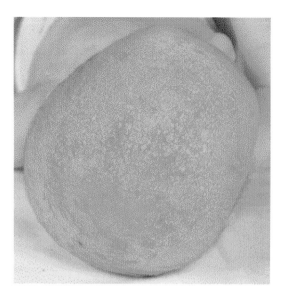

Figure 8–15. Seborrheic dermatitis ("cradle cap"). *Source:* Wolff K, Johnson RA, Suurmond D. *Fitzpatrick's Color Atlas and Synopsis of Clinical Dermatology*, 5th ed. New York, NY: McGraw-Hill; 2005.

of onset for atopic dermatitis is commonly after 3 months of age. Also there is ubiquitous pruritis in atopic dermatitis, which is uncommon in seborrheic dermatitis. The lesions of atopic dermatitis have varying responses to treatment with frequent relapses, while the lesions of seborrheic dermatitis are self-limited and respond well to treatment. The distribution of these 2 disorders is similar although atopic dermatitis is commonly found on the extremities.[39]

The exact etiology of seborrheic dermatitis is not known although hormonal fluctuations may be involved since the condition does seem to occur in locations with a high density of sebaceous glands. Some have suggested that the yeast *Malassezia furfur*, previously known as *Pityrosporum ovale*, causes the condition.[41] Generalized seborrheic dermatitis associated with failure to thrive and diarrhea should prompt an investigation for immunodeficiency.[40]

Infantile seborrheic dermatitis is commonly a self-limited condition, usually resolving in several weeks to months. Given the benign nature of the condition, a conservative approach to treatment is warranted beginning with reassurance and watchful waiting. In a 10-year follow-up prospective study in infants with seborrheic dermatitis, 85% of the children were free of skin disease. However, seborrheic dermatitis persisted in 8% of the subject children; the link between infantile and adult seborrheic dermatitis still remains unclear. In addition, 6% of the children in this study were later diagnosed with atopic dermatitis. This illustrates the difficulty in distinguishing these 2 conditions.[42] If cosmesis is a concern or the condition persists despite watchful waiting, several successful treatment options exist. The scales on the scalp can often be removed with a soft brush after softening the lesions with white petroleum jelly applied daily or by soaking the scalp overnight with olive or vegetable oil and then shampooing in the morning. Tar-containing shampoos can be recommended as first-line treatment when baby shampoo has failed.[40] These can be used several times a week. Selenium sulfide shampoos are probably safe, but rigorous safety data in infants are lacking; the use of salicylic acid is not recommended because of concerns for systemic absorption.[40] In cases where tar-containing shampoos have failed, the use of topical antifungal creams and shampoos has been supported. Ketoconazole cream applied to the scalp 3 times weekly or Ketoconazole shampoo, left on the scalp for 3 min and then rinsed, 3 times weekly has been effective. Small trials showed no systemic drug levels or change in liver function after 1 month of use.[43-45] Hydrocortisone 1% cream applied every other day or daily is an effective treatment for infantile seborrheic dermatitis, but Ketoconazole may be more effective in preventing recurrences.[46] When using steroid creams, limit the surface area to reduce the risk of systemic absorption and adrenal suppression.

Infectious Conditions of the Neonatal Skin

Herpes Simplex Virus (HSV)

Grouped vesicles on an erythematous base (Figure 8–16) should alarm all caretakers of neonates of the potential serious disease of herpes simplex infection. Most neonates are exposed to the virus during vaginal delivery. However, infection may occur in utero, by transplacental or ascending infection, or postnatally from relatives or attendants. While some infants with neonatal HSV will not have skin lesions, approximately half of neonates infected with HSV will have skin lesions.[47] Any area of the skin may be involved with scalp monitor sites, torso, and oral lesions being the most frequent sites.[48] Herpes simplex virus-positive papules and vesicles may be present on the skin at birth, but the onset after birth is more common, with 6 days as a mean age of onset.

Clinical signs and symptoms of neonatal HSV infection can develop within a few days to 4 weeks after birth. The infection in newborns usually develops in 3 main patterns: lesions localized to the skin, eyes and mouth (40%); disease localized to the CNS (35%); and fulminant, disseminated disease involving multiple organs (25%). Skin lesions are the most common and are found in all 3 forms. In a review of the natural history of neonatal HSV infection in the era of acyclovir therapy, skin lesions were noted at the time of presentation or developed during the acute HSV disease in 61% of patients with disseminated disease, 68% with CNS disease, and 83% with skin, eye, and mouth disease.[49] The lesions of neonatal HSV consist of 1- to 3-mm erythematous papules and vesicles, most commonly grouped and on an erythematous base, that usually evolve into pustules, crusts, and erosions. If HSV lesions are noted on the skin of a newborn they usually appear as superficial erosions and the infant is commonly premature, with low birth weight and microcephaly suggesting an intrauterine infection. Neonatal

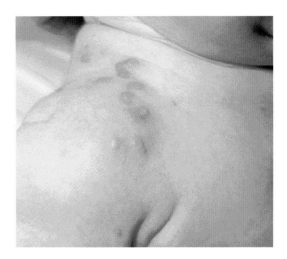

Figure 8–16. Herpes simplex vescicles. *Source:* Wolff K, Johnson RA, Suurmond D. *Fitzpatrick's Color Atlas and Synopsis of Clinical Dermatology*, 5th ed. New York, NY: McGraw-Hill; 2005.

HSV infection commonly disseminates and, therefore, aggressive investigation and treatment are highly recommended. Neonates with disseminated HSV infection may appear septic with vascular instability, hypothermia, hepatic dysfunction, disseminated intravascular coagulation, and respiratory failure. CNS disease may present with fever, lethargy, and focal seizures. If lesions that are suspicious for HSV infection are found on a neonate's skin or oral mucosa, a full septic workup including blood, urine, and cerebral spinal fluid cultures is recommended with the administration of IV acyclovir. Ninety percent of infants with initial herpetic skin lesions treated with IV acyclovir 30 mg/kg/day had no sequelae.[50] IV antibiotics will also most likely be started until all cultures are negative.

Varicella-Zoster Virus (VZV)

Neonatal varicella is a serious disease caused by the VZV, a member of the herpesvirus family. Newborns born to mothers exposed to VZV or mothers who have clinical disease within 2 weeks of delivery are at greatest risk for infection. The risk of infection and the case fatality rate are significantly increased when symptoms of maternal infection occur less than 5 days prior to delivery.[51] This interval does not allow sufficient time for the development of maternal IgG and subsequent passive transfer to protect the infant. In these cases a high incidence of disseminated varicella occurs and, when the rash appears in infants between 5 and 10 days of age, the mortality rate may be as high as 20%.[52] Postnatally acquired varicella occurring after 10 days of age is usually mild.[53]

The clinical picture of neonatal varicella is variable. The disease may be mild and resemble chickenpox found in older children or may be disseminated disease similar to that seen in immunocompromised patients. Fever may develop within the first few days after birth. Numerous vesicles on an erythematous base occur with a generalized distribution. In mild cases the lesions crust over and heal by 7 to 10 days. If disseminated disease occurs, varicella pneumonia, hepatitis, and meningoencephalitis are the most common.

The diagnosis of varicella is usually made clinically based upon the characteristic skin lesions and the history of the mother's exposure to VZV or lesion outbreak. VZV can be cultured from vesicular fluid but the virus takes several weeks to grow. Multiple diagnostic tests exist for detecting VZV including direct fluorescent antigen (DFA) and polymerase chain reaction (PCR), both of which are quite sensitive. DFA provides the most rapid test.

In the past, postexposure prophylaxis for newborns that have been exposed to VZV was accomplished through the administration of varicella-zoster immune globulin (VZIG). However a new product, VariZIG, a purified human immune globulin preparation made from plasma containing high levels of antivaricella antibodies, is replacing VZIG since the supply of VZIG is nearly depleted due to a discontinuation of production by its manufacturer. VariZIG became available in 2006. The administration of VariZIG to newborns with a significant exposure risk to VZV should follow

the same recommendations as that for VZIG: neonates whose mothers have signs and symptoms of varicella around the time of delivery (5 days before and 2 days after), premature infants born at greater than 28 weeks of gestation who are exposed during the neonatal period and whose mothers do not have signs of immunity, and premature infants born at less than 28 weeks of gestation or who weigh less than 1000 g at birth and were exposed during the neonatal period, regardless of maternal history of varicella or vaccination.[54,55] VariZIG should be administered within 96 hours of exposure since its efficacy is not known after this time interval.[55] The recommended dose is 125 units (one vial) IM. If VZIG or VariZIG cannot be administered within 96 hours of exposure, then administration of IV immunoglobulin should be considered. The treatment for neonatal varicella infection lies in the use of IV acyclovir, which reduces the risk of mortality in severe varicella. Newborns with severe infection should be treated with IV acyclovir 30 mg/kg/day in 3 divided doses for 10 days.[56,57]

Bacterial Infections

Bacterial infection in neonates may present with vesiculobullous or pustular lesions. The 2 gram-positive cocci, *Staphylococcus aureus* and group A beta hemolytic *Streptococcus*, are the major organisms responsible for the majority of skin and soft tissue infections in children and adults, and neonates are no exception. *S aureus* invades skin and causes impetigo, folliculitis, cellulitis, and furuncles. The toxins of *S aureus* cause the lesions of bullous impetigo and staphylococcal scalded skin syndrome. Streptococci invade traumatized skin and cause impetigo, erysipelas, cellulitis, and lymphangitis.

Impetigo (Figure 8–17) is a common, contagious, superficial skin infection. Because up to 60% of infants become colonized with *S aureus* in the first few weeks of life, this organism is an important cause of these

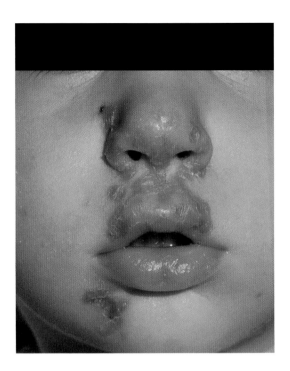

Figure 8-17. Impetigo. *Source:* Wolff K, Johnson RA, Suurmond D. *Fitzpatrick's Color Atlas and Synopsis of Clinical Dermatology*, 5th ed. New York, NY: McGraw-Hill; 2005.

superficial skin infections.[58] There are 2 distinct clinical entities: bullous impetigo and nonbullous impetigo. Both disorders begin as very thin vesicles whose roofs consist only of stratum corneum, the outer noncellular portion of the epidermis. Vesicles and bullae are circumscribed elevations of the skin containing serum. Vesicles are lesions up to 0.5 cm in diameter and bullae are more than 0.5 cm in diameter. It was once thought that bullous impetigo was secondary to *S aureus* and nonbullous impetigo was primarily a streptococcal infection. It is now known that *S aureus* is the primary pathogen in both bullous and nonbullous impetigo.[59]

Unlike nonbullous impetigo that originates as small vesicles or pustules that rupture to expose a red, moist base and evolve to reveal honey-yellow, firmly adherent crusts with minimal surrounding erythema, the vesicles of bullous impetigo enlarge rapidly to form bullae in which the contents turn from clear to cloudy. Neonatal lesions of impetigo are flaccid, well-demarcated bullae found most commonly in areas of trauma, such as the diaper area, circumcision wound, axillae, and periumbilical skin; however, lesions may appear anywhere on the body. The bullae may evolve to erosions and a collarette of scale around erosion is characteristic of *S aureus*.[60] The diagnosis is confirmed with demonstration of gram-positive cocci in clusters on Gram stain of the vesicular fluid and isolation of *S aureus* on culture. With small, localized lesions in a well-appearing, normothermic neonate, treatment may include local cleansing of the skin and the application of topical mupirocin. If lesions are extensive or the infant appears ill, then a blood culture and a full septic evaluation is recommended with the institution of parenteral antibiotics. Drug sensitivities should be checked and therapy adjusted due to the increasing prevalence of methicillin-resistant *S aureus* (MRSA).

The epidermis consists of several layers. The stratum corneum is the outer noncellular portion of the epidermis. The stratum lucidum or clear layer lies immediately beneath the stratum corneum. Next is the stratum granulosum or granular layer of the epidermis. It is in this layer that newborns are susceptible to the dissemination of *S aureus* epidermolytic toxins that produces the skin condition of staphylococcal scalded skin syndrome. The toxins cause cleavage of desmoglein 1 complex in the stratum granulosum, an important protein in desmosomes or site of adhesion between 2 cells. This complex consists of organelles that help anchor keratinocytes to each other.[61] The result is extensive distribution of fragile, dense bullae that often are no longer intact by the time of presentation.[62]

Staphylococcal scalded skin syndrome (Figure 8–18) commonly occurs in infants 3

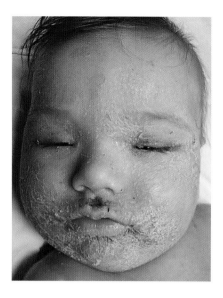

Figure 8–18. Staphylococcal scalded skin syndrome. *Source:* From Wolff K, Goldsmith LA, Katz SI, et al. *Fitzpatrick's Dermatology in General Medicine*, 7th ed. New York, NY: McGraw-Hill; 2008.

to 7 days of age, rarely being seen at birth,[63] with an abrupt onset of generalized, blanching erythema often beginning around the mouth. Within 24 hours bullae appear, particularly in areas of mechanical stress including flexural areas. Gentle pressure with traction applied to the bullae results in separation of the upper epidermis and wrinkling of the skin known as Nikolsky sign. Subsequent exfoliation of large sheets of skin occurs within 48 hours. The lesions commonly affect the head, neck, buttocks, groin, axillae, and the periumbilical area of the abdomen.[62] Affected infants are febrile and irritable, and often have conjunctivitis although the mucous membranes are not commonly involved. Since the cleavage plane of the blisters is intraepidermal, scarring does not occur. Look-alike conditions are toxic shock syndrome (TSS) and toxic epidermal necrolysis (TEN). However these 2 conditions are rarely seen in the neonatal period.

If staphylococcal scalded skin syndrome is suspected, the infant should be isolated and cultures obtained from blood, urine, nasopharynx, umbilicus, abnormal skin, and any suspected focus of infection. Intact bullae are usually sterile. Diagnosis is usually clinical. Treatment consists of the combination of immediate administration of IV fluid and electrolyte replacement, much like that provided for burn therapy, and penicillinase-resistant penicillin such as nafcillin. Therapy should be adjusted based upon local patterns of sensitivity. Supportive skin care should be provided using topical lubrication emollients, such as creams and ointments, to improve barrier function and decrease pain and associated discomfort.

Group A streptococcal skin infections may mimic those caused by staphylococci, although they are less common. Affected newborns may present with pustules and honey-colored crusts, often associated with a moist umbilical cord stump or omphalitis,[64] redness and induration of the umbilical region. If streptococcal disease is suspected, Gram stain and culture of skin lesions should be obtained. Gram-positive cocci in chains will differentiate from staphylococcal infections. Cultures of blood, urine, and CSF are obtained to rule out disseminated disease. Although the majority of omphalitis infections are caused by *S aureus* and IV antistaphylococcal antibiotic should be administered, treatment of culture positive group A streptococcal skin infection can be adequately accomplished using parenteral penicillin. However, if there is evidence of invasive infection, IV ampicillin and cefotaxime should be administered.

Diaper Dermatitis

Intertrigo (Figure 8–19) is a dermatitis that occurs between folded surfaces of the skin, areas that retain warmth and moisture encouraging the growth of resistant microorganisms. This condition commonly occurs between the gluteal folds of the buttocks, the scrotum and

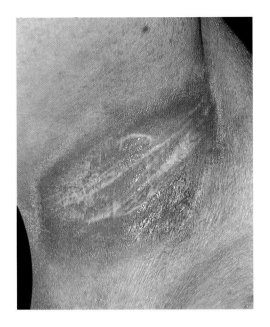

Figure 8–19. Intertrigo. *Source:* From Wolff K, Goldsmith LA, Katz SI, et al. *Fitzpatrick's Dermatology in General Medicine*, 7th ed. New York, NY: McGraw-Hill; 2008.

the thigh, the short neck and proximal trunk in young infants, posterior ear and postauricular head, and beneath pendulous breasts. An artificial intertriginous condition is created under a persistently wet diaper in an infant. This condition predisposes the diapered skin to the development of resistant *Candida* infection.[65] Diaper candidiasis appears as a bright red eruption with numerous pinpoint satellite papules and pustules. The intertriginous areas are predominantly involved and deeply erythematous. The urethral meatus is infected and the satellite lesions extend to the buttocks, bilateral adjacent thighs, and pubic region. *Candida* infection is a common complication of systemic antibiotic therapy, seborrheic dermatitis, psoriasis, and chronic irritant dermatitis. Treatment of this condition is the maintenance of dryness by frequent diaper changes or leaving the diaper off for short intervals of time. Diaper candidiasis responds well to topical antifungal medications such as

nystatin or clotrimazole applied twice a day for 10 days.[66] Low potency topical hydrocortisone applied twice a day for 3 to 4 days may rapidly improve the clinical condition but high-potency steroid agents can produce atrophy of the diapered skin in a short period of time and should be avoided. Several conditions of the diapered skin may mimic one another, often requiring follow-up physician visits to evaluate the effect of specific therapies.

Irritant contact dermatitis results from the diapered area being bathed in urine and stool and then wrapped in a plastic diaper. Although urine ammonia was once thought to be the prime instigator for the development of irritant diaper dermatitis, recent evidence points to feces as the principal culprit in the pathogenesis of this condition.[67] The epidermal barrier is disrupted after exposure to watery stools, especially after antibiotic use or viral infections such as *Rotavirus enteritis.* This often triggers a severe dermatitis resulting in a red, scaly, and erosive dermatitis that is usually confined to the convex surfaces of the perineum, lower abdomen, buttocks, and the inner, proximal thighs; the intertriginous areas are spared. This is in contrast to the intertriginous involvement of diaper candidiasis dermatitis (Figure 8–20). Gentle cleansing of the area with moist, nonmedicated tissue and the application of barrier pastes such as zinc oxide and lubricants such as petroleum usually result in clearing of the dermatitis.

When persistent intertriginous diaper dermatitis occurs, consider the possibility of seborrheic dermatitis and infantile psoriasis, particularly when there was no response to the therapy for diaper candidiasis. Seborrheic dermatitis in the diaper area appears as red, greasy, scaly patches that extend from the intertriginous creases to involve the genitals, perineum, suprapubic area, and thighs. The possible cause and treatment options of this condition have been described earlier in this chapter and this condition may clear without treatment in 2 to 3 months.

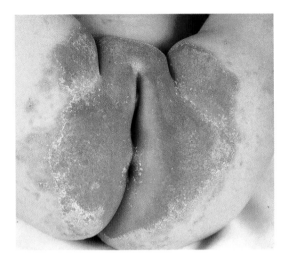

Figure 8–20. Candidal diaper diamatitis. *Source:* Wolff K, Johnson RA, Suurmond D. *Fitzpatrick's Color Atlas and Synopsis of Clinical Dermatology,* 5th ed., New York, NY: McGraw-Hill; 2005.

Infantile psoriasis usually begins as persistent diaper dermatitis. Lesions may disseminate to the trunk and extremities, but the condition may be present in the diaper area alone for months. The eruption is bright red, scaly, and well demarcated at the diaper line. Infants remain well and the eruption is usually asymptomatic. Skin biopsy is the only way to confirm the diagnosis.

The Red, Scaly Newborn

A postmature newborn may have prominent desquamation of the hands, feet, and lower trunk. When seen during the first few days of life when the infant's skin is bright red, an inexperienced observer may erroneously diagnose the condition as ichthyosis (a congenital disorder of keratinization characterized by dryness and fishskin-like scaling of the skin). Similarly, preterm newborns born at less than 32 weeks of gestation will have red, glistening skin that may be confused with ichthyosis. These skin conditions in these newborns are generally transient and resolve within the neonatal period.

Newborns with skin that appears to be encased in a thick, shiny, inelastic scale are referred to as collodion babies. The collodion membrane is excessively thick with stratum corneum and initially saturated with water. As the water content of this membrane dehydrates, multiple, deep fissures develop exposing bright red skin underneath. The presence of the collodion membrane does not necessarily predict the chronic condition of ichthyosis and spontaneous healing may occur.[68] Most collodion babies do have a form of ichthyosis and skin biopsy of the membrane is not diagnostic. Collodion babies should be observed closely for the danger of significant dehydration associated with high transepidermal water loss.[69]

REFERENCES

1. American Academy of Pediatrics. *American College of Obstetrics and Gynecologists; Guidelines for Perinatal Care.* 4th ed. Elk Grove Village, IL: Author; 1997.
2. Krengel S, Hauschild A, Schafer T. Melanoma risk in congenital melanocytic naevi: a systemic review. *Br J Dermatol.* 2006;155(1):1-8.
3. Kopf AW, Bart RS, Hennessey P. Congenital nevocytic nevi and malignant melanomas. *J Am Acad Dermatol.* 1979;1:123-130.
4. Berg P, Lindelof B. Congenital melanocytic naevi and cutaneous melanoma. *Melanoma Res.* 2003;13(5):441-445.
5. Swerdlow AJ, English JS, Qiao Z. The risk of melanoma in patients with congenital nevi: a cohort study. *J Am Acad Dermatol.* 1995;32:595-599.
6. Rhodes AR. Small congenital nevi (reply). *J Am Acad Dermatol.* 1982;7:687.
7. Kanzler MH. Management of large congenital nevocytic nevi: art vs. science. *J Am Acad Dermatol.* 2006;54(5):874-876.
8. Habif TB. Light-related diseases and disorders of pigmentation. In: Habif TB, ed. *Clinical Dermatology: A Color Guide to Diagnosis and Therapy.* 3rd ed. St. Louis, MO: Mosby-Year Book; 1996:597-626.
9. Jacobs AH, Walton RG. The incidence of birthmarks in the neonate. *Pediatrics.* 1976;58(2):218-222.

10. Jacobs AH, Cahn RL. Birthmarks. *Pediatr Ann.* 1976;5(12):743-758.

11. Drolet BA, Esterly NB, Frieden IJ. Hemangiomas in children. *N Engl J Med.* 1999;341(3):173-181.

12. Smolinski KN, Yan AC. Hemangiomas of infancy: clinical and biological characteristics. *Clin Pediatr (Phila).* 2005;44(9):747-766.

13. Illingworth RS. Thoughts on the treatment of vascular nevi. *Arch Dis Child.* 1976;51:138-140.

14. Sadan N, Wolach B. Treatment of hemangiomas of infants with high doses of prednisone. *J Pediatr.* 1996;128(1):141-146.

15. Edgerton MT. The treatment of hemangiomas: with special references to the role of steroid therapy. *Ann Surg.* 1976;183:517-532.

16. Esterly NB. Kasabach-Merritt syndrome in infants. *J Am Acad Dermatol.* 1983;8:504-513.

17. Nguyen CM, Yohn JJ, Huff C, et al. Facial port wine stains in childhood: prediction of the rate of improvement as a function of the age of the patient, size and location of the port wine stain and the number of treatments with the pulsed dye (585nm) laser. *Br J Dermatol.* 1998;138(5):821-825.

18. Helsing P, Mork NJ, Flage T. Pathological findings in the eye of children with facial nevus [Norwegian]. *Tidsskr Nor Laegeforen.* 2001;121(16):1911-1912.

19. Kramer U, Kahana E, Shorer Z, Ben-Zeev B. Outcome of infants with unilateral Sturge-Weber syndrome and early onset seizures. *Dev Med Child Neurol.* 2000;42(11):756-759.

20. Tallman B, Tan OT, Morelli JG, et al. Location of port-wine stains and the likelihood of ophthalmic and/or central nervous system complications. *Pediatrics.* 1991;87:323-327.

21. Meggyessy V, Mehes K. Association of supernumerary nipples with renal anomalies. *J Pediatr.* 1987;111(3):412-413.

22. Drolet B. Birthmarks to worry about. Cutaneous markers of dysraphism. *Dermatol Clin.* 1998;16(3):447-453.

23. Tavafoghi V, Ghandchi A, Hambrick GW, Udverhelyi GB. Cutaneous signs of spinal dysraphism. Report of a patient with a tail-like lipomas and a review of 200 cases in the literature. *Arch Dermatol.* 1978;114(4):573-577.

24. Guggisberg D, Hadj-Rabia S, Viney C, et al. Skin markers of occult spinal dysraphism in children: a review of 54 cases [published correction appears in *Arch Dermatol.* 2005;141(4):425]. *Arch Dermatol.* 2004;140(9):1109-1115.

25. Mazereeuw-Hautier J, Carel-Caneppele S, Bonafe JL. Cutis marmorata telangiectatica congenita: report of two persistent cases. *Pediatr Dermatol.* 2002;19(6):506-509.

26. Gerritsen MJ, Steijlen PM, Brunner HG, Rieu P. Cutis marmorata telangiectatica congenita: report of 18 cases. *Br J Dermatol.* 2000;142(2):366-369.

27. O'Connor NR, McLaughlin MR, Ham P. Newborn skin: part 1. Common rashes. *Am Fam Physician.* 2008;77(1):47-52.

28. Liu C, Feng J, Qu R, et al. Epidemiologic study of the predisposing factors in erythema toxicum neonatorum. *Dermatology.* 2005;210(4):269-272.

29. Carr JA, Hodgman JE, Freedman RI, Levan NE. Relationship between toxic erythema and infant maturity. *Am J Dis Child.* 1966;112(2):129-134.

30. Schachner L, Press S. Vesicular, bullous and pustular disorders in infancy and childhood. *Pediatr Clin North Am.* 1983;30(4):609-629.

31. Van Praag MC, Van Rooij RW, Folkers E, et al. Diagnosis and treatment of pustular disorders in the neonate. *Pediatr Dermatol.* 1997;14(2):131-143.

32. Chang MW, Jiang SB, Orlow SJ. Atypical erythema toxicum neonatorum of delayed onset in a term infant. *Pediatr Dermatol.* 1999;16(2):137-141.

33. Laude TA. Approach to dermatologic disorders in black children. *Semin Dermatol.* 1995;14(1):15-20.

34. Katsambas AD, Katoulis AC, Stavropoulos P. Acne neonatorum: a study of 22 cases. *Int J Dermatol.* 1999;38(2):128-130.

35. Paller A, Mancini AJ, Hurwitz S. *Hurwitz Clinical Pediatric Dermatology: A Textbook of Skin Disorders of Childhood and Adolescence.* 3rd ed. Philadelphia, PA: Elsevier Saunders; 2006:737.

36. Rivers JK, Frederiksen PC, Dibdin C. A prevalence survey of dermatoses in the Australian neonate. *J Am Acad Dermatol.* 1990;23:77.

37. Feng E, Janniger CK. Miliaria. *Cutis.* 1995;55(4):213-216.

38. Murphy WF, Langley AL. Common bullous lesions—presumably self-limited—occurring in utero in the newborn infant. *Pediatrics.* 1963;32:1099.

39. Williams ML. Differential diagnosis of seborrheic dermatitis. *Pediatr Rev.* 1986;7(7):204-211.

40. Janniger CK. Infantile seborrheic dermatitis: an approach to cradle cap. *Cutis.* 1993;51(4):233-235.

41. Tollesson A, Frithz A, Stenlund K. Malassezia furfur in infantile seborrheic dermatitis. *Pediatr Dermatol.* 1997;14(6):423-425.

42. Mimouni K, Mukamel M, Zeharia A, Mimouni M. Prognosis of infantile seborrheic dermatitis. *J Pediatr.* 1995;127(5):744-746.

43. Taieb A, Legrain V, Palmier C, et al. Topical Ketoconazole for infantile seborrheic dermatitis. *Dermatologica.* 1990;181(1):26-32.

44. Brodell RT, Patel S, Venglarcik JS, et al. The safety of Ketoconazole shampoo for infantile seborrheic dermatitis. *Pediatr Dermatol.* 1998;15(5):406-407.

45. Zeharia A, Mimouni M, Fogel D. Treatment with bifonazole shampoo for scalp seborrhea in infants and young children. *Pediatr Dermatol.* 1996;13(2):151-153.

46. Cohen S. Should we treat infantile seborrheic dermatitis with topical antifungals or topical steroids? *Arch Dis Child.* 2004;89(3):288-289.

47. Whitley R, Arvin A, Prober C, et al. A controlled trial comparing vidarabine with acyclovir in neonatal herpes simplex virus infection. *N Engl J Med.* 1991;324:444-449.

48. Parvey LS, Ch'ien LT. Neonatal herpes simplex virus infection introduced by fetal-monitor scalp electrodes. *Pediatrics.* 1980;65:1150.

49. Kimberlin DW, Lin CY, Jacobs RF, et al. Natural history of neonatal herpes simplex virus infections in the acyclovir era. *Pediatrics.* 2001;108:223.

50. Arvin Am. Antiviral treatment of herpes simplex infection in neonates and pregnant women. *J Am Acad Dermatol.* 1988;18:200-203.

51. Meyers JD. Congenital varicella in term infants: risk considered. *J Infect Dis.* 1974;129:215.

52. Stagno S, Whitley RJ. Herpesvirus infections of pregnancy. Part II. Herpes simplex virus and varicella-zoster virus infections. *N Engl J Med.* 1985;313:1327-1330.

53. Bailey JE, Toltzis P. Viral infections. In: Fanaroff AA, Martin RJ, eds. *Neonatal-Perinatal Medicine.* 7th ed. St. Louis: Mosby; 2002:755.

54. American Academy of Pediatrics. Varicella-Zoster infections. In: Pickering LK, ed. *Red Book: 2006 Report of the Committee on Infectious Diseases.* 27th ed. Elk Grove Village, IL, Author; 2006:711.

55. A new product (VariZIG) for postexposure prophylaxis of varicella available under an investigational new drug application expanded access protocol. *MMWR Morb Mortal Wkly.* 2006;55:209.

56. American Academy of Pediatrics. Antiviral drugs for non-human immunodeficiency virus infections. In: Pickering LK, ed. *Red Book: 2006 Report of the Committee on Infectious Diseases.* 27th ed. Elk Grove Village, IL, Author; 2006:785.

57. Kesson AM, Grimwood K, Burgess MA, et al. Acyclovir for the prevention and treatment of varicella zoster in children, adolescents and pregnancy. *J Paediatr Child Health.* 1996;32:211.

58. Speck WT, Driscoll JM, Polin RA, et al. Staphylococcal and streptococcal colonization of the newborn infant: effect of antiseptic cord care. *Am J Dis Child.* 1977;131:1005.

59. Barton LL, Friedman AD. Impetigo: a reassessment of etiology and therapy. *Pediatr Dermatol.* 1987;4:185-188.

60. Darmstadt GL, Lane AT. Impetigo: an overview. *Pediatr Dermatol.* 1994;11:293.

61. Patel GK, Finlay AY. Staphylococcal scalded skin syndrome: diagnosis and management. *Am J Clin Dermatol.* 2003;4:165.

62. Ladhani S, Joannou CL, Lochrie DP, et al. Clinical, microbial and biochemical aspects of the exfoliative toxins causing staphylococcal scalded skin syndrome. *Clin Microbiol Rev.* 1999;12(2):224.

63. Drolet BA, Esterly NB. The skin. In: Fanaroff AA, Martin RJ, eds. *Neonatal-Perinatal Medicine.* 7th ed. St. Louis: Mosby; 2002:1537.

64. Isenberg HD, Tucci V, Lipsitz P, et al. Clinical laboratory and epidemiological investigations of a Streptococcus pyogenes cluster epidemic in a newborn nursery. *J Clin Microbiol.* 1984;19:366.

65. Ferrazzini G, Kaiser RR, Hirsig Cheng SK, et al. Microbiologic aspects of diaper dermatitis. *Dermatology.* 2003;206:136-141.

66. Sires UI, Mallory SB. Diaper dermatitis: how to treat and prevent. *Postgrad Med.* 1995;98:79-86.

67. Prasad HR, Srivastava P, Verma KK. Diaper dermatitis: ammonia. *Indian J Pediatr.* 2003; 70:635-637.

68. Frenk E, Techtermann F. Self-healing collodion baby: evidence for autosomal recessive inheritance. *Pediatr Dermatol.* 1992;9:95.

69. Buyse L, Graves C, Marks R, Wijeyesekera K, Alfaham M, Finlay AY. Collodion baby dehydration: the danger of high transepidermal water loss. *Br J Dermatol.* 1993;129:86.

CHAPTER 9

Neonatal Infections

P. David Sadowitz, MD

LaLainia Secreti, MD

Jeff Lapoint, DO

Infections represent an important cause of morbidity and mortality in the first month of life. Up to 2% of infants may be infected in utero, and 12% to 28% of infants may develop infection in the first month of life.[1-3] Although the majority of neonates with fever have a benign, self-limited viral infection, the goal of evaluation and treatment in the emergency department (ED) is to rapidly and accurately identify and treat the child at high risk for serious bacterial infection, specifically defined as bacteremia, bacterial meningitis, and urinary tract infection (UTI). Fever (defined as a rectal temperature of 38 degrees Celsius) is the most common presentation of infection in the neonate and may be overlooked by parents as there may be no other symptoms to suggest infection. In the neonate without fever, the signs of a potential life-threatening infection can be subtle and consist of only poor feeding, lethargy, apnea, or hypothermia. Evaluation of the neonate with fever is complicated by the inability of the child to vocalize symptoms and the absence of localizing signs and symptoms in many neonates. The current approach for the evaluation and treatment of febrile neonates in the ED setting will be outlined in the following.

▶ PATHOPHYSIOLOGY

Many factors are responsible for the increased risk of life-threatening infection in the neonate. One of the most important is the immature immune system in the neonate. The neonate is initially protected against some bacterial pathogens, ie, encapsulated bacteria and GBS, from maternal IgG that is transported across the placenta.[4] The neonate does not produce effective quantities of IgG until the third month of life. There is no transplacental IgM antibody-mediated protection against *Escherichia coli* and other Enterobacteriacae.

The fetus begins to synthesize complement components in the first trimester. IgM production in the neonate increases rapidly from birth and in response to infection.[5] The presence of complement and IgM are thus available in response to bacterial pathogens such as *E coli* and Group B *Streptococcus* (GBS), although this response is diminished to some extent against GBS and enteric gram-negative organisms.

Neutrophil migration (chemotaxis) is impaired as the result of an immature neutrophil cytoskeleton and decreased expression of adhesion molecules on the surface of the neutrophil. In addition, neonatal neutrophils have decreased adhesion, deformability, and aggregation in response to infection. Neonatal neutrophils have a decreased ability to phagocytose GBS and gram-negative bacteria.[6] The neutrophil storage pool is only 20% to 30% of that seen in adults and is rapidly depleted in the face of infection. Neonates with neutropenia in the face of sepsis have an increased mortality. Normal levels of circulating monocytes are present; tissue macrophages are decreased at birth. Monocytes are delayed in their ability to develop an inflammatory response. Natural killer cells are present at birth and are able to destroy cells infected with viruses as well as antibody-coated cells (antibody directed-cell mediated cytotoxicity [ADCC]); however, this ability is impaired in comparison to adult natural killer cells. These defects partially explain the increased risk of disseminated herpes simplex infections in the neonate.

▶ PATHOGENESIS

In utero infection occurs as the result of transplacental passage of organisms from an infected mother (vertical transmission). Potential pathogens are summarized in Table 9–1.

Toxoplasmosis gondii, Treponema pallidum, Rubella, cytomegalovirus (CMV), and herpes simplex infection (TORCH) represent some of the more common infections present at birth. Clinical manifestations of disease may include congenital malformations, ie, microcephaly, hepatosplenomegaly, pneumonia, and petechiae.

▶ **TABLE 9–1. NEONATAL INFECTION: COMMON ETIOLOGIC AGENTS**

Transplacental	Intrapartum	Postpartum
Cytomegalovirus	Anaerobic bacteria	Adenovirus
Enterovirus	*Chlamydia*	*Candida*
Herpes simplex virus	Cytomegalovirus	Coagulase negative and
Mycobaterium tuberculosis	Enteric bacteria (*Escherichia coli*)	positive staphylococci
Parvovirus B19	Group B streptococci	Cytomegalovirus
Rubella virus	*Haemophilus influenza*	Echoviruses
Toxoplasma gondii	Hepatitis B	Enteric bacteria (*Escherichia coli*)
Treponema pallidum	Herpes simplex virus	HIV
Varicella-zoster virus	Human immunodeficiency virus	Influenza A, B
	Listeria monocytogenes	*Listeria* monocytogenes
	Mycobacterium tuberculosis	*Mycobacterium tuberculosis*
	Mycoplasma	Parainfluenza
	Neisseria meningitidis	Pseudomonas
		Respiratory syncytial virus
		Staphylococcus aureus

Intrapartum infection usually occurs within 7 days of birth, and is caused by transmission of infectious agents to the neonate via the blood stream in mothers with bacteremia or viremia and at delivery as the neonate moves through the birth canal. The neonate is exposed to multiple life threatening organisms including human immunodeficiency virus (HIV), herpes simplex virus (HSV), hepatitis B virus (HBV), and aerobic and anaerobic bacteria in the vaginal canal, which includes GBS, enteric organisms, gonococci, and chlamydiae. Prolonged rupture of membranes (PROM) greater than 18 hours increases the incidence of chorioamnionitis, increasing the likelihood of GBS infection. The risk of neonatal infection is also increased with traumatic delivery or maternal bleeding (placenta previa or abruption placentae).

Postpartum infections occur after the first 7 days of life through person-to-person contact and can be transmitted through breast feeding (HIV, CMV). Neonates are also susceptible to environmental viral pathogens such as respiratory syncytial virus, parainfluenza virus, influenza virus, and adenovirus.

▶ CLINICAL PRESENTATION

FEVER

The rectal temperature represents the gold standard for detection of fever in the neonate. A temperature of 38° Celsius or above is defined as fever. Tympanic temperatures and axillary temperatures are notoriously inaccurate in this setting and should not be used.[7,8] Regarding parental reporting of fever, retrospective studies have shown that >90% of neonates with rectal temperatures above 38° Celsius had fever in the hospital setting. Bundling may minimally elevate skin temperatures but almost never raises the rectal temperature.[9] Temperatures above 38.5° Celsius should never be attributed to bundling.

▶ HISTORY

A thorough history is an essential component in evaluating the neonate presenting to the ED with fever. The presence of associated symptoms such as cough, vomiting, or diarrhea may give important clues as to the organism responsible for infection. The birth history is especially significant due to the increased risk of vertically transmitted infection to the newborn and would include a history of maternal fever, prolonged rupture of membranes, the presence of maternal sexually transmitted diseases such as herpes, chlamydia infection, and gonorrhea, the presence of GBS in the maternal genital tract, and the infant's nursery course.

The use of antibiotics pre- and postdelivery and the presence of sick contacts in the home are also important historical points.

▶ PHYSICAL EXAMINATION

The vital signs including oximetry, pulse, BP, and perfusion should be immediately obtained. The presence of respiratory distress, grunting, cyanosis, irritability, lethargy, poor perfusion, floppy tone, skin lesions (petechiae, vesicles), joint erythema or swelling, and inflammation of the umbilical cord or mucous membrane lesions consistent with herpetic infection are red flags suggestive of life-threatening infection. (Table 9–2) Immediate resuscitation (ABCs) with broad-spectrum antibiotic administration must be readily available following this initial evaluation.

▶ **TABLE 9–2. INITIAL SIGNS AND SYMPTOMS OF INFECTION IN NEWBORN INFANTS**

General	Cardiovascular System	Gastrointestinal System
Fever	Pallor, mottling, cold	Abdominal distension
Temperature instability	Tachycardia	Vomiting
"Not doing well"	Hypotension	Diarrhea
Poor feeding (poor suck)	Bradycardia	Hepatomegaly
Edema		Periumbilical discharge
	Respiratory System	
Central Nervous System	Apnea, dyspnea	**Hematologic System**
Irritability, lethargy	Tachypnea, retractions	Jaundice
Tremors, seizures	Flaring, grunting	Splenomegaly
Hyporeflexia, hypotonia	Cyanosis	Pallor
Abnormal Moro reflex		Petechiae, purpura
Irregular respirations	**Renal System**	Bleeding
Full fontanel	Oliguria	
High-pitched cry		

▶ DIAGNOSTIC TESTING

Several risk stratification strategies have been devised in an attempt to determine which febrile neonates are at high risk for bacterial disease given the limited data supplied by the history and physical examination. All of these studies used laboratory data to supplement the information obtained from the history and physical examination, and included the CBC with complete white cell differential, urinalysis and urine Gram stain, and, in some cases, CSF studies (CSF cell count, Gram stain). These treatment strategies include the Rochester criteria,[10] the Philadelphia criteria,[11] and the Boston criteria,[12] and are outlined in Table 9–3.

Jaskiewicz and colleagues in a prospective study using the Rochester criteria found that 2 of 222 neonates who met criteria for a low risk of bacterial infection had serious bacterial disease.[10] In this study the negative predictive value (NPV) was 98.9%, which means that 1.1% of neonates classified as low-risk patients had bacterial infections. In a retrospective study, Ferrara found that 6% of neonates classified as low risk for bacterial infection by the Rochester criteria had serious bacterial infections.[13] Baker et al characterized neonates into low- and

high-risk groups for bacterial infection on the basis of the Philadelphia criteria. The infants in the high-risk group had a significant risk for bacterial infection (18.6%); however, 4.6% of the neonates in the low-risk group also had bacterial infections.[1] Finally, Kadish and colleagues applied both the Philadelphia criteria and the Boston criteria in a retrospective review of the febrile neonate and found that 4% of low-risk neonates had bacterial infection.[3]

LABORATORY TESTING CURRENTLY USED TO EVALUATE FEBRILE NEONATES

Because the physical examination and history alone are poor predictors of invasive bacterial disease, diagnostic testing is essential in helping identity the neonates at risk for life-threatening infection. The commonly used ancillary tests and their utility and limitations are discussed in the following.

Blood Culture

Isolation of bacteria from the blood remains the most specific method used to diagnose

▶ TABLE 9-3. **RISK STRATIFICATION FOR FEBRILE NEONATES**

	Rochester Criteria	Philadelphia Criteria	Boston Criteria
Age	<60 days	29-60 days	28-89 days
Temperature	>38.0°	>38.2°	>38.0°
History and Physical Exam	Term infant No antibiotics No underlying disease Home with mother Normal exam	History not given Normal exam	No immunizations within 48 h No antibiotics within 48 h Normal exam
Laboratory (Defines Lower Risk Patients)	WBC >5000/μL WBC <15,000/μL Absolute band count <1500/μL UA <5WBC/hpf	WBC <15,000/μL Band-neutrophil ratio <0.2 UA <10 WBC/hpf Urine Gram stain negative CSF <8 WBC/hpf Chest x-ray normal	WBC <20,000/μL UA <10 WBC/hpf CSF<10 WBC/hpf Chest x-ray normal
Reported Statistics	Sensitivity 92% NPV 98.9%	Sensitivity 98% NPV 99.7%	Sensitivity—Not available NPV—Not available

Abbreviations: CSF, cerebral spinal fluid; NPV, negative predictive value; UA, urinalysis; WBC, white blood cells.

sepsis in the febrile neonate.[14] It is important to carefully disinfect the skin and collect an appropriate volume of blood in order to accurately detect bacteria in the blood stream. Neonates with implanted vascular disease such as a Hickman catheter should have line and peripheral cultures drawn and include quantitative cultures.

Complete Blood Count (CBC)

Virtually all studies to date rely on the CBC, absolute neutrophil count, and band/neutrophil ratio as a standard part of evaluating the neonate with fever. Many studies have demonstrated that infants greater than 1 month of age with a WBC <15,000/μL and an absolute band count <1500/μL have a lower risk of bacterial infection. Given the fact that many febrile neonates with a normal WBC have bacterial sepsis or meningitis, the CBC and differential on their own are not sufficient to exclude life-threatening infection in this age group.[15,16]

Urine Studies

Urinary tract infections represent the most common bacterial cause of fever in the neonate. In a large prospective study of 1025 infants less than 60 days of age, UTI was diagnosed in 9% of the infants and 21% of uncircumcised males.[17] Although the urinalysis and urine Gram stain are useful screens for detecting UTI, 20% of neonates with a UTI will have a normal urinalysis.[18-20] Urine culture and sensitivity is mandatory in this setting and specimens should be obtained by bladder catheterization or suprapubic aspiration. Bagged urine specimens should be avoided due to the high percentage of contaminated specimens obtained using this technique.[21-23]

Lumbar Puncture

A lumbar puncture should be performed in all febrile neonates given the limited information obtained from the history and physical examination, and the inability of laboratory evaluations such as the CBC to exclude patients with bacterial meningitis.[16] CSF should be sent for culture, Gram stain, and cell count. Appropriate studies should be done to exclude the possibility of herpetic infection (polymerase chain reaction [PCR] for herpes or culture for herpes).

NEW APPROACHES TO IDENTIFY BACTERIAL DISEASE

The ideal early diagnostic test for identifying bacterial infection in the neonate would have a sensitivity of 100% and be readily available within a short time frame. To date no such test is available and our current methods for evaluating the febrile neonate use a combination of tests. Some of the newer diagnostic modalities that may aid in the evaluation of the febrile neonate in the future are discusse dint he following

C-Reactive Protein (CRP)

This protein is synthesized 6 to 8 hours following exposure to damaged tissue or an infective agent with a half-life of 19 hours. The sensitivity for predicting early-onset sepsis (first week of life) is only 47% but increases to 93% to 100% in late-onset sepsis (after 7 days of age).[24,25] The combination of the CRP in conjunction with a CBC and differential had a sensitivity of 97% for predicting early-onset sepsis.[25]

Procalcitonin

Procalcitonin is an acute phase reactant produced by monocytes and hepatocytes within 4 hours after exposure to bacterial endotoxin with a peak at 20 hours postexposure.[26] Several studies have demonstrated that neonates with sepsis or necrotizing enterocolitis have a marked increase in procalcitonin levels.[27] Elevated procalcitonin concentration is superior to any single, currently available acute phase reactant for determining bacterial sepsis with a sensitivity ranging from 87% to 100% in both early- and late-onset sepsis.[27] At present this test is not readily available in hospital laboratories.

Cell Surface Markers

Neutrophil cell surface proteins CD11b and CD64 appear to be promising early markers for detecting early- and late-onset sepsis.[28,29] CD11b is a subunit of the integrin adhesion molecule normally expressed at low levels on neutrophils. In blood culture-proven sepsis, there is a 2- to 4-fold increase in expression of this molecule within a few hours after exposure to bacterial antigens with sensitivity between 86% and 100% in identifying early-onset sepsis. The presence of an elevated CD64 had a sensitivity of 97% and a specificity of 90% in predicting early-onset sepsis.[30] The presence of an elevated neutrophil CD64 in combination with an elevated CRP had a sensitivity of 100% in predicting bacterial sepsis in febrile neonates who subsequently had a positive blood culture.[30] The utility of this testing modality awaits further prospective testing and standardization, and is dependent on availability of flow cytometry, which is not present in many hospitals.

Polymerase Chain Reaction (PCR) Testing

During the past decade there have been many reports of nucleic amplification techniques using PCR to detect the presence of bacterial genomes in the blood. This modality has the potential to be a rapid and sensitive modality for detecting bacterial disease in the neonate and may revolutionize our ability to detect bacterial infection at an early stage. PCR testing has the potential to detect small numbers of bacteria in the patient well before any other testing modality would indicate signs of bacterial infection. The potential sensitivity and specificity of PCR testing is unmatched by any available ancillary test for bacterial infection. To date the primary target of PCR testing for bacterial infection is the 16S rRNA gene, which is highly conserved across all bacterial genomes.[31] Within this gene, there are bacterial species divergent regions that can be targeted to diagnosis the specific bacteria responsible for infection. Golden et al demonstrated 100% sensitivity and 100% specificity in detecting GBS in blood specimens from which a bacterial pathogen was identified by culture.[32] In this study the test was able to detect 100 copies of the GBS genome. The second major benefit of PCR testing is the ability to amplify bacterial genomic specimens and identify the presence of antibiotic resistance genes that are known and have been previously described.[33] In the future we may have the ability to detect bacterial infection and antibiotic resistance patterns within 1 hour of obtaining a blood sample from the patient. Obviously, further study will be needed to confirm the accuracy of this

diagnostic modality and to make the technology available and adaptable in the hospital setting. Given these data and the inability to totally exclude the possibility of bacterial infection with currently available testing, all febrile neonates require a complete sepsis evaluation. This evaluation should include a CBC with differential, blood culture, urinalysis, urine Gram stain and urine culture, and examination of the CSF with cell count, Gram stain, and culture. PCR and cultures for herpes simplex should be obtained if there is a history or maternal genital herpetic lesions, or if CSF pleocytosis is present. A chest x-ray should be obtained if there are clinical signs to suggest pneumonia. Stool cultures should be sent when diarrhea is present along with appropriate testing for rotavirus. Hospitalization and administration of parental antibiotics is indicated for 48 to 72 hours pending culture results. Ampicillin-cefotaxime or ampicillin- gentamycin are the antibiotic combinations generally used in this age group. Acyclovir should be given in cases where herpetic infection is suspected (Table 9–4).

► TABLE 9–4. **EVALUATION AND MANAGEMENT OF FEBRILE NEONATES (TEMP >38°C)**

Evaluation	Management
Detailed history Complete physical exam	Admission for IV antibiotics until culture results available

Laboratory
CBC with differential
Blood culture
CSF cell count, glucose, protein
CSF Gram stain and culture
CSF PCR for herpes or enterovirus
  if indicated
Chest x-ray if indicated
Stool cultures and exam for rotavirus
  (diarrhea)
	Antimicrobial Agents
	  Ampicillin and cefotaxime
	    Ampicillin 100 mg/kg IV q12h <1 wk
	    Cefotaxime 50 mg/kg IV q8h <1 wk
	    Ampicillin 50-100 mg/kg IV q6h >1 wk
	    Cefotaxime 50 mg/kg IV q6h >1 wk
	  Ampicillin and Gentamycin
	    Gentamycin 2.5 mg/kg IV q12h <1 wk
	    Gentamycin 2.5 mg/kg/ IV q8h >1 wk
	  Acyclovir
	    Acyclovir 20 mg/kg IV q8h

► MANAGEMENT

CURRENT THERAPEUTIC STRATEGIES FOR THE FEBRILE NEONATE

In the most recent, large-scale, prospective study of febrile neonates conducted by the Pediatric Research in Office Settings (PROS) Network of the American Academy of Pediatrics, the rate of bacteremia was 3%, 1.2% of febrile neonates had bacterial meningitis, and 4.1% had both bacteremia and meningitis, while 9.9% of febrile neonates had UTI.[34,35]

While medical advances from the past 20 years have decreased the mortality of neonatal CNS infections, the morbidity and long-term sequelae from meningitis have remained relatively unchanged to this day.[36-38] The current conservative standard of clinical practice is partially born from this fact, as well as the inability to identify all febrile neonates with meningitis on the basis of history, physical examination, and current laboratory evaluation. The emergency physician caring for the pediatric population commonly encounters the "rule out meningitis/sepsis" patient. Current practice dictates that infants who present with a fever during the first 28 days of life will be admitted following a sepsis/meningitis workup as noted previously.[39,40] Understanding the epidemiology, pathophysiology, and clinical signs and symptoms of meningitis can aid the emergency physician when faced with atypical presentations of this entity.

BACTERIAL MENINGITIS

Epidemiology

While the morbidity of meningitis has remained relatively constant over recent decades, the incidence and mortality of bacterial meningitis has declined significantly. There are multiple reasons for this decline including prenatal GBS surveillance and subsequent use of peripartum antibiotic prophylaxis, and vaccine development for both Haemophilus influenzae and Streptococcus pneumoniae. Bacterial meningitis is more common during the first 2 years of life and especially during the first month of life. Factors that contribute to the increased risk of meningitis in the neonate include an immature immune system and exposure to a wide set of pathogens via the birth process and from potential nosocomial infections. The current incidence of neonatal bacterial meningitis in the United States has been reported to range from 0.25 of 1000 neonates to 0.32 of 1000 neonates.[41,42] Various historical factors appear to carry higher risk for infections including meningitis, and may aid the clinician in establishing a higher pretest probability in the neonatal patient. Low birth weight,[43,44] prematurity,[45] premature rupture of membranes,[46] maternal infections (herpes, UTI), and neonatal hypoxia have all been associated with an increased risk of infection that include meningitis. As with sepsis, neonatal meningitis can present in the first week of life (early onset) while late-onset meningitis occurs after the first week of life. Meningitis can occur in the absence of sepsis but is more commonly seen in conjunction with sepsis. Several studies have suggested that 25% of septic neonates have concomitant meningitis.[47] Early-onset disease is historically believed to result from vertical transmission from the mother with late-onset meningitis resulting from vertical transmission and infection spread from outside contacts.

In a study monitoring cases of neonatal meningitis from 1979 to 1998, GBS was the most common pathogen (50% of neonates with meningitis) and *E coli* was found in approximately 25% of cases.[48] *Listeria* is a significant, if less common, pathogen responsible for meningitis and most antibiotic regimens include ampicillin/cefotaxime to provide *Listeria* coverage. Other important but less frequently isolated bacteria are in listed in Table 9–1.

Pathophysiology

The immature immune system of the neonate is characterized by inefficient functioning of the complement, opsonizing, and phagocytic processes necessary for cellular and humoral defense mechanisms against encapsulated bacteria and it is responsible in part for the increased risk of meningitis in the neonate[49,50] here have been several proposed avenues for bacterial violation of the blood brain barrier including transmission via the choroid plexus and through skull defects along the path of the olfactory nerves[51]

The basic model to explain the pathophysiology of meningitis involves host exposure to immunogenic particles on bacterial cell walls (peptidoglycan, endotoxins, and lipopolysaccharides), causing activation of the host immune response and release of cytokines and acute phase reactants resulting in local infiltration of leukocytes into the meningeal space, increased permeability of the blood brain barrier, and subsequent direct cellular toxicity to the brain tissue.[52] One study conducted by Tuomanen et al was able to reproduce clinical meningitis in an animal model using only immunogenic bacterial particles without the presence of live bacteria.[53]

Clinical Manifestations

Clinical signs and symptoms are nonspecific and often mirror septicemia.[53] One of the common initial presenting features of a meningitis neonate is temperature instability. While high fever has been a hallmark of bacterial infection, this is not often seen in neonatal meningitis. Hypothermia is often present, but more commonly in the premature infant.[54] Neurologic complaints include irritability, poor feeding, seizures, and lethargy[54] (Table 9–2). In rare cases the initial complaint of respiratory distress and diarrhea have also been reported. Evaluation of the asymptomatic patient (afebrile, happy, playful, normal feeding, and no irritability) with a high-risk stratification for sepsis/meningitis secondary to prematurity, hypoxia, very low birth weight, and galactosemia should be carefully evaluated at the discretion of the individual clinician.

Diagnosis

A high index of suspicion is necessary in the evaluation of the neonate in the ED. A full septic work up is indicated on all febrile neonates and classically consists of blood culture, urine culture, and CSF culture from lumbar puncture with examination of CSF cell count, CSF Ggram stain, CSF culture, glucose, and protein. Several studies have found the normal values for neonatal CSF to differ from those of adults and can vary with gestational age and birth weight.[55-58]

Treatment should be administered immediately once the appropriate cultures have been obtained and should not be withheld until the laboratory results are available. The most common entities responsible for causing sepsis and meningitis in the neonate are discussed below.

GBS MENINGITIS

Group B *streptococcus* is gram-positive cocci that colonizes the gastrointestinal tract and genital tract in adults and the respiratory tract in newborn infants; it is responsible for life-threatening sepsis and meningitis in the neonate.[59] Infants acquire the organism in utero and during the birth process. After birth, infants can acquire the organism from household contacts. Early-onset disease (sepsis-meningitis) is defined as occurring during the first 7 days and represents maternally acquired disease, whereas late-onset disease occurring after 7 days is felt to represent extrauterine infection. The incidence of early-onset disease has decreased over the past 25 years from 1.8 in 1000 live births in 1990, to 0.34 cases in 1000 live births in 2004.[60] The decrease is due in large part to effective screening of pregnant woman for GBS and treating colonized woman with antibiotics. The incidence of late-onset disease has remained unchanged over the past 25 years at 0.35 cases in 1000 live births.[60] GBS serotypes are defined by the presence of specific polysaccharides and proteins on the cell surface. In the United States, serotypes IA, III, and V account for most infections in the neonatal population.[60,61] In early-onset disease these 3 serotypes account for 74% to 98% of documented infections with GBS.[61] Similar results are described for late-onset disease (83% to 94% of GBS infections). The type III serotype is responsible for most late-onset disease and is more likely to cause meningitis.[61]

HERPES INFECTIONS

Clinical Presentation

Herpes simplex virus (HSV) can cause life-threatening, disseminated, multi-organ and CNS infection in the neonate. Infected infants have 1 of 3 clinical presentations: infection localized to the skin, eyes, and mucous membranes; meningitis; and multi-organ disseminated disease.[62,63] Many infants with HSV acquired in the neonatal period have a normal physical examination and no manifestations of infection. The peak incidence of CNS disease occurs between 10 and 17 days of life but can occur any time during the first 4 weeks of life. The initial signs of infection are often nonspecific and may rapidly progress to hypotension, apnea, and disseminated intravascular coagulation.

Diagnostic Testing

Diagnostic testing should include culture of skin or mouth lesions with polymerase chain reaction assay of the CSF.[64] Disseminated infections typically present in the first week of life.

Management

Acyclovir administration should be promptly administered if there is any clinical suspicion for HSV infection. The current recommendations for treatment are acyclovir given at 20 mg/kg/dose IV q8h for 14 days if the disease is limited to the skin, eyes, and mouth, and 21 days for meningitis or disseminated infection.[65]

ENTEROVIRAL INFECTIONS

Epidemiology & Pathophysiology

Human enteroviruses are found throughout the world and are transmitted between individuals via the fecal-oral route. The nonpolio enteroviruses viruses, including Echovirus and Coxsackievirus, are responsible for a wide spectrum of clinical presentations and disease in all patients including neonates. Coxsackievirus serotypes 2 through 5 and echovirus 11 are most frequently associated with overwhelming and life-threatening infections in the neonate.[66] The majority of women (70%) with infected newborns have a febrile viral illness during the week of delivery.[67] Transmission of the virus to the infant may occur via infected cervical secretions or from maternal viremia.[68]

Clinical Presentation

Many neonates with enteroviral infection will only have fever, rash, asymptomatic hepatitis, or aseptic meningitis with complete recovery; however, some infants will develop life-threatening myocarditis or fulminant live failure. Most infants acquire this infection in utero and during the birth process. Symptoms of illness typically develop between days 3 and 7 of life and may include fever, irritability, and poor feeding, which resolves in a few days in many infants.[69] Some infants (1 of 3) who have these early symptoms will develop generalized infection with life-threatening complications. Systemic enteroviral infections typically occur in 2 specific clinical entities. Neonatal hepatitis caused by enteroviral infection usually presents in explosive and life-threatening fashion characterized by sudden onset of hepatomegaly with jaundice, significant bleeding due to live failure, and coagulation factor deficiency and shock.[67] The second entity is myocarditis with heart failure as manifested by cardiomegaly, tachypnea, and hepatomegaly.

Management

The current management of infants with enteroviral infections with bleeding and fulminate liver failure is vigorous supportive care combined with transfusion of fresh frozen plasma, red cells, and platelets combined with administration of vitamin K (1 mg IV). Administration of diuretics and isotropic agents may be required in patients with heart failure. Experimental therapies include the use of IV IgG with reported improvement in one case.[70]

▶ SUMMARY

Although sepsis and meningitis are uncommon occurrences in the neonatal period, these entities remain a significant risk for morbidity and mortality in this population. A focused and accurate history including the maternal history and the perinatal clinical history, and a careful physical examination will dictate the need for septic workup with prompt institution of appropriate antibiotic and antiviral therapy.

References

1. Baker MD, Bell LM. Unpredictability of serious bacterial illness in febrile infants from birth to 1 month of age. *Arch Pediatr Adolesc Med.* 1999;153(5):508-511.

2. Chiu CH, Lin TY, Bullard MJ. Identification of febrile neonates unlikely to have bacterial infections. *Pediatr Infect Dis J.* 1997;16(1):59-63.

3. Kadish HA, Loveridge B, Tobey J, et al. Applying outpatient protocols in febrile infants 1-28 days of age can the threshold be lowered? *Clin Pediatr.* 2000;39(2):81-88.

4. Lin F-YC, Phillips JB III, Azimi PH, et al. Level of maternal antibody required to protect neonates against early onset disease caused by Group B streptococcus IA: A multicenter, epidemiology study. *J Infect Disease.* 2001;184:1022.

5. Lewis DB, Wilson CB. Developmental immunology and the role of host defenses to neonatal susceptibility to in infection. In: Remington JS, Klein JO, eds. *Infectious Diseases of the Fetus and Newborn Infant.* 5th ed. Philadelphia, PA: WB Saunders; 2001:25-138.

6. Levy O. Impaired innate immunity at birth: deficiency of bacteriacidal/permeability-increasing protein (BPI) in the neutrophils of newborns. *Pediatr Res.* 2002;51:667.

7. Craig JV, Lancaster GA, Taylor S, et al. Infrared ear thermometry compared with rectal thermometry in children: a systemic review. *Lancet.* 2002;360:603-609.

8. Craig JV, Lancaster GA, Williamson PR, et al. Temperature at the axilla compared with rectal thermometry in children: a systemic review. *Br Med J.* 2000;329:1174-1178.

9. Grover G, Berkowitz CD, Lewis RJ, et al. The effects of bundling on infant temperatures. *Pediatrics.* 1994;94:669.

10. Jaskiewicz JA, McCarthy CA, Richardson AC, et al. Febrile infants at low risk for serious bacterial infection: an appraisal of the Rochester criteria and implications for management. *Pediatrics.* 1994;94(3):390-396.

11. Baker MD, Bell LM, Avner JR. Outpatient management without antibiotics of fever in selected infants. *N Engl J Med.* 1993;329:1437-1441.

12. Baskin MN, O'Rourke EJ, Fleisher GR. Outpatient treatment of febrile infants 28 to 89 days if age with intramuscular administration of ceftriaxone. *J Pediat.* 1992;120:22-27.

13. Ferrera PC, Bartfield JM, Snyder HS. Neonatal fever: Utility of the Rochester criteria in determining low risk for serious bacterial infections. *Am J Emerg Med.* 1997;15(3):299-302.

14. Ng PC. Diagnostic markers of infection in neonates. *Arch Dis Child Fetal Neonatal Ed.* 2004;89:F229-F235.

15. Bonsu BK, Harper MB. Identifying febrile young infants with bacteremia: Is the peripheral white cell count an accurate screen? *Ann Emerg Med.* 2003;42(2):216-225.

16. Bonsu BK, Harper MB. Utility of the peripheral white blood cell count for identifying sick young infants who need lumbar puncture. *Ann Emerg Med.* 2003;41(2):206-214.

17. Zorc JJ, Levine DA, Platt SL, et al. Clinical and demographic factors associated with urinary tract infections in young febrile infants. *Pediatrics.* 2005;116:664.

18. Bachur R, Harper MB. Reliability of the urinalysis for predicting urinary tract infections in young febrile children. *Arch Pediatr Adolesc Med.* 2001;155:60-65.

19. Gorelick MH, Shaw KN. Screening tests for urinary tract infections in children: a meta-analysis. *Pediatrics.* 1999;104(5):E54.

20. Shaw KN, McGowan KL, Gorelick MH, et al. Screening for urinary tract infection in infants in the emergency department: which test is best? *Pediatrics.* 1998;101(6):e1.

21. Committee on Quality improvement, Subcommittee on Urinary Tract Infection. Practice Parameter. The diagnosis, treatment and evaluation of the initial urinary tract infection in febrile infants and young children. *Pediatrics.* 1999;103(4):843-852.

22. McGillivray D, Mok E, Mulronney E, et al. A head-to-head comparison: "clean-void" bag catheter urinalysis in the diagnosis of urinary tract infection in young children. *J Pediatr.* 2005;147(4):451-456.

23. Schroeder AR, Newman TB, Wasserman RC, et al. Choice of urine collection methods for the diagnosis of urinary tract infection in young, febrile infants. *Arch Pediatr Adolesc Med.* 2005;159(10):915-922.

24. Fowlie PW, Schmidt B. Diagnostic tests for bacterial infection from birth to 90 days: a systemic review. *Arch Dis Child Fetal Neonatal Ed.* 1998;78:F92-F98.

25. Garland SM, Bowman ED. Reappraisal of C-reactive Protein as a screening tool for diagnosis for neonatal sepsis. *Pathology.* 2003;35:240-243.

26. Dandona P, Nix D, Wilson MF, et al. Procalcitonin increase after endotoxin injection in normal subjects. *J Clin Endocrinol Metab.* 1994;79:1605-1608

27. Guibourdenche J, Bedu A, Petzold L, et al. Biochemical markers of neonatal sepsis: value of Procalcitonin in the mergency setting. *Ann Clin Biochem.* 2002;39:130-135.

28. Fjaertoft G, Hakansson L, Ewald U, et al. Neutrophils from term and and preterm newborn express the high affinity Fc gamma-receptor I (CD64) during bacterial infections. *Pediatr Res.* 1999;45:871-876.

29. Weirich E, Rabin RL, Maldonado Y, et al. Neutrophil CD11b expression as a diagnostic marker for early-onset neonatal infection. *J Pediatr.* 1998;132:445-451.

30. Ng PC, Li G, Chui KM, et al. Neutrophil CD64 is a sensitive diagnostic marker for early-onset neonatal infection. *Pediatr Res.* 2004;56:796-803.

31. Maiwald M. Broad-range PCR for the detection and identification of bacteria. In Persing DH, Tenover FC, Versalovic J, eds. *Molecular Microbiology: Diagnostic Principles and Practice.* 2nd ed. Washington, DC: American Society of Microbiology; 2004:379-390.

32. Golden SM, Stamilio DM, Faux BM, et al. Evaluation of a real-time fluorescent PCR assay for the rapid detection of Group B Streptococci in neonatal blood. *Diagn Microbiol Infect Dis.* 2004;50:7-13.

33. Jaffe RI, Lane JD, Albury SV, et al. Rapid extraction from and direct identification in clinical samples of methicillin-resistant staphylococci using the PCR. *J Clin Microbiol.* 2000;38:3407-3412.

34. Pantell R, Newman T, Bernzweig J, et al. Management and outcomes of care of fever in early infancy. *JAMA.* 2004;291:1203-1212.

35. Newman T, Bernzsweig J, Takayama J, et al. Urine testing and urinary tract infections in febrile infants seen in office settings: The Pediatric Research in Office Settings' Febrile Infant Study. *Arch Pediatr Adolesc Med.* 2002;156:44-54.

36. Bell AH, Brown D, Halliday HL, et al. Meningitis in the newborn—a 14 year review. *Arch Dis Child.* 1989;64:873-874.

37. Harvey D, Holt DE, Bedford H. Bacterial meningitis in the newborn: a prospective study of mortality and morbidity. *Semin Perinatol.* 1999;23:218-225.

38. Wegner JD, Hightower AW, Facklam RR, Gaventa S, Broome CV. Bacterial Meningitis Study Group. Bacterial meningitis in the United States, 1986: report of a multistate surveillance study. *J Infect Dis*. 1990;162;1316-1323.

39. Berger JE ed, Deitschel CH Jr, ed. Committee on Medical Liability, American Academy of Pediatrics. *Medical Liability for Pediatricians*. 6th ed. 2004:163, 169.

40. Karcz A, Holbrook J, Auerbach BS, et al. Preventability of malpractice claims in emergency medicine: a closed claims study. *Ann Emerg Med*. 1990;19(8):865-873.

41. Bell AH, Brown D, Halliday HL, et al. Meningitis in the newborn—a 14 year review. *Arch Dis Child*. 1989;64:873-874.

42. de Louvois J. Acute bacterial meningitis in the newborn. *J Antimicrob Chemother*. 1994;34(Suppl A):61.

43. Escobar GJ, De-kun L, Armstrong MA, et al. for the Neonatal Infection Study Group. Neonatal sepsis workups in infants ≥2000 grams at birth: a population-based study. *Pediatrics*. 2000;106(2):256-263.

44. Fanaroff AA, Korones SB, Wright LL, et al. The incidence, presenting features, risk factors and significance of septicemia in low birth weight infants. *Pediatr Infect Dis J*. 1998;17(7):593-598.

45. Voora S, Srinivasan G, Lilien LD, et al. Fever in full-term newborns in the first four days of life. *Pediatrics*. 1982;69:40-44.

46. St. Geme Jr JW, Murray DL, Carter J, et al. Perinatal infection after prolonged rupture of membranes: an analysis of risk and management. *J Pediatr*. 1984;104:608-613.

47. Feigin RD. Diagnosis and management of meningitis. *Pediatr Infect Dis J*. 1992;11(9):785-814.

48. Klinger G, Chin CN, Beyene J, Perlman M. Predicting the outcome of neonatal bacterial meningitis. *Pediatrics*. 2000;106:477-482.

49. Schelonka RL, Infante AJ. Neonatal immunology. *Semin Perinatol*. 1998;22:2-14.

50. Berger M. Complement deficiency and neutrophil dysfunction as risk factors for bacterial infection in newborns and the role of granulocyte transfusion in therapy. *Rev Infect Dis*. 1990;12(Suppl 4):S1401-S1409.

51. Weber JR, Tuomanen EI. Cellular damage in bacterial meningitis: an interplay of bacterial and host driven toxicity. *J Neuroimmunol*. 2007;184(1–2):45-52.

52. Volpe JJ. Bacterial and fungal intracranial infections. In: Volpe JJ, ed. *Neurology of the Newborn*. 4th ed. Philadelphia, PA: WB Saunders Co.; 2001:774-781.

53. Tuomanen E, Liu H, Hengstler B, Zak O, Tomasz A. The induction of meningeal inflammation by components of the pneumococcal cell wall. *J Infect Dis*. 1985;151:859–868.

54. Pong A, Bradley JS. Bacterial meningitis and the newborn infant. *Infect Dis Clin North Am*. 1999;13:711.

55. Anderson SG, Gilbert GL. Neonatal gram negative meningitis: A 10-year review, with reference to outcome and relapse of infection. *J Paediatr Child Health*. 1990;26:212-216.

56. Palazzi DL, Klein JO, Baker CJ. Bacterial sepsis and meningitis. In: Remington JS, Klein JO, Wilson CB, Baker CJ, eds. *Infectious Diseases of the Fetus and Newborn Infant*. 6th ed. Philadelphia, PA: Elsevier Saunders; 2006:247.

57. Sarff LD, Platt LD, McCracken GH. Comparison of high risk neonates with and without meningitis. *J Pediatr*. 1976;88:473-477.

58. Gerdes JS. Diagnosis and management of bacterial infections in the neonate. *Pediatr Clin North Am*. 2004;51(4):939-959.

59. Edwards MS, Nizet V, Baker CJ. Group B Streptococcal Infections. In: Remington JS, Klein JO, Wilson CB, Baker CJ, eds. *Infectious Diseases of the Fetus and Newborn Infant*. 6th ed. Philadelphia, PA: Elsevier Saunders; 2006:403.

60. Centers for Disease Control and Prevention (CDC). Early-onset and late-onset neonatal group B streptococcal disease—United States 1996-2004. *MMWR Morb Mortal Wkly Rep*. 2005;54:1205-1208.

61. Lin FY, Clemons JD, Azimi PH, et al. Capsular polysaccharide types of group B streptococcal isolates from neonates with early-onset systemic infection. *J Infect Dis*. 1998;177:790.

62. Kimberlin DW, Lin CY, Jacibs RF, et al. Natural history of neonatal herpes simplex infections in the acyclovir era. *Pediatrics*. 2005;115:795.

63. Kohl S. Neonatal herpes simplex infection. *Clin Perinatol*. 1997;24:129.

64. Kimberlin DW, Lakeman FD, Arvin AM, et al. Application of the polymerase chain reaction to the diagnosis and management of neonatal

herpes simplex virus disease: National Institute of Allergy and Infectious Diseases Collaborative Study Group. *J Infect Dis*. 1996;174:1162.

65. American Academy of Pediatrics. Herpes simplex. In: Pickering LK, ed. *Red Book: 2006 Report of the Committee on Infectious Diseases*. 27th ed. Elk Grove Village, IL: Author; 2006:361.

66. Kinney JS, McCray E, Kaplan JE, et al. Risk factors associated with echovirus 11 infection in a hospital nursery. *Pediatr Infect Dis*. 1986;5:192.

67. Modlin JF. Perinatal echovirus infection: insights from a literature of 61 cases of serious infection and 16 outbreaks in nurseries. *Rev Infect Dis*. 1986;8:918.

68. Reyes MP, Osrea EM, Roskamp J, Lerner AM. Disseminated echovirus 11 disease following antenatal maternal infection with a virus-positive cervix and virus-negative gastro-intestinal tract. *J Med Virol*. 1983;12:155.

69. Kaplan MH, Klein SW, McPhee J, Harper RG. Group B coxsackievirus infections in infants younger than three months of age: a serious childhood illness. *Rev Infect Dis*. 1983;5:1019.

70. Johnston JM, Overall JC, Jr. Intravenous immunoglobulin in disseminated neonatal echovirus 11 infection. *Pediatr Infect Dis J*. 1989;8:254.

CHAPTER 10

Hematologic Emergencies in the Neonate

P. David Sadowitz, MD

Trisha Tavares, MD

The neonatal period is marked by a series of rapid physiologic changes in the hematopoietic and coagulation pathways as the infant adapts to the extrauterine environment. For a variety of reasons the neonate is at significant for risk for life-threatening anemia or hemorrhage during this time. This chapter summarizes the key diagnostic and therapeutic pathways needed to carefully evaluate the neonate presenting to the emergency department (ED) with anemia or bleeding.

▶ ANEMIA

The newborn period is characterized by a rapid transition from the hypoxic environment present in the uterus to the extra-uterine setting. This physiologic change leads to rapid alterations in several organ systems including the pulmonary, cardiovascular, and hematopoietic systems. In the absence of the hypoxia present within the uterus, neonatal erythrocyte production rapidly decreases during the first

several days after birth with changes in hemoglobin concentration in the first month of life, which are summarized in Table 10–1.[1-3]

Anemia is defined as the inability of circulating red cells to meet the oxygen demands of the body. The etiology of anemia can result from 1 of 3 causes: failure of red cell production, hemolysis, or blood loss. The need for rapid diagnosis and treatment dictates that an organized workup be rapidly and precisely undertaken. The key historical elements, physical examination findings, and diagnostic

▶ TABLE 10–1. HEMOGLOBIN AND HEMATOCRIT CHANGES AFTER BIRTH

Age	Hemoglobin	Hematocrit
Birth	18.4 g/dL	58
Day 3	17.8 g/dL	55
Day 7	17.0 g/dL	54
Day 14	15.6 g/dL	46
Day 21	14.2 g/dL	43
Day 28	12.7 g/dL	36

testing in the neonate with anemia are out-lined below and summarized in Table 10–2.

HISTORY

The history can be a powerful and useful tool in the diagnosis and treatment of neonatal anemia. A complete maternal history is vital in this setting. Maternal conditions predating the pregnancy are important to note and would include a history of any bleeding disorders or collagen vascular disease such as lupus. Important events during the pregnancy would include bleeding from the vagina during pregnancy, placenta previa, placental abruption,

▶ **TABLE 10–2. KEY FINDINGS IN THE NEONATE WITH ANEMIA**

History	Laboratory Evaluation	Physical Examination
Family history	CBC/differential/platelet count	ABCs
Ethnicity	Red cell morphology	Jaundice
Maternal history (ie, infections, chronic diseases, medications)	Reticulocyte count	Petechiae
	Coombs test	Hepatosplenomegaly
Obstetrical history	PT/PTT/TT	
Neonatal disease (eg, malignancy, hemophilia)		

Coombs Negative	Coombs Positive
Elevated Reticulocyte Count	ABO-Rh incompatibility
Red Cell Morphologic Abnormalities	Maternal autoimmune hemolytic
Spherocytes	anemia
Stomatocytes	
Elliptocytes	
Fragmented red cells	
Infection	
CBV, Enterovirus, herpes, HIV	
Bacterial infection	
Syphilis	
Toxoplasmosis	
Red Cell Enzyme Deficiency	
G6PD deficiency	
Pyryvate kinase deficiency	
Miscellaneous	
Galactosemia	
Hemoglobinopathy (alpha chain and gamma chain)	
Decreased Reticulocyte Count	
Bone Marrow Failure	
Blackfan diamond syndrome	
Fanconi aplastic anemia	
Sideroblastic anemia	
Leukemia, metastatic tumor	
Nutrition	
Maternal vitamin B12 deficiency	
Chronic blood loss (fetal)	
Maternal iron deficiency	

caesarian section or twin delivery. Other important questions to ask regarding the delivery would include early cord clamping or sudden traumatic birth.[4] The family history and ethnicity may be significant in determining the etiology of neonatal anemia. For example, there is a high prevalence of G6PD deficiency in populations from the Mediterranean region and in the Black population in Africa, while populations from Southeast Asia have a high incidence of alpha thalassemia, which could produce anemia in the neonate. The presence of anemia in other family members in conjunction with jaundice, gallstones, and splenectomy might suggest the diagnosis of hereditary spherocytosis. The age at which anemia presents in the neonate gives an important clue to the cause of the anemia. Severe anemia in the first 1 to 2 days of life is almost always the result of hemorrhage or severe ABO-Rh incompatibility. Anemia presenting after the first 2 days of life is usually caused by hemolysis from ABO and Rh incompatibility and is characterized by jaundice and anemia.

PHYSICAL EXAMINATION

A careful physical examination may give important clues to the etiology of the anemia. A rapid assessment of vital signs (ABCs) is imperative, as the presence of tachycardia, tachypnea, and hypotension may indicate a rapid loss of circulating blood volume from hemolysis or acute blood loss and requires immediate resuscitative efforts. Skin examination may reveal the presence of pallor or jaundice that can be seen with blood loss and hemolytic anemia, respectively. The presence of hepatosplenomegaly can be seen with hemolytic processes but also is seen with congenital viral infection and malignancies. Abnormalities involving the extremities such as absent thumbs or absent radii are seen with Fanconi aplastic anemia, characterized by marrow dysfunction with deficient production of red cells.[5-10]

DIAGNOSTIC TESTS

The initial laboratory evaluation should include a complete CBC with red cell indices, white cell count with differential, platelet count, prothrombin time (PT), partial thromboplastin time (PTT), and thromboplastin time (TT) if bleeding is present, blood type and Coombs test, reticulocyte count, bilirubin (direct and indirect), and a careful review of the smear for morphologic red cell abnormalities. If the reticulocyte count is elevated, a hemolytic process or hemorrhage represents the most likely etiology. If the reticulocyte count is low in the face of severe anemia, this finding suggests a failure of the marrow to produce adequate numbers of red cells.

A second consideration in the neonate with low or absent reticulocytes is the presence of a marrow infiltrative process such as leukemia. A positive Coombs test identifies infants with antibody-mediated destruction of the red cells. These antibodies are produced in the mother (IgG subclass), cross the placenta, and bind to the fetal red cells with resultant destruction of these cells. In most case these antibodies are produced in response to ABO or Rh incompatibilities between the mother and fetus. On rare occasions the mother may have unrecognized autoimmune hemolytic anemia, which leads to transfer of maternal antibody to the neonate and hemolytic anemia.

The smear should be carefully examined for morphologic abnormalities. If there are numerous spherocytes on the smear and if the Coombs test is negative, the diagnosis of hereditary spherocytosis is suggested (Figure 10–1). Numerous elliptocytes on the peripheral smear suggests the diagnosis of hereditary elliptocytosis (Figure 10–2).

The presence of hypochromic red cells seen on smear with a corresponding low MCV <95 fl suggests chronic fetal-maternal hemorrhage but can also be seen with alpha thalassemia trait. Infants with sudden onset of severe anemia, normal red cell indices, and

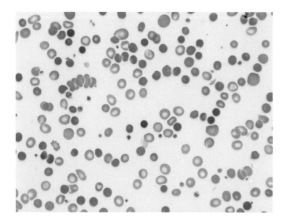

Figure 10–1. Spherocytes.

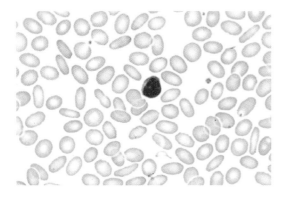

Figure 10–2. Elliptocytes. *Source:* From Lichtman MA, Beutler E, Kipps TJ, et al. Williams' Hematology, 7ed, 2006, New York, NY: McGraw-Hill.

absence of jaundice have hemorrhage until proven otherwise. Typically infants with hemorrhage present to the ED with pallor and signs of impending hypovolemic shock, which include tachycardia, tachypnea, delayed capillary refill, skin mottling, and hypotension. The usual sites for hemorrhage include the head (cephalohematoma), liver, spleen, and, rarely, lung. In today's world the diagnosis of nonaccidental trauma (NAT) must be considered in the neonate presenting to the ED with hypovolemic shock and evidence of hemorrhage. Infants with jaundice and hemolytic

anemia may be infected by a variety of organisms including cytomegalovirus, herpes, toxoplasmosis, syphilis, or bacterial agents. As discussed previously, disseminated intravascular coagulation (DIC) can present in this setting with anemia as a byproduct. The most common entities associated with anemia are briefly discussed below and are summarized in Table 10–3.

DIFFERENTIAL DIAGNOSIS

Decreased Red Cell Production

Neonates with anemia caused by decreased red cell production represent a minority of patients. The hallmark of this diagnosis is a low or absent reticulocyte count in the presence of anemia.

Congenital Viral Infection

Parvovirus B19 is a single-stranded DNA virus that can produce disease in adults and children and is the etiologic agent in erythema infectiosum ("fifth disease").[11,12] Parvovirus B19 preferentially infects rapidly dividing cells and is cytotoxic for erythroid progenitor cells.[12-18] Maternal infection with parvovirus B19 during pregnancy may lead to fetal loss with the greatest in the first 20 weeks of the pregnancy.[17,18] Infection of the fetal red cells can produce severe anemia and lead to nonimmune hydrops fetalis. The diagnosis of parvovirus B19 infection can be accurately established by polymerase chain reaction (PCR) for the parvovirus genome.[19-21] This diagnosis should be considered in the neonatal period in an infant with anemia and absent reticulocyte count. Transfusion support may be required in neonates with severe anemia until red cell production resumes.

Congenital Marrow Dysfunction

Diamond-Blackfan anemia (DBA) is a heterogeneous mix of pure red cell aplasias

▶ TABLE 10–3. **ETIOLOGY OF NEONATAL ANEMIA**

Bleeding	Increased Red Cell Destruction	Decreased Red Cell Production
Prior to Delivery	**Immune Mediated**	**Infection**
Acute and chronic fetal maternal hemorrhage	ABO incompatibility	HIV
Acute and chronic fetal-placental hemorrhage	Rh incompatibility	Parvovirus
	Minor blood group incompatibility	Rubella
Acute and chronic twin-twin hemorrhage	Maternal autoimmune hemolytic anemia	Cytomegalovirus
Traumatic amniocentesis	Drug-induced hemolytic anemia	Bacterial
Umbilical vein sampling in utero	**Anatomic**	**Nutrition**
	Hemolysis on abnormal heart valves	Maternal vitamin B12 deficiency
Maternal trauma	Central line-induced hemolysis	Maternal iron deficiency
At Delivery	Renal artery stenosis	Maternal folate deficiency
Placenta abruption	Aortic stenosis	**Marrow Dysfunction**
Placenta previa	**Infection**	Diamond-Blackfan anemia
Velamentous cord insertion	HIV	Fanconi aplastic anemia
Rupture of a normal or abnormal umbilical cord	CMV	Congenital leukemia
	Rubella	Congenital neuro-blastoma with marrow replacement
Hemorrhage Following Delivery	Herpes	
	Toxoplasmosis	
Cephalohematoma	Syphilis	
Subgaleal hematoma	Bacterial	
Intracranial bleed	**DIC**	
DIC	Bacterial/viral/fungal infections	
Liver, spleen, adrenal, or renal trauma	Microangiopathic hemolytic anemia	
	Cavernous hemangioma (Kasabach-Merritt syndrome)	
Pulmonary hemorrhage	**Red Cell Membrane Abnormalities**	
Line accidents (umbilical, arterial)	Hereditary spherocytosis	
	Hereditary elliptocytosis	
Neonate with hemophilia-factor deficiencies	Hereditary stomatocytosis	
	Red Cell Enzyme Deficiencies	
	G6PD deficiency	
	Pyryvate kinase deficiency	
	Hemoglobinopathy	
	Alpha thalassemia syndromes	
	Gamma thalassemia	
	Metabolic Abnormalities	
	Galactosemia	
	Drug Induced	
	Depicted	
	Sulfa drugs (G6PD deficiency)	

that typically presents in the first year of life and is characterized by the presence of a macrocytic anemia, reticulocytopenia, and a marrow devoid of red cell precursors.[22,23]

Thirty-five percent of patients will have the diagnosis established in the first month of life on presentation to the primary care physician or ED.[23] Physical abnormalities are present in one-third of patients and include short stature, thumb abnormalities, congenital heart disease, short or webbed neck, cleft palate, and ocular abnormalities.[23,24] The pathogenesis of DBA is uncertain. Most investigators believe that the erythroid progenitor cell is unable to proliferate.[22,24-32] The diagnosis should be suspected in the neonate with macrocytic anemia, reticulocytopenia, and the morphologic abnormalities noted previously.

Fanconi Aplastic Anemia

Fanconi aplastic anemia is an autosomal recessive marrow disorder leading to marrow failure and increased risk for malignancy.[5-10] To date 13 genes have been identified, which are widely dispersed among several chromosomes including the X chromosome.[31] Many of the normal genes have tumor suppressor activity that includes maintaining genomic stability, promoting DNA repair, and maintaining apoptosis.[32] Characteristic morphologic changes are seen in two-thirds of neonates, including elfin facies, skin hyperpigmentation, café-au-lait spots, renal abnormalities, and thumb-radius abnormalities. The diagnosis is confirmed by the presence of increased chromosomal breakage in lymphocytes in the presence of DNA cross-linking agents such as mitomycin C or diepoxybutane. Five percent of children are diagnosed in the first year of life and the diagnosis should be suspected in the neonate with macrocytic anemia and the described physical abnormalities.

Malignancy

Congenital malignancies such as leukemia or metastatic neuroblastoma may present with anemia and low reticulocyte count. Typically these patients have hepatosplenomegaly on physical examination. Nucleated red cells may be present on the peripheral smear and immature white cells will be present in neonates with leukemia (Figure 10–3).

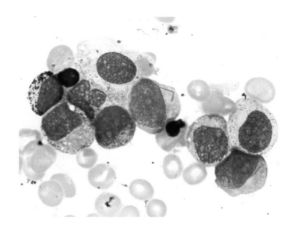

Figure 10–3. Leukemic cells and nucleated red cells.

Bleeding

The neonate can experience bleeding prior to birth, during delivery, and following delivery (Table 10–4). Selected entities are briefly discussed below.

Bleeding Prior to Delivery

Fetal-maternal bleeding occurs in 50% of pregnancies and can occur throughout the pregnancy, but in the vast majority, the bleeding is insignificant and does not result in anemia for the newborn. Approximately 1 of 400 pregnancies have significant bleeding (>30 mL) resulting in significant anemia in 30% of affected infants and most commonly occurs just prior to birth.[33,34] The source of the bleeding is typically via the placenta and chorionic villi.

Twin-twin transfusion can occur in up to 20% of twin gestations. This entity occurs as the result of placental anastamoses that allows rapid transfer of blood between the twins. There is a significant risk of mortality in this setting; this syndrome causes 15% of prenatal mortality in twins.[35,36]

Bleeding During Delivery

Obstetrical complications can lead to life-threatening bleeding and anemia. Placental

▶ TABLE 10-4. **ETIOLOGY OF NEONATAL BLEEDING**

Prior to Birth	Bleeding at Delivery	Internal Hemorrhage
Fetal-Maternal	**Rupture Normal Umbilical Cord**	Intracranial
Traumatic amniocentesis	Precipitous delivery	Cephalohematoma
Chorioangioma of the	Cord entanglement	Subgaleal hematoma
placenta	**Rupture Abnormal Umbilical Cord**	Adrenal-retroperitoneal
Use of oxytocin	Varices	Liver rupture
Manual placenta extraction	Aneurysm	Splenic rupture
Spontaneous	Aberrant vessels in the cord	Pulmonary
Fetal-Placental	Velamentous cord insertion	
Placental hematoma	**Placental Laceration During C-Section**	
Cesarean section	**Placenta Previa**	
Tight nuchal cord	**Abruptio Placenta**	
Twin-Twin Bleed	**Vasa Previa**	

rupture and cord malformations have also been associated with severe intrapartum bleeding. Velamentous insertion of the cord complicates 1% of all pregnancies and is associated with an increased risk of bleeding. In this entity the vessels exit the umbilical cord and insert into the placenta with no protection from the cord. These vessels are therefore fragile and subject to tearing during delivery.[37,38] Placenta previa, vas previa (placental vessels lying across the cervical os), and placental abruption carry an increased risk for bleeding and vas previa is associated with a high mortality rate.[39,40]

Birth-Process Bleeding
The birth process itself can be a traumatic event and lead to internal hemorrhage in the newborn. Subgaleal bleeding and cephalohematoma are the most common sites of birth-process hemorrhage. Subgaleal bleeds can extend throughout the soft tissues of scalp and produce life-threatening anemia, while cephalohematoma is well contained by the periosteum and rarely produces life-threatening bleeding.[41] Intracranial bleeding is uncommon in full-term deliveries but can occur and should be suspected in the apneic, lethargic newborn with a tense fontanel. Emergent CT scan is indicated in these settings. Less common sites of internal

hemorrhage include liver, spleen, adrenal glands, and lungs.

Bleeding After Birth
Nonaccidental trauma must be included in the differential diagnosis of the neonate who presents to the ED with unexplained bruising or internal bleeding involving the CNS, liver, spleen, or lung. DIC, hemophilia and other bleeding disorders will be discussed separately.

Anemia—Hemolytic

Hemolytic anemia in the first few weeks of life is a common entity and can occur as the result of intrinsic red cell defects or, more commonly, as the results of factors extrinsic to the red cell. In either case, the hallmark of hemolysis is a shortened red cell life span (normally 60-90 days in the newborn), elevated reticulocyte count, morphologic abnormalities (spherocytes, fragmented red cells) seen on the peripheral smear, and jaundice (Figure 10–4).

In the neonate, hemolysis can be divided into 3 major categories: immune mediated red cell destruction, intrinsic red cell defects, and factors extrinsic to the red cell (ie, such as sepsis).

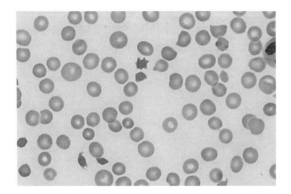

Figure 10–4. Fragmented red cells.
Source: From Lichtman MA, Beutler E, Kipps TJ, et al. Williams' Hematology, 7ed, 2006, New York, NY: McGraw-Hill.

Immune-Mediated Red Cell Destruction

Hemolytic disease of the newborn is caused by the destruction of fetal and neonatal red cells by maternal IgG antibodies. These antibodies are produced when fetal red cells enter the maternal circulation and express antigens not found on maternal red cells.[42] There are many antigens that have the potential to stimulate an antibody response in the newborn and include the antigens in the ABO, Rh, Kell, and Duffy systems. The vast majority of immune-mediated red cell destruction occurs in response to ABO and Rh incompatibility between the infant and the mother and are discussed below.

ABO Incompatibility

This entity was first described by Halbrecht in 1944.[43] In general the hemolysis induced by fetal-maternal ABO incompatibility is not severe, as the level of IgG antibody in the maternal circulation against the A and B antigens on the fetal cells is not markedly elevated, thus the amount of antibody transferred to the infant is low. Hemolysis in this setting is minimal to moderate, and is typically seen only when the mother is type O and the infant is either A or B. The

incidence of ABO mismatch with the fetus in a mother with blood type O is 15%. Only 20% of infants will become significantly jaundiced for the reasons noted previously.[44,45]

Clinically apparent jaundice appears on the first day of life in 20% of infants with ABO incompatibility.[44] Anemia and subsequent pallor are rarely seen. Typically the physical examination is normal except for jaundice and possibly mild hepatomegaly. The peripheral smear is remarkable for the presence of spherocytes and the Coombs test is positive.[46] It is important to note that the direct Coombs test is positive only 40% of the time, thus it is vital to obtain the indirect Coombs test to detect small amount of antibody bound to the red cell membrane. Treatment for infants with hyperbilirubinemia involves admission to the hospital for phototherapy.

Rh Hemolytic Disease

The widespread availability and use of Rhogham in Rh-negative women has dramatically decreased the incidence of this potentially life-threatening cause of hemolytic anemia. Prior to advent of Rhogham, 1% of women developed significant sensitization to the Rh antigen leading to severe anemia and hydrops in the developing fetus.[47] Sensitization of the Rh-negative mother rarely occurs (1 in 1000 pregnancies) in the Rhogham era.[48] Nevertheless this entity still appears and need immediate recognition to prevent potential life-threatening anemia.

This entity was first described in 1934 by Diamond who noted a condition characterized by fetal hydrops, anemia, and circulating erythroblasts.[49] Weiner and coworkers discovered the Rh system in 1940 and found that 15% of the population was Rh negative.[50] Subsequent studies revealed that this antigen was responsible for many transfusion reactions and was the most common entity associated with the development of severe hemolytic disease of the fetus and newborn.

The antigens of the Rh system are found at 3 loci: Dd, Cc, and Ee.[51] Most significant antibody responses are related to the Dd system.[51] In infants with the DD or Dd phenotype born to a mother with the dd genotype, the presence of fetal red cells can induce an antibody response. The risk of sensitization in the first pregnancy ranges from 11% to 16% and the risk increases in subsequent pregnancies.[52,53] Because the antibody generated is of the IgG subclass, subsequent pregnancies have a much higher risk of severe hemolysis due to the heightened antibody response on re-exposure to the antigen with subsequent pregnancies. Severe hemolysis can occur in the fetus leading to hydrops and fetal demise.

Fifty percent of infants with Rh incompatibility have mild disease with a normal physical examination other than jaundice. Phototherapy may be required; tranfusional support is rarely required. Moderately severe hemolysis develops in 30% of infants in this setting. These infants have a normal physical examination at birth except for jaundice and rapidly increasing bilirubin that necessitates immediate hospitalization and treatment with phototherapy. Severely affected infants present at birth with severe anemia and varying degrees of hydrops and are managed in the neonatal nursery with exchange transfusion. It is important to note that severely affected infants who undergo exchange transfusion may continue to require tranfusional support for weeks due to ongoing destruction of red cells including the transfused red cells. These infants may present to the ED in the first 6 weeks of life with severe anemia and decreased reticulocyte count due to the persistent presence of maternal antibody that destroys the immature red cells in vitro.

Hereditary Spherocytosis

Hereditary spherocytosis is an autosomal dominant condition characterized by defects in the membrane surface proteins––spectrin and ankyrin––producing a red cell membrane that is less deformable leading to red cell membrane loss, spherocyte formation, and premature red cell destruction in the spleen.[54] This entity is present in 1 in 4000 births in the Caucasian population; the frequency in the Black population is significantly less.[54]

Many children remain asymptomatic for years; however, neonates can present with jaundice, anemia, and splenomegaly. Fifty percent of neonates with hereditary spherocytosis have jaundice in the neonatal period.[55]

The diagnosis can be strongly suspected in the neonate with a positive family history of hereditary spherocytosis, jaundice on physical examination in an otherwise well-appearing infant, spherocytes on the peripheral blood smear, and a negative Coombs test.

Little intervention is required in the neonatal period other than phototherapy for jaundice. Most children with hereditary spherocytosis will eventually require splenectomy. Gallstones and subsequent need for cholecystectomy may occur during childhood due to ongoing red cell hemolysis.

Glucose-6-Phosphate Dehydrogenase Deficiency (G6PD Deficiency)

G6PD deficiency is an X-linked trait and represents the most common inherited red cell enzyme defect affecting nearly 500 million people worldwide.[56] This entity is most commonly seen in Africa but is present throughout the world. G6PD is most prevalent in regions of the world where malaria is endemic. G6PD-deficient red cells are not able to produce an adequate quantity of reduced glutathione; thus, in the presence of oxidant stress, the red cells will hemolyze.

Many infants in the newborn period will develop jaundice if G6PD deficiency is present.[57] Presently the pathophysiology of jaundice in this setting is unclear. Management of neonatal jaundice in G6PD deficiency is no different than the management of infants with immune-mediated red cell destruction. Phototherapy is used if indicated and exchange transfusion is rarely required. Testing for G6PD deficiency should be considered in all jaundiced infants who do not have immune-mediated red cell destruction, especially in populations with a high prevalence of this entity.

Nonaccidental Trauma (NAT)

Neonates with unexplained bruising and petechiae need a careful evaluation to exclude an underlying bleeding disorder such as hemophilia, thrombocytopenia, or DIC. In the absence of these entities, NAT must be considered, especially in the setting of unexplained subarachnoid or intracranial bleeding or unexplained facial bruising. Evaluation would include a complete skeletal survey, bone scan, dilated eye examination, and CT and MRI of the brain.

SUMMARY

Neonates presenting to the ED with symptoms of anemia need a complete and focused history, a careful physical examination, and appropriate laboratory testing to determine the etiology of the anemia. Transfusional support may be required to support the cardiovascular system and may be life-saving in some neonates.

▶ BLEEDING IN THE NEONATE

For a variety of reasons the neonate is at increased risk for potentially life-threatening bleeding. Maternal diseases and medication use, the fragility of newborn vessels, trauma associated with birth, physiologic coagulation factor deficiencies present at birth, along with hypoxia and sepsis are all contributing factors toward bleeding in this group of children.

PHYSIOLOGY OF NEONATAL CIRCULATION

The platelet-endothelial cell interaction represents the initial hemostatic response to damaged endothelium. This response is diminished in neonates due in part to decreased production of thromboxane, which promotes vasoconstriction and adherence of platelets to the vessel wall. Neonatal endothelium and vessels are more fragile and susceptible to injury than in older children. Several soluble proteins are present in the plasma, which is activated in the presence of endothelial cell injury generating fibrin, which then binds to the platelet complex adherent to the damaged endothelium. Many of these proteins are present in diminished concentration in the neonate and include factor 11, and the vitamin K-dependent factors 2, 7, 9, and 10.[58] These deficiencies lead to prolongation of both the PT and PTT, and place the neonate at risk for bleeding. In the normal neonate the levels of factors promoting fibrinolysis and inhibiting thrombus formation are diminished and include decreased levels of antithrombin III, plasminogen, protein S, and protein C.[58] Most neonates who are otherwise healthy will not experience bleeding or thrombus formation. Table 10–5 summarizes the reference values for the coagulation tests and factors in the first month of life.[59]

HISTORY

A complete and accurate history is often the key to the diagnosis in the bleeding neonate and the important historical elements are summarized in Table 10–6. The key information needed includes the presence of maternal infection or disease, medication use in the mother, trauma during the birth process, family history of bleeding disorders, the presence of fever or other signs of systemic illness in the infant, and history of vitamin K administration.

▶ TABLE 10–5. **REFERENCE VALUES FOR COAGULATION TESTS, FACTOR LEVELS, AND ANTICOAGULANTS IN THE FIRST MONTH OF LIFE AND IN ADULTS**

Coagulation Tests	5 Days Old	30 Days Old	Adult
PT (sec)	12.4 (10-15.3)	11.8 10-14.3)	12.4 (10.8-13.9)
INR	0.89 (0.53-1.48)	0.79 (0.53-1.26)	0.89 (0.64-1.17)
PTT (sec)	42.6 (25.4-59.8)	40.4 (32-55.2)	33.5 (26.6-40.3)
Factor Levels (U/mL)			
Factor 2	0.63 (0.33-0.93)	0.68 (0.34-1.02)	1.08 (0.70-1.46
Factor 7	0.89 (0.35-1.43)	0.90 (0.42-1.38)	1.05 (0.67-1.43)
Factor 8	0.88 (0.50-1.54)	0.91 (0.50-1.57)	0.99 (0.50-1.49)
Factor 9	0.53 (0.15-0.91)	0.51 (0.21-0.81)	1.09 (0.55-1.63)
Factor 10	0.49 (0.19-0.79)	0.59 (0.31-0.87)	1.06 (0.70-1.52)
Factor 11	0.55 (0.23-0.87)	0.53 (0.27-0.79	0.97 (0.67-1.27)
Anticoagulants (U/mL)			
Protein C	0.42 (0.20-0.64)	0.43 (0.21-0.65)	0.96 (0.64-1.28)
Protein S	0.50 (0.22-0.78)	0.63 (0.33-0.93)	0.92 (0.60-1.24)
Antithrombin III	0.56 (0.30-0.82)	0.59 (0.37-0.81)	1.05 (0.79-1.31)

▶ TABLE 10–6. **HISTORICAL AND PHYSICAL EXAMINATION KEYS IN EVALUATING THE BLEEDING NEONATE**

Maternal Factors	Neonatal Factors
Maternal Disease	**Neonatal Birth**
SLE	**Complications**
ITP	Birth trauma
Malignancy	Prematurity
Maternal Medica-	Hypoxia
tion Use	Hypotension
Aspirin	Respiratory distress
Motrin	syndrome
Pregnancy Compli-	**Neonatal Physical**
cations	**Abnormalities**
Preeclampsia	Fever
Abruptio placentae	Absent radii/thumbs
Maternal Infection	Hepatosplenomegaly
Family History	Hemangiomas
of Bleeding	**Neonatal Infection**
Disorders	**Vitamin K**
	Administration
	Nonaccidental
	Trauma (NAT)

PHYSICAL EXAMINATION

The bleeding infant requires a careful and rapid assessment to determine if the bleeding is secondary to an underlying disease process or if it is related to a primary bleeding disorder. Once the initial assessment of the infant is completed, 2 groups of infants are identified. The first group is comprised of the "sick" infant who needs immediate therapy prior to availability of laboratory testing, while infants in the second group appear clinically well and do not require emergent treatment. Table 10–7 lists the common clinical and laboratory findings and possible diagnoses in each group of patients.

The presence of shock, hypoxia, fever, hypotension, hypothermia, acidosis, and perinatal infection suggests that bleeding is secondary to DIC. Hepatosplenomegaly in the bleeding neonate suggests the diagnosis of congenital viral infection or leukemia. The presence of congenital abnormalities involving the skin, face, heart, radius, or thumbs should suggest the possibility of Fanconi aplastic anemia, Wiskott-Aldrich syndrome, and

▶ TABLE 10–7. **CLINICAL AND LABORATORY FINDINGS IN THE BLEEDING NEONATE**

Platelet Count	PTT	PT	Potential Diagnoses
Well Neonate			
Decreased	Normal	Normal	**Antibody-Mediated Conditions**
			Maternal ITP
			Alloimmune thrombocytopenia
			Rare Conditions
			Marrow hypoplasia
			Leukemia
			Metastatic malignancy
Normal	Prolonged	Prolonged	Vitamin K deficiency
Normal	Prolonged	Normal/prolonged	Inherited factor deficiencies (hemophilia)
Normal	Normal	Normal	Trauma
			Anatomic abnormalities (hemangioma)
			Platelet functional abnormalities
Sick Neonate			
Decreased	Increased	Increased	Disseminated intravascular coagulation
Decreased	Normal	Normal	**Platelet Consumption**
			Catheter related
			Infection
			NEC
			Renal vein thrombosis
			Kasabach-Merritt syndrome
Normal	Increased	Increased	Vitamin K deficiency
Normal	Normal	Normal	**Compromised Vascular Integrity**
			Hypoxia
			Acidosis
			Prematurity

thrombocytopenia absent radii syndrome (TAR syndrome). Well-appearing infants with stable vital signs and no observable physical abnormalities typically have a primary bleeding disorder. Diagnostic considerations in this group include immune thrombocytopenia, hemophilia, vitamin K deficiency, von Willebrand disease, or a localized vascular lesion.

Type of Bleeding

The presence of petechiae, bruising, or GI tract bleeding is most commonly associated with thrombocytopenia. Localized bleeding following trauma as manifested by cephalohematoma, postcircumcision bleeding, or hematoma formation at injection sites points toward the diagnosis of a specific factor deficiency.

DIAGNOSTIC TESTS

The CBC with platelet count, PT, and PTT often help identify the reason for bleeding. The platelet count can be accurately measured using an automated electronic cell counter and quickly estimated by viewing a well-prepared peripheral smear. Under microscopic review with an oil immersion lens at 100x, each platelet represents 10-15,000 platelets. A child with 10 or more platelets in each field would have a platelet count. >100,000/μL. It is important to recognize causes of "false" thrombocytopenia, which commonly occurs and should be suspected in a clinically well neonate with no evidence of bleeding. Difficult blood draws with slow blood flow and the presence of antibodies that are activated by the anticoagulant EDTA can both cause platelet clumping and a falsely low platelet count.

The PTT and PT provide a measure of the soluble clotting proteins and thus represent a valuable screening test for blood coagulation. The PTT measures the intrinsic pathway, which contains all of the clotting factors except for factors 7 and 13. The PT measures the extrinsic pathway and does not measure factors 13, 12, 11, 9, and 8. The presence of a normal PT and PTT effectively rules out a coagulation factor deficiency as a cause of bleeding.

Prolongation of the PTT and PT can occur for several reasons. This can occur when the level of 1 or more factors is decreased by 40%. Reduced levels of the so-called contact factors such as factor 12, prekallikrein, and high molecular weight kininogen can prolong the PTT without causing increased bleeding, as these factors are not the primary factors needed in activation of the coagulation cascade. Several technical factors can produce false prolongations of the PT and PTT. A long, difficult blood draw can release tissue thromboplastin and trigger production of small fibrin clots, which will prolong the PT and PTT. The presence of heparin in a catheter from which blood is drawn will markedly elevate the PTT with minimal effect on the PT. The presence of a hematocrit >65% or an inadequate amount of blood placed in the citrate tube used for the PT and PTT will increase the ratio of citrate to plasma and prolong the PT and PTT.

In cases where the PT and PTT are truly prolonged, the fibrinogen and fibrin split products should be obtained. The presence of elevated fibrin split products and decreased fibrinogen with a prolonged PT and PTT establishes the diagnosis of DIC.

DIFFERENTIAL DIAGNOSIS AND MANAGEMENT

Disseminated Intravascular Coagulation (DIC)

DIC represents the most common and potentially life-threatening cause of impaired hemostasis in the neonate. This entity is characterized by endothelial damage from a variety of factors (Table 10–8) with activation of the coagulation cascade, consumption of clotting factors, intravascular thrombi formation,

▶ **TABLE 10–8. DISSEMINATED INTRAVASCULAR COAGULATION: ETIOLOGIC FACTORS**

Endothelial Cell Injury
    Bacterial infection
    Viral infection
    Fungal Infection
    Acidosis
    Hypoxemia
    Vascular catheters
    Cavernous hemangioma
Red Cell/Platelet Injury
    Hemolytic disease of the newborn
Tissue Injury/Release of Tissue Factor
    Birth asphyxia
    Respiratory distress syndrome
    Meconium aspiration
    Congenital leukemia
    Neuroblastoma
    Pre-eclampsia
    Abruption placentae
    Severe brain injury
    Necrotizing enterocolitis
    Crush injury
Congenital Thrombotic Disorders
    Protein S deficiency
    Protein C deficiency
    Antithrombin III deficiency

and hemorrhage.[60] When DIC is present the underlying disease state must be identified, as DIC is always a secondary event. Table 10–8 summarizes the entities most commonly associated with DIC.

The initial pathophysiologic event in most cases of DIC involves injury to the endothelial cell and surrounding tissue, which activates both the intrinsic and extrinsic coagulation systems with production of intravascular thrombi and depletion of coagulation factors. The fibrin clot present in the microcirculation produces a microangiopathic hemolytic process as the red cells are impaled on the fibrin clots. Fibrin formation activates the fibrinolytic system producing plasminogen that cleaves fibrinogen and fibrin clot, producing fibrin degradation products. The fibrin degradation products interfere with platelet aggregation and impair fibrin polymerization. The fibrin clot impairs oxygen delivery to end organs causing ischemic injury.

Clinical Presentation

DIC occurs in a variety of settings, which are summarized in Table 10-8. The main causes of DIC in neonates are briefly discussed below. Neonatal viral infections (rubella, herpes, enterovirus, and cytomegalovirus) and bacterial infections (gram-negative organisms and Group B streptococcal infections) are responsible for most cases of infection-triggered DIC.[61] Abruptio placentae, pre-eclampsia, and eclampsia may cause fetal anoxia and anoxic-tissue injury triggering DIC.[62] Necrotizing enterocolitis and respiratory distress syndrome are 2 neonatal conditions characterized by hypoxic tissue injury leading to the release of tissue factor that triggers DIC. Congenital deficiency of the antithrombotic factors protein C, S, or antithrombin III deficiency can lead to DIC. The presence of large hemangiomas can lead to Kasabach-Merritt syndrome where platelets, fibrinogen and coagulation factors are consumed within the hemangioma.

The clinical presentation of DIC will vary depending on the underlying entity triggering DIC. Typically the neonate with DIC may present with oozing from punctures, bruising, and purpura, and can present with internal bleeding (CNS, GI tract). Thrombosis of peripheral or central vessels may occur with tissue necrosis, organ dysfunction, or stroke if the vessels of the CNS are involved.

Laboratory Findings

These are characteristic and support this diagnosis in the setting of an ill-appearing infant with 1 or more of the clinical presentations noted above. The laboratory abnormalities include prolongation of the PT and PTT, decreased fibrinogen, increased fibrin split products (variable in the first month of life), and a decreased platelet count (<100,00/μL). The D-dimer (antigen produced when plasminogen cleaves fibrin) is elevated in >90% of neonates with DIC and is the most sensitive single test available for the diagnosis of DIC.[63-65] Microangiopathic changes are seen in the red cells, which are fragmented by fibrin strands in the capillary beds leading to the production of schistocytes. The neutrophils often demonstrate toxic granulations especially in the setting of sepsis. Immature myeloid elements are often seen in the setting of sepsis, hypoxia or shock.

Treatment

Treatment must be directed toward the underlying disease process that triggered DIC. Simple replacement of the missing coagulation factors, platelets, and blood represents inadequate therapy as consumption of factors will continue until the underlying disease process is identified and treated.

In the setting where sepsis is suspected, appropriate broad-spectrum antibiotic coverage should be instituted. In the child who is stable with minimal bleeding or bruising, tranfusional support is not required if the PT, PTT, and platelet count are minimally decreased.

In the child with obvious bleeding who is ill with unstable vital signs, immediate resuscitation efforts should be employed to include tranfusional support with fresh frozen plasma (15-20 mL/kg), platelets (single donor and leuko-depleted-irradiated, and red cells.[66] Clearly infants with a platelet count less than 10,000/µL with bleeding or infants with a PT greater than 30 (INR >2) who are bleeding should receive platelets or FFP, respectively. Cryoprecipitate contains fibrinogen, von Willebrand factor, and factor 8 coagulant. Infusion of 10 mL/kg of body weight will temporarily restore the factor 8 activity and fibrinogen to near normal levels. The advantage of cryoprecipitec is the small volume that needs to be infused, as each bag is only 25-30 mL. The disadvantage of cryoprecipitate is the absence of the vitamin K dependent factors 2, 7, 9, and 10, which are present in FFP and are often depleted in the infant with DIC.

It is important to remember that the goal of tranfusional therapy with FFP, cryoprecipitate, and platelets in the setting of DIC is to control bleeding. The tests results will not be normalized due to the ongoing consumption of coagulation factors until the underlying disease state is controlled. Reasonable transfusion goals are to achieve a platelet count >50,000 µL and a fibrinogen >100 mg/dL.

Anticoagulation therapy in theory is a logical approach to prevent the life-threatening effects of DIC. Two approaches have been studied to date. The first approach is the use of exogenous anticoagulants such as heparin. To date there are no controlled trials that support the routine use of heparin in DIC. Heparin use is absolutely contraindicated when CNS bleeding or liver failure is present in the setting of DIC. Heparin may be useful in the setting of significant, life-threatening thrombi in the absence of bleeding. Replacement of the naturally occurring anticoagulants antithrombin III and protein C are attractive options given the decreased levels of these anticoagulants in patients with DIC. Antithrombin III infusions have been used to treat adults with sepsis and DIC with no proven benefit. There are no large studies in children to suggest a benefit for the use of antithrombin III in this setting.[67] Protein C infusions have proven useful to treat DIC in specific settings. Clearly protein C infusions have been life saving in neonates with DIC secondary to protein C deficiency in the newborn period.[68] Protein C infusions have also been used in children with DIC associated with meningococcal sepsis with significant decreases in morbidity and mortality including a reduced amputation rate. Recombinant soluble thrombomodulin is currently under investigation in treating patients with DIC. Thrombomodulin inhibits the coagulation cascade by binding to and inactivating thrombin and by activating protein C. A recent phase 3 clinical trial in Japan demonstrated improved survival in patients with DIC from sepsis or malignancy.[69]

Hemorrhagic Disease of the Newborn

The normal newborn has diminished levels of the vitamin K-dependent factors that are 3-60% of normal adult values in the first 2 months of life.[70] The deficiency of factors 2, 7, 9, and 10 is directly related to the immaturity of the liver and deficiency of vitamin K in the newborn. Vitamin K is an essential factor required for activation of factors 2, 7, 9, and 10 and proteins S and C. In the absence of vitamin K, these factors are not functional. Vitamin K administration at birth leads to rapid activation of these factors. Without vitamin K administration, the levels of the vitamin K-dependent factors are markedly decreased for the first 6 to 8 weeks of life. The administration of vitamin K, 1 mg IM at birth, activates the vitamin K-dependent factors and markedly diminishes the risk of life-threatening bleeds that were commonplace in the era prior to routine administration of vitamin K.

The infant diet represents the most important source of vitamin K. Proprietary formulas contain 50 μg/L of vitamin K. The other source of vitamin K in the neonate is production of vitamin K in the intestinal tract by certain strains of bacteria including *Escherichia coli.* In contrast to the formula-fed infant, the breast-fed infant receives milk with little vitamin K (5 μg/L) and the intestinal flora in breast-fed infants is not efficient in producing vitamin K. In the absence of vitamin K administration at birth, the breast-fed infant is very susceptible to bleeding as the result of vitamin K deficiency. Three forms of vitamin K deficiency have been described. Early hemorrhagic disease of the newborn is a rare entity occurring in utero or in the first 24 hours following birth. Invariably the mother is on medication, which adversely affects vitamin K metabolism leading to significant depletion of this essential vitamin in the newborn. This list of medications associated with this complication includes warfarin, isoniazid, rifampin, dilantin, and barbiturates.[71] Clinically, infants in this setting can have mild bleeding or life-threatening intracranial or pulmonary hemorrhage.

Classic hemorrhagic disease of the newborn presents in the first 2 to 5 days following birth and occurs in 1% to 2 % of infants prior to routine administration of vitamin K at birth.[72] Affected infants typically have bruising or GI bleeding. Less common presentations include bleeding from the umbilicus or circumcision site. Massive, life-threatening intracranial bleeding has been reported. Late-onset disease occurs after 3 weeks of age and is usually associated with a disease state characterized by intestinal malabsorption or poor dietary intake (breast milk with decreased vitamin K content). The entities associated with late onset hemorrhagic disease include cystic fibrosis, chronic diarrhea, biliary atresia, hepatitis, and celiac disease.

Treatment of bleeding in this setting includes rapid administration of vitamin K, 1 mg IV with transfusion of 15-20 mL/kg of fresh frozen plasma (FFP).

Factor Deficiencies

Congenital deficiencies of fibrinogen and factors 2, 7, 8, 9, 10, 11, and 13 have been described and may present as life-threatening bleeding in the first month of life. Factors 8 and 9 deficiency represent more than 90% of the reported bleeding episodes due to factor deficiency in this age group.

Hemophilia

Hemophilia is an X-linked trait characterized by a variable decrease in the activity of factors VIII and IX in the blood, which can lead to life-threatening spontaneous bleeding. In the United States, hemophilia A (factor VIII deficiency) occurs in 1 in 5000-10,000 males while hemophilia B (factor IX deficiency) is found in 1-25,000-30,000 males.[73] Approximately one-third of patients have a negative family history for hemophilia and thus represent de novo mutations.[74] Maternal factor 8 and 9 do not cross the placenta. It is vital to remember that only 50% of patients with severe hemophilia bleed in the neonatal period. The most common bleeding site in the neonate is the circumcision site. Intracranial bleeds, scalp hematomas, and umbilical cord stump bleeding can also occur. The level of factor present determines the severity of hemophilia A and B. Mild hemophilia is defined by the presence of >5% factor activity in the patient's plasma. Patients with moderate hemophilia have 1% to 5% factor activity, and patients with severe hemophilia have <1% factor activity in the plasma. Of patients with diagnosed hemophilia A, approximately 60% have severe disease (<1% factor activity), 30% have moderate disease (1% to 5% factor activity), and 10% have mild hemophilia (>5% activity). In any given kindred, the severity of hemophilia is relatively constant.[75] Patients with severe hemophilia can bleed spontaneously; spontaneous bleeding is rare in patients with moderate or mild hemophilia.

In normal neonates, factor VIII levels at birth are normal, but factor IX levels are decreased as noted previously. The PTT is 50% longer in normal term infants when compared to values in normal adults (Table 10–5). Specific factor assay for factors 8 and 9 represent the definitive test for the diagnosis of hemophilia. Hemophilia A can be diagnosed with certainty, as can severe and moderate hemophilia B. Circumcision can routinely be performed if the child has been appropriately replaced with factor.

Infused factor VIII has a biologic half-life of 8 to 12 hours; 1 U/kg of infused VIII raises the plasma level of factor 8 activity by 1.5-2%. Infused factor IX has a biologic half-life of 18-24 hours; 1 U/kg of infused IX raises the plasma level by 1%. In an emergent setting with an unstable bleeding neonate with a prolonged PTT and in the absence of a specific factor assay, FFFP 15 mL/kg can be given IV immediately. If available, solvent detergent-treated FFP (purified product with decreased potential of viral transmission) should be administered. Due to the potential risk of viral transmission (hepatitis, HIV) in blood products, and the availability of recombinant factors, every attempt should be made to obtain a specific diagnosis on a STAT basis so that a specific recombinant factor can be infused. If there is a known family history of hemophilia A or B, and the patient is theoretically at risk, then a presumptive diagnosis of either VIII or IX deficiency can be made, and the patient treated with a recombinant factor as long as blood has been obtained for factor assays. Patients with the diagnosis of factor VIII deficiency would receive 50 U/kg IV; a patient with factor 9 deficiency would receive 100 U/kg IV.

Thrombocytopenia

Effective hemostasis in the newborn is dependent on the interaction among platelets, blood vessels, and the plasma coagulation proteins. Impaired platelet function or thrombocytopenia (platelet count <150,000/μL) can lead to hemorrhage in the neonate and should be suspected in infants that present with petechiae, bruising, or mucosal bleeding.[76]

It is essential to obtain a complete history from the mother regarding a maternal bleeding disorder, underlying maternal disease (ie, systemic lupus), and any maternal medications that might cross the placenta leading to platelet dysfunction in the neonate and bleeding (this would include aspirin and Motrin). The details of the birth history are also important regarding the presence of maternal infection at delivery or birth asphyxia.

Classic thrombocytopenic bleeding most frequently presents with cutaneous and mucosal petechiae and cutaneous bruising. Significant bleeding rarely occurs until the platelet count falls below 50,000/μL. Spontaneous intracranial bleeding can be seen in neonate with platelet counts <10,000 μL. Thrombocytopenia in the neonate has been reported in 1% to 2% of healthy appearing newborns and 20% to 30% of sick preterm infants. It occurs as the result of increased platelet destruction, platelet sequestration, or decreased platelet production.[77-79] Table 10–9 summarizes the causes of thrombocytopenia in the neonate.

Neonatal Alloimmunization Thrombocytopenia

Neonatal alloimmunization thrombocytopenia represents the single most common cause of thrombocytopenia in an otherwise healthy neonate and occurs in approximately 1 in 1000 newborns.[80] The thrombocytopenia occurs as the result of maternal sensitization to paternal antigens present on the fetal platelets that are not expressed on maternal platelets. These antibodies, which are of the IgG class, can cross the placenta and produce thrombocytopenia in the fetus and significant bleeding in utero.[81] The typical newborn with this entity is a well- appearing child with mucosal or cutaneous petechiae born after a

▶ TABLE 10–9. **NEONATAL THROMBOCYTOPENIA**

Increased Destruction	Decreased Production
Immune Mediated	**Bone Marrow Replacement**
Neonatal alloimmune thrombocytopenia	Congenital leukemia
(fetal maternal platelet incompatibility)	Neuroblastoma
Unrecognized maternal ITP	Osteopetrosis
Maternal collagen vascular disease	**Bone Marrow Aplasia**
Maternal Factors	Fanconi aplastic anemia
Hyperthyroidism	Thrombocytopenia absent radii
Preeclampsia	Wiskott-Aldrich syndrome
Maternal medications	Amegakaryocytic thrombocytopenia
Nonimmune	Trisomy 13 and 18
Asphyxia	
Aspiration	
Respiratory distress syndrome	
Necrotizing enterocolitis	
Neonatal thrombosis	
Hemangiomas (Kasabach-Merrittt syndrome)	
Splenomegaly	
Infection	
Portal hypertension	
Storage disease (Gaucher, Nieman-Pick)	
Unknown	
Hyperbilirubinemia	
Phototherapy	
Polycythemia	
Rh hemolytic disease	
Total parenteral nutrition	

normal pregnancy and delivery. Life threatening bleeding (CNS) is the initial presentation in 15% of neonates in this setting.[82] It is important to note that alloimmune thrombocytopenia can present in the first pregnancy and that there is no screening process to test for this potential problem. This is in contrast to the standardized testing and available treatment with Rhogham to prevent Rh sensitization in Rh-negative mothers. Treatment modalities would include transfusion of maternal leuko-depleted, irradiated platelets (15 mL/kg), IV IgG (1 g/kg) or IV solumedrol 1 mg/kg IV q6h.[83] A CT scan or ultrasound of the brain is indicated to rule out intracranial hemorrhage.[76]

Autoimmune Thrombocytopenia

Autoimmune thrombocytopenia occurs in children born to mothers with an underlying immune-mediated destruction thrombocytopenia such as maternal ITP or systemic lupus. Children born in this setting are typically well appearing with some cutaneous and occasional mucosal petechiae. The platelet count may be normal at birth in contrast to infants with alloimmune thrombocytopenia, and generally the platelet count normalizes within 3 weeks of birth. These IgG antibodies are produced by the mother in response to specific platelet antigens present on both the maternal and fetal platelets. At present there is no way to predict the severity of the thrombocytopenia in the infant, as there is no correlation between the maternal platelet count and the platelet count in the infant. The thrombocytopenia in autoimmune thrombocytopenia is usually less severe than in alloimmune thrombocytopenia. Only 10% to 15% of affected infants will have platelet counts less than 50,000/μL.[84] ICH can occur but is extremely rare. Treatment modalities would include IV IgG and IV steroid as outlined previously for alloimmune thrombocytopenia. A CT scan of the brain should be performed. Platelet transfusions are not a useful treatment modality given that the antibody will react with and destroy all platelets.

Infection-Thrombocytopenia

Thrombocytopenia occurring in the first few days after birth in a "sick" neonate is usually associated with a perinatal infection and/or DIC as discussed previously.

Kasabach-Merritt Syndrome

First described in 1940 as a consumptive coagulopathy in conjunction with the presence of a capillary hemangioma,[85] this entity is associated with a kaposiform hemangioendothelioma, which is a form of giant hemangioma and not a simple capillary hemangioma.[86]

Platelets are sequestered and trapped in this vascular malformation leading to thrombocytopenia. Lesions are noted at birth in 50% of patients. Visceral lesions occur in the trunk, extremities, and cervical facial area and often require imaging studies for detection (Figure 10–5).

This entity should be considered in the neonate with bleeding in the setting of severe thrombocytopenia and fragmented red cells (microangiopathic red cell changes such as schistocytes and helmet cells). Treatment is directed at hastening resolution of the hemangioma while supporting hemostasis by transfusion of the appropriate blood products. Therapeutic modalities include embolization,

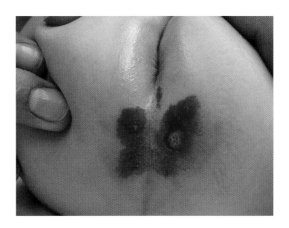

Figure 10–5. Hemangioma of the buttock.

surgery, steroids, interferon, and chemotherapeutic agents such as vincristine and cyclophosphamide, which all are designed to hasten resolution of the hemangioma.[87,88]

Necrotizing Enterocolitis (NEC)

Thrombocytopenia is a frequent finding in neonates with NEC and can result in significant bleeding. The primary mechanism for thrombocytopenia in NEC is platelet destruction.[89]

Thrombocytopenia Absent Radii (TAR) Syndrome

TAR syndrome is an autosomal recessive condition characterized by severe thrombocytopenia with bilateral absent radii. Despite the absent radii, the thumbs are present.[90] Absence or hypoplasia of the ulna and humerus may also be present. Atrial septal defect or tetralogy of Fallot are present in 30% of neonates with TAR syndrome.[90] Severe thrombocytopenia is present in 60% of patients with TAR syndrome in the neonatal period (platelet count <10,000/μL), which leads to significant mortality in the neonatal period as the result of CNS hemorrhage.[91] Prophylactic platelet transfusions are usually needed for the first several months of life to prevent life-threatening bleeding. Marrow production of platelets usually normalizes after the first year of life.

Congenital Leukemia

Congenital leukemia should be suspected when the CBC reveals abnormal immature WBCS in conjunction with thrombocytopenia. These patients often have cutaneous leukemic cell infiltrates and hepatosplenomegaly. Neuroblastoma may also present in the neonatal period with thrombocytopenia, skin infiltration with neuroblastoma cells, abdominal mass, or intrathoracic mass.

Table 10–10 summarizes the evaluation of the thrombocytopenic neonate prior to transfusion of platelets or blood.

► SUMMARY

The bleeding neonate is at significant risk for life-threatening morbidity and death. A rapid, focused and accurate history including the maternal history and the perinatal clinical course, a careful physical examination, and appropriate laboratory testing are essential in providing appropriate treatment in this

► **TABLE 10–10. EVALUATION AND TREATMENT OF NEONATAL THROMBOCYTOPENIA**

History	Laboratory	Physical Examination
Family history	CBC/platelet count	ABCS
Maternal history	PT, PTT, TT	Petechiae, bruising
(ITP, CVD, chronic disease)	Maternal CBC	Pallor
Maternal medications	Red cell morphology	Hepatomegaly
Obstetrical history		Splenomegaly
(birth asphyxia)		Absent radii
Neonatal disease		Skin nodules (leukemia,
(leukemia, sepsis)		neuroblastoma)

Well-Appearing Neonate	Ill-Appearing Neonate
Normal Maternal Platelet Count	Sepsis
Alloimmune thrombocytopenia	DIC
Treatment:	Kasabach-Merritt
Maternal platelet transfusion	Malignancy
(irradiated)	*Treatment:*
IV IgG	Treat underlying condition
IV steroids	Transfusion of platelets, FFP, blood as
Pediatric hematology consultation	indicated
	Pediatric hematology consultation
Decreased Maternal Platelet Count	
Maternal ITP	
Maternal CVD	
Treatment:	
IV IgG	
IV Steroids	
Pediatric hematology consultation	

setting prior to administration of any blood products.

REFERENCES

1. Matoth Y, Zaizov R, Varsano I. Postnatal changes in some red cell parameters. *Acta Paediat Scand.* 1971;60(3):275.

2. Zaizov R, Mamoth Y. Red cell values on the first day of life during the last 16 weeks of gestation. *Am J Hematol.* 1976;1(2):275.

3. Oski FA. Normal blood values in the newborn period. In: Nathan DG, Oski FA, eds. *Nathan and Oski's Hematologic Problems in the Newborn.* 3rd ed. Philadelphia: WB Saunders; 1982:12.

4. Linderkamp O, Nelle M, Kraus M, Zilow EP. The effect of early and late cord-clamping on blood viscosity and other hemorrheological parameters in full term neonates. *Acta Pediatrica.* 1992;81:745.

5. Alter BP. Fanconi's anemia and its variability. *Br J Haematol.* 1993;85:9.

6. D'Andrea AD, Grompe M. Molecular biology of Fanconi anemia: implications for diagnosis and therapy. *Blood.* 1997;90:1725.

7. Tischkowitz M, Dokal I. Fanconi anaemia and leukaemia—clinical and molecular aspects. *Br J Haematol.* 2004;126:176.

8. D'Andrea AD, Grompe M. The Fanconi anaemia/BRCA pathway. *Nat Rev Cancer.* 2003;3:23.

9. Levitus M, Waisfisz Q, Godthelp BC, et al. The DNA helicase BRIP1 is defective in Fanconi anemia complementation group. *J Nat Genet.* 2005;37:934.

10. Levran O, Attwooll C, Henry RT, et al. Addendum: the BRCA1-interacting helicase BRIP1 is deficient in Fanconi anemia. *Nat Genet.* 2005;37:1296.

11. Anderson LJ. Role of parvovirus B19 in human disease. *Pediatr Infect Dis J.* 1987;6:711.

12. Anderson MJ, Higgins PG, Davis LR, et al. Experimental parvoviral infection in humans. *J Infect Dis.* 1985;152:257.

13. Young N, Mortimer P. Viruses and bone marrow failure. *Blood.* 1984;63:279.

14. Anand A, Gray ES, Brown T, et al. Human parvovirus in Pregnancy and hydrops fetalis. *N Engl J Med.* 1987;316:183.

15. Schwartz TF, Roggendorf M, Hottentrager B, et al. Human parvovirus B19 infection in pregnancy. *Lancet.* 1988;2:566.

16. Jordan J. Identification of human parvovirus B19 infection in idiopathic non-immune hydrops fetalis. *Am J Obstet Gynecol.* 1996;174:37.

17. Enders M, Weidner A, Zoellner I, et al. Fetal morbidity and mortality after acute parvovirus B19 infection in pregnancy: Prospective Evaluation of 1018 cases. *Prenat Diagn.* 2004;24:513.

18. Petrikovsky BW, Baker D, Schneider E. Fetal hydrops secondary to human parvoviral infection in early pregnancy. *Prenat Diagn.* 1996;16:342.

19. Torok TS, Wang QY, Gary GW, et al. Prenatal diagnosis on intrauterine infection with parvovirus B19 by the polymerase in reaction technique. *Clin Infect Dis.* 1992;14:149.

20. Clewley JP. Polymerase chain reaction assay of parvovirus B19 DNA in clinical specimens. *J Clin Microbiol.* 1989;27:2647.

21. Yamakawa Y, Oka H, Hori S, et al. Detection of Human Parvovirus B19 DNA by nested polymerase chain reaction. *Obstet Gynecol.* 1995;86:126.

22. Willig TN, Gazda H, Sieff CA. Diamond-Blackfan anemia. *Curr Opin Hematol.* 2000;7:85.

23. Ball SE, McGuckin CP, Jenkins G, Gordon-Smith EC. Diamond-Blackfan anaemia in the U.K.: analysis of 80 cases from a 20-year birth cohort. *Br J Haematol.* 1996;94:645.

24. Alter B. Inherited bone marrow failure. In: Nathan DG, Orkin SH, Ginsberg D, Look AT, eds. *Nathan and Oski's Hematology of Infancy and Childhood.* 6th ed. Philadelphia: WB Saunders; 2003:280.

25. Gazda HT, Sieff CA. Recent insights into the pathogenesis of Diamond-Blackfan anaemia. *Br J Haematol.* 2006;135:149.

26. Bagnara GP, Zauli G, Vitale L, et al. In vitro growth and regulation of bone marrow enriched CD34+ hematopoietic progenitors in Diamond-Blackfan anemia. *Blood.* 1991;78:2203.

27. Ohene-Abuakwa Y, Orfali KA, Marius C, Ball SE. Two-phase culture in Diamond Blackfan anemia: localization of erythroid defect. *Blood.* 2005;105:838.

28. Ebert BL, Lee MM, Pretz JL, et al. An RNA interference model of RPS19 deficiency in Diamond-Blackfan anemia recapitulates defective hematopoiesis and rescue by dexamethasone:

identification of dexamethasone-responsive genes by microarray. *Blood.* 2005;105:4620.

29. Flygare J, Karlsson S. Diamond-Blackfan anemia: erythropoiesis lost in translation. *Blood.* 2007;109:3152.

30. Abkowitz JL, Sabo KM, Nakamoto B, et al. Diamond-Blackfan anemia: In vitro response of erythroid progenitors to the ligand for c-kit. *Blood.* 1991;78:2198.

31. Taniguchi T, D'Andrea AD. Molecular pathogenesis of Fanconi anemia: recent progress. *Blood.* 2006;107:4223.

32. Redi S, Schindler D, Hanenberg H, et al. Biallelic mutations in PALB2 cause Fanconi anemia subtype FA-N and predispose to childhood cancer. *Nat Genet.* 2007;39:162.

33. Scott JR, Warenski JC. Tests to detect and quantitate fetal maternal bleeding. *Clin Obstet Gynecol.* 1982;25:277.

34. Medearis Al, Hensleigh PA, Parks DR, Herzenber LA. Detection of fetal erythrocytes in maternal blood post partum with the fluorescence-activated cell sorter. *Am J Obstet Gynecol.* 1984;148:290.

35. Lopriore E, Vandenbussche FP, Tiersma ES, et al. Twin-to-twin transfusion syndrome: new perspective. *J Pediatr.* 1995;127:675.

36. Leung WC, Jouannic JM, Hyett J, et al. Procedure-related complications of rapid amniodrainage in the treatment of polyhydramnios. *Ultrasound Obstet Gynecol.* 2004;23:154.

37. Heinonnen S, Ryynanen M, Kirkinen P, Saarikoski S. Perinatal diagnostic evaluation of velamentous umbilical cord insertion: clinical, Doppler, and ultrasound findings. *Obstet Gynecol.* 1996;87:112.

38. Feldman DM, Borgida AF, Trymbulak WP, et al. Clinical implications of velamentous cord insertion in triplet gestations. *Am J Obstet Gynecol.* 2002;186:809.

39. Lee W, Lee VL, Kirk JS, et al. Vasa previa: prenatal diagnosis, natural evolution and clinical outcome. *Obstet Gynecol.* 2000;95:572.

40. Oyelese Y, Smulian JC. Placenta previa, placenta accretia, and vasa previa. *Obstet Gynecol.* 2006;107:927.

41. Chadwick LM, Pemberton PJ, Kurinczuk JJ. Neonatal subgaleal hematoma: associated risk factors, complications and outcome. *J Paediatr Child Health.* 1996;32:228.

42. Halbrecht I. Role of hemagglutinins anti-A and anti-B in pathogenesis of jaundice of the newborn (icterus neonatorum precox). *Am J Dis Child.* 1944;64:248.

43. Desjardins L, Blajchman MA, Chintu C, et al. The spectrum of ABO hemolytic disease of the newborn. *J Pediatr.* 1979;95:447.

44. Grundbacher FJ. The etiology of ABO hemolytic disease of the newborn. *Transfusion.* 1980;20:563.

45. Zipursky A. Isoimmune hemolytic diseases. In: Nathan DG, Oski FA, eds. *Hematology of Infancy and Childhood.* Philadelphia: WB Saunders; 1987:44-73.

46. Bowman JM. Hemolytic disease (erythroblastosis fetalis). In: Creasy RK, Resnick R, eds. *Maternal-Fetal Medicine: Principles and Practice.* Philadelphia: WB Saunders; 1994:711-743.

47. Chavez GF, Mulinare J, Edmonds LD. Epidemiology of Rh hemolytic disease of the newborn in the United States. *JAMA.* 1991;265:3270.

48. Diamond LK, Blackfan KD, Baty JM. Erythroblastosis fetalis and its association with universal edema of the newborn. *J Pediatr.* 1932;1:269.

49. Landsteiner K, Wiener AS. An agglutinable factor in human blood recognized by immune sera for rhesus blood. *Proc Soc Exp Biol Med.* 1940;43:223.

50. Race RR. The Rh genotype and Fisher's theory. *Blood.* 1948;3:27.

51. Chown B. Anemia from bleeding of the fetus into the mother's circulation. *Lancet.* 1954;1:1213.

52. Nevanlinna HR. Factors affecting maternal Rh immunization. *Ann Med Exp Biol.* 1953;31:1.

53. Miraglia del Gludice E, Francese M, Nobilli B, et al. High frequency of de novo mutations in ankyrin gene (ANK1) in children with hereditary spherocytosis. *J Pediatr.* 1998;132:117.

54. Eber SW, Armbrust R, Schroter W. Variable clinical severity of hereditary spherocytosis: Relation to erythrocyte spectrin concentration, osmotic fragility, and autohemolysis. *J Pediatr.* 1990;117:409.

55. Beutler E. G6PD deficiency. *Blood.* 1994;84:3613.

56. Huang CS, Hung KI, Huang MJ, et al. Neonatal jaundice and molecular mutations in

glucose-6-phosphate dehydrogenase deficient newborn infants. *Am J Hematol.* 1996;51:19.

57. Fessas PH, Doxiadis SA, Valaes T. Neonatal jaundice in glucose-6-phosphate dehydrogenase deficient infants. *Brit Med J.* 1962;2:1359.

58. Andrew M, Paes B, Milner R, et al. Development of the human coagulation system in the full-term infant. *Blood.* 1988;72:1651.

59. Andrew M, Paes B, Johnston M. Development of the hemostatic system in the neonate and young infant. *Am J Pediatr Oncol.* 1990;12:95.

60. Levi M. Disseminated intravascular coagulation. *Crit Care Med.* 2007;35:2191.

61. Kreuz W, Veldman A, Fischer D, et al. Neonatal sepsis: a challenge in hemostasis. *Semin Thromb Hemost.* 1999;25:531.

62. Woods WG, Luban NL, Hilgartner MW, Miller DR. Disseminated intravascular coagulation in the newborn. *Am J Dis Child.* 1979;133:44.

63. Taylor FB, Toh CH, Hoots WK, Wada H, Levi M; Scientific Subcommittee on Disseminated Intravascular Coagulation (DIC) of the International Society on Thrombosis and Haemostasis (ISTH). Towards definition, clinical and laboratory criteria and a scoring system for disseminated intravascular coagulation. *Thromb Haemost.* 2001;86:1327.

64. Bakhtiari K, Meijers JC, de Jonge E, Levi M. Prospective validation of the International Society of the Thrombosis and Haemostasis scoring system for disseminated intravascular coagulation. *Crit Care Med.* 2004;32:2416.

65. Toh CH, Hoots WK. The Scoring System of the Scientific and Standardization Committee for Disseminated Intravascular Coagulation of the International Society on Thrombosis and Haemostasis: a five year overview. *J Thromb Haemost.* 2007;5:604.

66. Williams MD, Chalmers EA, Gibson BE. The investigation and management of neonatal haemostasis and thrombosis. *Br J Haematol.* 2007;5:604.

67. Hanada T, Abe T, Takita. Antithrombin III concentrates for the treatment of disseminated intravascular coagulation in children. *Am J Pediatr Hematol Oncol.* 1985;7:3.

68. Dreyfus M, Magny JF, Bridey F, et al. Treatment of homozygous protein C deficiency and neonatal purpura fulminans with a purified protein C concentrate. *N Engl J Med.* 1991;325:1565.

69. Saito H, Maruyuma I, Shimazaki S, et al. Efficacy and safety of recombinant human soluble thrombomodulin (ART-123) in disseminated intravascular coagulation: results of a phase III, randomized, double-blind clinical trial. *J Thromb Haemost.* 2007;5:31.

70. Motohara K, Endo F, Matsuda I. Effect of vitamin K administration on acarboxy Prothrombin (PIVKA-II) levels in newborns. *Lancet.* 1985;2:242.

71. Cornelissen M, Steegars-Theunissen R, Kollee L, et al. Increased incidence of neonatal vitamin K deficiency resulting from maternal anticonvulsant therapy. *Am J Obstet Gynecol.* 1993;168:923.

72. Sutor AH. Vitamin K deficiency bleeding in infants and children. *Semin Thromb Hemost.* 1995;21:317.

73. Hoyer LW. Hemophilia A. *N Engl J Med.* 1994;330:38.

74. Lawn RM. The molecular genetics of hemophilia: blood clotting factors VIII and IX. *Cell.* 1985;42:405.

75. White GC II, Rosendaal F, Aledort LM, et al. Definitions in hemophilia. Recommendation of the scientific subcommittee on factor VIII and factor IX of the scientific and standardization of the International Society on Thrombosis and Haemostasis: Factor VIII and Factor IX Subcommittee. *Thromb Haemost.* 2001;85:560.

76. Sola MC, Del Vecchio A, Rimsza LM. Evaluation and treatment of thrombocytopenia in the neonatal intensive care unit. *Clin Perinatol.* 2000;27:655.

77. Dreyfus M, Kaplan C, Verdy E, et al. Frequency of immune thrombocytopenia in newborns: a prospective study. Immune Thrombocytopenia Working Group. *Blood.* 1997;89:4402.

78. Saino S, Jarvenpaa AL, Renlund M, Riikonen S. Thrombocytopenia in term infants: a population-based study. *Obstet Gynecol.* 2000;95:441.

79. Christensen RD, Henry E, Wiedmeier SE, et al. Thrombocytopenia among extremely low birth weight neonates: data from a multihospital healthcare system. *J Perinatol.* 2006;26:348.

80. Bussel JB, Zabusky MR, Berkowitz RL, et al. Fetal alloimmune thrombocytopenia. *N Engl J Med.* 1997;337:22.

81. Murphy MF, Bussel JB. Advances in the management of alloimmune thrombocytopenia. *Br J Haematol.* 2007;136:366.

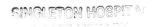

82. Ghevaert C, Campbell K, Walton J, et al. Management and outcome of 200 cases of fetomaternal alloimmune thrombocytopenia. *Transfusion.* 2007;47:901.

83. Bassler D, Greinacher A, Okascharoen C, et al. A systematic review and survey of the management of unexpected neonatal alloimmune thrombocytopenia. *Transfusion.* 2008;48:92.

84. Burrows RF, Kelton JG. Pregnancy in patients with idiopathic thrombocytopenic purpura: assessing the risks for the infant at delivery. *Obstet Gynecol Surv.* 1993;48:781.

85. Kasabach HH, Merritt KK. Hemangioma with extensive purpura. *Arch Dis Child.* 1940;59:1063.

86. Blei F. New clinical observations in hemangiomas. *Semin Cutan Med Surg.* 1999;18:187.

87. Blei F, Karp N, Rofsky N, et al. Successful multimodal therapy for kaposiform hemangioendothelialoma complicated by Kasabach-Merritt phenomenon: case report and review of the literature. *Pediatr Hematol Oncol.* 1998;15:295.

88. Hall GW. Kasabach-Merritt syndrome: pathogenesis and management. *Br J Haematol.* 2001;112:851.

89. Ververidis M, Kiely EM, Spitz L, et al. The clinical significance of thrombocytopenia in neonates with necrotizing enterocolitis. *J Pediatr Surg.* 2001;36:799.

90. Jones KL. *Smith's Recognizable Patterns of Human Malformation.* 6th ed. Philadelphia: Elsevier Saunders; 2006.

91. Hedberg VA, Lipton JM. Thrombocytopenia with absent radii. A review of 100 cases. *Am J Pediatr Hematol Oncol.* 1988;10:51.

CHAPTER 11

Selected Topics in Neonatal Pharmacology

Jeanna Marraffa, PharmD

Jamie Nelsen, PharmD

▶ MANAGEMENT OF NEONATAL SEIZURES

Seizures are a reported complication in approximately 0.1% to 2% of neonates.[1-3] The natural history of neonatal seizures is unknown; however, significant mortality and long-term disability[4] have persuaded most clinicians to practice conservatively and manage clinical and electrographically documented seizures pharmacologically. As is the case with most drug therapy in this particular cohort, randomized, placebo-controlled trials demonstrating the superiority of 1 anticonvulsant versus another are lacking and it remains unclear if any particular therapy is decidedly better than observation alone.

Preliminary animal data have even suggested anticonvulsants may have deleterious effects on the developing brain,[5-7] although lack of long-term controlled trials limits the ability to extrapolate risk in humans.

INITIAL PHARMACOLOGIC APPROACH

Despite inconclusive data demonstrating improved response rates with phenobarbital (PHB) compared to other anticonvulsants, PHB is often used as the first-line anticonvulsant to manage neonatal seizures.[8-10] Unfortunately, neonatal seizures are often refractory to single drug therapy and approximately half of treated patients will need a second-line agent.[9,11,12] For patients with continued seizures despite additional therapy, a trial of IV pyridoxine may be reasonable. Due to the often-observed resolution of clinical but not electrographic seizures in neonates,[4,9,12-14] drug therapy should be accompanied by EEG monitoring regardless of clinical response observed with any of the agents discussed.[15] Certainly seizures caused by a specific metabolic disturbance should be addressed before anticonvulsant therapy is initiated. Because many pediatric neurologists are reluctant to prescribe continuous anticonvulsant therapy for newborns after symptoms of brain injury have resolved or the underlying disease process has been identified and treated,[16] this review will focus on pharmacologic considerations during the acute management period.

PHENOBARBITAL

Therapeutic PHB plasma concentrations are considered to be in the range of 20-40 mg/L.[9,17,18] Assuming drug distribution in neonates approximates 1 L/kg,[10,19] an initial PB loading dose of 20 mg/kg should be administered IV at a rate of 1-2 mg/min to avoid rate-related hypotension. Intramuscular dosing has shown to be 90% to 100% bioavailable,[10,19,20] and the initial loading dose need not be adjusted for this route of administration. If seizures persist, additional doses of PHB up to 40 mg/kg may be administered before considering initiating a second agent. Plasma concentrations >40 mg/L have not been associated with improved success and increase the risk for drug toxicity.[18,21] The best time to sample PHB concentrations in an acute scenario is undefined. If PHB is administered IV, a sample should be obtained at least 1 hour after the infusion to avoid the drug's distribution phase, although clearance is generally slow in this population and obtaining a level 12 to 24 hours following initial seizure control

to determine a maintenance dose is generally recommended. If the patient continues to seize after the initial load, it is impractical to wait to redose pending a drug level. Initial maintenance doses are typically initiated at 2.5-4 mg/kg per day.[17,19]

Despite its accepted utility as a first-line agent, PHB has a moderate success rate in seizure termination when evaluated via EEG. Painter et al found that only 43% of patients treated with PHB had both clinical and electrographic seizure resolution. This is consistent with other reports.[14,21] Phenobarbital exerts its antiseizure effect by enhancing chloride influx through the gamma-aminobutyric acid (GABA) receptor.[22] Excessive CNS depression and diminished feeding occur with increasing plasma concentrations, particularly at PHB concentrations >50 mg/L. Interestingly, Boylan et al[13] found that PHB administration actually increased electrographic seizures following PHB administration, although this was not a consistent effect and the sample size was small. This finding reiterates the need for EEG monitoring in the acute management period.

HYDANTOINS

Phenytoin (PHT) antagonizes voltage-dependent sodium channels, thereby blocking high-frequency, repetitive firing, resulting in its anticonvulsant activity.[22] Therapeutic PHT concentrations are considered to be in the range of 15-25 mg/L.[9,19] As expected, drug distribution in neonates is considerably larger than in adult patients, approximately 1.2 L/kg vs 0.7 L/kg, respectively.[19] An initial loading dose of 20 mg/kg of PHT should be administered IV at a rate not exceeding 1 mg/min to avoid rate-limiting hypotension and cardiac depression. The pharmaceutic characteristics of PHT do not make the drug amenable to IM administration, which may be painful and cause localized tissue damage. If seizures persist despite an initial load, additional doses of 5 mg/kg, up to a total of 30 mg/kg, may be administered before considering additional therapy. If maintenance therapy is initiated, current evidence suggests poor oral bioavailability,[19,23] and high oral doses, 30-40 mg/kg day, may be necessary in conjunction with close therapeutic drug monitoring.[24]

Although the overwhelming majority of experience with managing seizures has come from using PHT, fosphenytoin (FPT), a prodrug of PHT, may be a more desirable agent due to its side-effect profile. The pharmacologic activity of FPT is derived almost entirely from its conversion to PHT via hydrolyses. FPT may be administered as an initial dose of 30 mg/kg IV at a rate not to exceed 0.5-3 PHT equivalents/min (approximately 1.5 mg/kg of FPT is equivalent to 1 mg/kg of PHT).[25] When administered IM, bioavailability of FPT is approximately 100% and no dose adjustments need to be made.

BENZODIAZEPINES

Benzodiazepines (BDZs) enhance inhibitory tone via their effect on GABA-mediated chloride transmission.[22] Despite their well-recognized role as first-line therapy for acute seizure termination in adults, BDZs are generally reserved for add-on therapy in neonates and their efficacy has been poorly documented in controlled studies using EEG monitoring. An initial loading dose of lorazepam (LZP) of 0.05 mg/kg given over 2-5 minutes, repeated up to a total of 0.15 mg/kg, has been shown to be an effective adjunct agent in seizure termination. Similarly effective, diazepam (DZP) may be administered 0.25 mg/kg IV over 2-5 minutes, followed by an IV infusion starting at 0.3 mg/kg/h. If IV access is limited, DZP may be administered rectally, 0.5 mg/ kg.[26] Either agent may be administered IM. Compared to LZP, DZP has a quicker redistribution from the central compartment and a longer half-life predisposing to drug accumulation, which may

make LZP a more desirable agent, although the 2 drugs have never been formally compared in this scenario. Current literature suggests midazolam (MDZ) may have limited utility in this setting, and that response is largely dose dependent. Castro Conde et al found that MDZ effectively controlled refractory seizures in 77% of neonates as documented by EEG.[27] The doses used in this study were considerably higher than comparative evaluations that found no benefit,[28] 0.15 mg/kg IV bolus, followed by an infusion of 0.06 mg/kg/h titrated up to a maximum dose of 1 mg/kg/h.

Generally BZD therapy is well tolerated in neonates, although compared to other anticonvulsants, respiratory depression may be a more common finding.[29,30] Paridoxical movement disorders have been described in several case reports detailing myoclonic activity in the minutes following BZD administration.[31-33] These findings have not been documented in concordance with EEG monitoring and the clinical significance of this adverse event is unknown. In all cases these movement disorders dissipated over the ensuing hours with drug discontinuation.

PYRIDOXINE

Pyridoxine (vitamin B6), is a water-soluble vitamin that is rapidly metabolized to its active form, pyridoxal, in vivo. Pyridoxal is an important cofactor in the synthesis of GABA, a primary inhibitory amino acid.[34] Pyridoxine-dependent seizures are a result of inborn errors of metabolism and are an infrequent but well-described cause of intractable seizures in neonates. Diagnosis is often delayed and treatment in the acute setting is empiric. In patients with refractory seizures not responding to PHB, PHT or BZD, pyridoxine 100 mg IV should be administered. The dose may be repeated up to 500 mg. If a response is noted, an oral pyridoxine dose of 5 mg/kg per day should be initiated and titrated to response.[35]

Side effects related to the acute administration of pyridoxine have not been described.

► APPROACH TO THE SEPTIC NEONATE

Emergent antibiotic therapy for the treatment of neonates with suspected sepsis and/or meningitis is largely empiric and the initial choice of therapy is based on knowledge of probable pathogens and perinatal history. Antibiotics should be initiated immediately after appropriate cultures and IV access has been obtained.[36] The most common bacterial organisms responsible for neonatal sepsis include Group B *Streptococcus* (GBS), *Escherichia coli*, *Staphylococcus* spp. coagulase positive and negative, and *Listeria monocytogenes*.[37,38] The choice of antibiotic treatment for neonatal sepsis must be driven by hospital-specific guidelines based on prevalent organisms and their susceptibility patterns. Ampicillin plus ceftazidime is the initial therapy of choice for a neonate with sepsis or meningitis of unknown etiology, unless pertinent history dictates otherwise.[38] Empiric vancomycin therapy should be withheld, unless strong evidence indicates an infection attributable to gram-positive microorganisms and the prevalence of infections attributable to methicillin-resistant *S aureus* (MRSA) in the hospital is significant.[39] An uncommon cause of meningitis that should be considered in all cases is herpes simplex, in which case acyclovir should be started promptly. Continued antibiotic therapy should be guided by culture and susceptibility results, as well as the type and location of the infection.[36,40]

PENICILLINS

Penicillins are time-dependent antimicrobial agents that mitigate their effect by inhibiting cell wall synthesis.[41] Ampicillin plus an aminoglycoside is the initial treatment of choice for a neonate with presumptive invasive GBS infection.[42] Although resistance of GBS strains to both penicillin G and ampicillin remain universally low, penicillin G should be reserved until GBS has been identified as the cause of the infection and when clinical and microbiologic responses have been documented.[42] Compared to penicillin G, ampicillin has a broader spectrum of antimicrobial activity, including *Haemophilus infulenzae* and *E coli*. In neonates suspected of having GBS meningitis, experts have advocated using higher doses of penicillins due to poor penetration across meninges.[36,38,41,42] Both penicillin G and ampicillin are generally well tolerated, although rare reports of neurotoxicity thought to be mediated by gamma-aminobutyric acid inhibition have been reported. In neonates with age-adjusted renal impairment, the dosing interval of penicillins may be extended to mitigate accumulation, although formal guidelines have not been adopted.

CEPHALOSPORINS

Cephalosporins are structurally similar to penicillins in that they contain a ß-lactam ring, although modifications of substituent groups off the ß-lactam ring confer a different spectrum of antibacterial activity. Third-generation cephalosporins, including cefotaxime, differ from first-generation agents in that they are generally less active against gram-positive cocci, but much more active against gram-negative rods. Cefotaxime has the added advantage of having the greatest activity against *S aureus* and *Streptococcus pyogenes*.[41] In patients with presumed meningitis, cefotaxime therapy should be added to ampicillin plus an aminoglycocide. Although cefotaxime has increased penetration of meninges compared to conventional therapies and resultantly increases the proportion of patients who will have sterile cerebral spinal fluid cultures 48-72 hours into treatment, improved morbidity and mortality have not been demonstrated.[38,43] Ceftriaxone, another third-generation cephalosporin, has a spectrum of activity similar to cefotaxime although the toxicity profile in neonates is significant. Approximately 50% of ceftriaxone is removed via biliary excretion and consequently can cause substantial displacement of bilirubin at concentrations obtained during therapeutic use. Theoretically, the drug may increase the risk of kernicterus and should be used with caution in high-risk neonates with jaundice.[44] Recently the manufacturer revised the ceftriaxone (Rocephin, Roche Laboratories Inc) labeling to reflect a specific contraindication in neonates concomitantly receiving calcium-containing products, including parenteral nutrition, due to complexation and precipitation of a ceftriaxone-calcium salt in lung and kidneys resulting in fatality.[45]

AMINOGLYCOCIDES

Aminoglycosides inhibit bacterial protein synthesis and are used primarily to treat gram-negative bacterial infections. Neonates presenting with sepsis of unknown etiology should empirically receive an aminoglycocide in combination with a penicillin antibiotic.

Gentamicin, due in part to demonstrated synergistic activity against GBS, staphylococcal species, and enterocci,[41,46] has traditionally been the most common empirically prescribed aminoglycocide. For optimal bactericidal activity, peak gentamicin levels (drawn ~30 min postinfusion) should be targeted to achieve ~8 mg/L. To minimize the potential for ototoxicity and nephrotoxicity, trough levels (immediately prior to next dose) should be <2 mg/L. In an effort to reduce the potential for drug toxicity, once-daily dosing using higher doses (4-5 mg/kg) and longer dosing intervals (24 hours) has been advocated in term neonates.[47] The dosing reflected in Table 11–1 is consistent with American Academy of Pediatrics (AAP) dosing

guidelines.[48] The incidence of aminoglycoside nephrotoxicity in neonates is not well defined but is thought to be considerably lower than in the adult population. Although reversible tubular dysfunction has been shown in many studies involving neonates, persistent glomerular filtration impairment has not been conclusively shown in prospective studies.[49]

VANCOMYCIN

Vancomycin is a glycopeptide antibiotic that acts similarly to penicillins by inhibiting bacterial cell wall synthesis.[41] Vancomycin is primarily active against gram-positive bacteria, but due to increasing resistance, empiric use in septic neonates is typically reserved for cases in which there is strong suspicion that the infection is attributable to a gram-positive organism and the prevalence of infections attributable to MRSA in the hospital is significant. Vancomycin exhibits concentration-independent killing, and specific peak plasma concentrations have not been correlated with efficacy. The appropriate dosing regimen of vancomycin is best determined by volume of distribution and ability to clear drug. The volume of distribution of vancomycin changes with the amount of body water and is larger in premature neonates, ranging from 0.57–0.69 L/kg in term neonates to as high as 0.97 L/kg in premature neonates.[49] Vancomycin clearance increases with postconceptional age. Determination of dosing frequency should be guided by trough concentrations, ideally in the range of 5-15 mg/L.[50] If serum trough concentrations are <5 mg/L, increasing the dosing frequency is advised. Vancomycin has been associated with various adverse effects including eosinophilia, thrombocytopenia, ototoxicity, and nephrotoxicity.[46] The occurrence of nephrotoxicity, similar to aminoglycocides, appears to be rare and reversible. Unlike aminoglycocides, however, the relationship between ototoxicity and nephrotoxicity and serum drug concentrations is unclear.[51] Red man syndrome

▶ TABLE 11–1. SUGGESTED ANTIBIOTIC DRUGS AND DOSING FOR THE YOUNG INFANT

Drug	Indication	BW <1200 g	< 7 days BW 1200-2000 g	< 7 days BW >2000 g	≥ 7 days BW 1200-2000 g	≥ 7 days BW >2000 g
Acyclovir, IV	Sepsis/ meningitis	20 mg/kg q8h	20 mg/kg q8h	20 mg/kg q8h	20 mg/kg q8h	20 mg/kg q8h
Ampicillin, IV/ IM	Sepsis	50 mg/kg q12h	50 mg/kg q12h	50 mg/kg q8h 100 mg q8h	50 mg/kg q8h	50 mg/kg q6h 100 mg q8h
	Meningitis					
Cefotaxime, IV/ IM	Meningitis	50 mg/kg q12h	50 mg/kg q 12 h	50 mg/kg q 8-12h	50 mg/kg q 8 h	50 mg/kg q6-8h
Penicillin G, IV/ IM	Sepsis	125,000 U/kg q12h	125,000 U/kg q8-12h	150,000 U/kg q8h	100,000-125,000 U/kg q 6 h	100,000-125,000 U/kg q 6 h
	Meningitis	125,000 U/kg q 12 h	125,000 U/kg q 8-12 h	150,000 U/kg q8 h	100,000-125,000 U/kg q 6 h	100,000-125,000 U/kg q 6 h
Gentamicin, IV/ IM	Sepsis/ meningitis	2.5 mg/kd q 24h	2.5 mg/kg q12h	2.5 mg/kg q12h	2.5 mg/kg q 8-12 h	2.5 mg/kg q8h
Tobramycin, IV/ IM	Sepsis/ meningitis	2.5 mg/kd q24h	2.5 mg/kg q12h	2.5 mg/kg q12h	2.5 mg/kg q8-12h	2.5 mg/kg q8h
Vancomycin, IV	Sepsis/ meningitis	15 mg/kg q24h	10-15 mg/kg q12-18h	10-15 mg/kg q8-12h	10-15 mg/kg q8-12h	10-15 mg/kg q6-8h

is a histamine-mediated, infusion-related phenomenon characterized by a erythematous rash that is self-limiting. This reaction does not prohibit further therapy, but does warrant reducing the rate of infusion.

ACYCLOVIR

Acyclovir is an antiherpesvirus agent that inhibits viral DNA synthesis via its action on herpes simplex virus (HSV), thymidine kinase, and DNA polymerase.[41] Parenteral acyclovir is the treatment of choice for neonatal HSV infections.[52] The currently recommended dose of acyclovir in neonates, regardless of gestational age, is 60 mg/kg per day in 3 divided doses for 14 to 21 days. Acyclovir is generally well tolerated in neonates.[53] Neurotoxicity and renal insufficiency, secondary to drug crystallization and deposition in proximal renal tubules, have been observed in approximately 1% to 5% of adult patients.[41] Baker et al described inadvertent administration of 220 mg/kg of acyclovir in an 11-day-old patient.[54] The patient was observed to have a transient increase in serum creatinine, which resolved with adequate hydration. Neurotoxicity, including tremors, myoclonus, seizures, or coma were not observed. This is consistent with other reports of inadvertent overdose.[55]

▶ SEDATION AND ANALGESIA IN THE YOUNG INFANT

The importance of adequate and appropriate pain management in neonates has garnered significant attention in the last decade. It is becoming increasingly apparent that inadequately controlled pain may have long-term consequences on subsequent child development, although this concern is wholly based on animal data.[56-58]

A comprehensive review of pain management in neonates is beyond the scope of this chapter. The following discussion will focus on acute pharmacologic treatment of pain related to interventional procedures. The approach to pain management for minor procedures involves a variety of nonpharmacologic pain-prevention techniques (nonnurtive sucking, skin-to-skin contact, facilitated tucking, swaddling), oral sucrose administration, and topical anesthetics.[59] Effective pain control should be guided by ongoing pain assessment. A number of scales to assess pain have been developed and validated to varying degrees. These scales may vary given differences in types of pain (procedural, postoperative, ventilation) and the gestational age of the patient. Regardless of the scale used, attention should be paid to physiologic indicators of pain including, but not limited to, changes in heart rate, respiratory rate, blood pressure, oxygen saturation, and palmar sweating.[59] Behavioral indicators of pain, including changes in facial expressions, body movements, and crying, although helpful when present, may often be absent for a variety of reasons.

ACETAMINOPHEN

Acetaminophen is a commonly used analgesic for fever reduction and mild procedural pain in neonates, although there is insufficient evidence that it has any benefit in reducing pain associated with heel prick[66] or reducing opioid requirements after surgery.[67] Acetaminophen mediates its effects though cyclooxygenase (COX) inhibition, although it has reduced activity in the presence of inflammation and its major use is as an antipyretic.[41] Acetaminophen may be administered orally or rectally, 10-15 mg/kg every 6 to 8 hours.[68] The most concerning toxicity of acetaminophen is its potential for hepatotoxicity. Hepatotoxicity is dependent on the balance between: (1) rate of formation of N-acetyl-p-benzoquinoneimine (NAPQI), acetaminophen's toxic metabolite; (2) capacity of nontoxic pathways of acetaminophen elimination; and (3) endogenous glutathione stores. Neonates can produce hepatotoxic metabolites (eg, NAPQI), although they have decreased enzyme activity compared with older infants. Despite reduced capacity for NAPQI formation, neonates are still at risk for hepatotoxicity when acetaminophen is used chronically, as neonates have markedly reduced clearance of the parent drug, which varies with gestational age.[68,69]

NONSTEROIDAL ANTIINFLAMATORY DRUGS (NSAIDs)

Despite extensive use for patent ductus arteriosus closure in preterm neonates, there are no studies investigating NSAIDs for the purpose of analgesia in neonates.[68] As a class, NSAIDs inhibit COX enzymes (COX-1 and COX-2), which are responsible for prostaglandin generation. Adverse effects associated with NSAID use include a reduction in glomerular filtration rate (~20%), gastrointestinal bleeding, neutrophil dysfunction, and bronchoconstriction.[68,70]

LOCAL ANESTHETICS

When compared to placebo, topically applied local anesthetics have been shown to reduce acute pain in neonates during most commonly performed medical procedures, with the exception of heel lances.[71] Local anesthetics can be injected SC or applied topically on intact skin. Several preparations of topical anesthetics are currently available. Lidocaine-prilocaine cream (equal parts 2.5%) has been demonstrated to reduce pain from various cutaneous procedures compared to placebo, although it takes approximately 60 min for onset of clinical effect, which may therefore limit applicability in providing emergent care.[71] Lehr and Taddio have reviewed available clinical data evaluating the analgesic efficacy of local anesthetics used for various procedures.[71] Interestingly,

2 more-recent trials found local anesthetics provided no benefit in reducing pain caused by venipuncture when compared to or added to oral sucrose.[62,72]

Local anesthetics are not routinely used for lumbar puncture and their benefit for this purpose has demonstrated inconsistent efficacy in pain relief. Lidocaine 1%, 0.1-0.4 mL/kg SC, lidocaine-priolcaine cream, and liposomal lidocaine 4%, are all reasonable options if warranted given the clinical situation. Compared to lidocaine-prilocaine cream, liposomal lidocaine cream has a quicker onset of action (30 min), although in emergent situations SC lidocaine should be used.[71]

KETAMINE

Ketamine is an N-methy-D-aspartate antagonist resulting in dissociative analgesia.[41] Despite extensive clinical use in children for induction and maintenance anesthesia, minimal data exist describing its use in neonates, and its use as a sedative and/or analgesic cannot be advocated at this time. In preterm neonates, pain associated with tracheal suctioning was moderately reduced with 1 mg/kg of IV ketamine, although changes in heart rate and blood pressure were not attenuated even with 2 mg/kg.[73] Ketamine causes mild increases in blood pressure, heart rate, and bronchodilation.[41]

▶ SUCROSE

A growing body of literature advocates concentrated oral sucrose as an effective modality of minimizing neonatal pain and this intervention is currently endorsed by both the AAP and the American College of Emergency Physicians.[59,60] In conjunction with nonpharmacologic pain reduction measures, oral sucrose administration is a reasonable first-line approach to minor pain-provoking interventions, including heel stick and venipuncture.[61,62] Fernadez et al demonstrated that oral sucrose eliminated EEG changes associated with procedural pain.[63] Typically 0.05-0.5 mL of a 24% solution is administered via a syringe onto the tongue or by dipping a pacifier into the sucrose solution and onto the tongue or cheek. The onset of action is almost immediate with maximal analgesia observed at 120 sec.[64] The duration of effect is ~5 to 10 min. There appears to be no difference between the analgesic properties of sucrose or glucose.[65]

► PHARMACOLOGIC CONSIDERATIONS IN NEONATAL ABSTINENCE SYNDROMES

In utero exposure to drugs may result in neonatal withdrawal upon delivery, commonly referred to as neonatal abstinence syndrome (NAS). The use of both prescription and illicit drugs in women of childbearing age is common. The National Household Survey on Drug Abuse reports nearly 4.1 million women of child-bearing age abuse drugs of which approximately 4.1% are believed to continue drug use during pregnancy (Substance Abuse and Mental Health Services Administration. Results from the 2006 National Survey on Drug Use and Health: National Findings 2006). Many substances are implicated in causing withdrawal symptoms including opioids, ethanol, barbiturates, caffeine, tobacco, benzodiazepines, and, most recently, the serotonin reuptake inhibitors (SSRIs).[74-82] Stimulants, including cocaine, are more likely to cause symptoms in neonates consistent with continued drug effect rather than withdrawal symptoms.[83,84]

The clinical presentation of NAS varies with individual xenobiotics, the frequency, timing and dose of the last maternal use, and both mother and neonatal metabolism. CNS irritability is a common finding in NAS, secondary to opioid and nonopioid withdrawal. Seizures can be present in up to 11% of neonates withdrawing from opiates[85] and represent a true neonatal emergency. The mechanism for the seizure activity remains unclear. Indications for drug therapy are seizures, poor feeding, vomiting, and diarrhea with resultant hypovolemia, inability to sleep, and fever.

In a neonate presenting with signs of withdrawal, it is imperative to rule out other causes of irritability including infectious or metabolic disorders.

This section will focus on the major culprits of NAS and the acute management of the neonate in opioid withdrawal. The management of withdrawal syndromes is primarily supportive and a full discussion is outside the scope of this chapter.

OPIOID WITHDRAWAL

Newborns exposed to opioids in utero have approximately a 50% to 90% incidence of developing signs of withdrawal.[85-87] Although tolerance can develop with chronic use of any opioid, withdrawal from heroin and methadone has been most rigorously described. Though the incidence of withdrawal secondary to heroin is reported to be less than that of methadone, logic states that methadone maintenance programs in opiate-addicted pregnant women should be employed. Methadone has been shown to be associated with increased compliance and prenatal care.[88] There are conflicting data on whether higher doses of methadone are associated with increased incidences of NAS. Berghella et al[76] and McCarthy et al[88] all performed retrospective studies on pregnant women on methadone-maintenance programs and found no difference in the severity, duration, or treatment of NAS in high- versus low-dose methadone. Withdrawal signs secondary to heroin generally occur within 24 hours of birth and nearly always by 72 hours of birth. Methadone withdrawal generally begins at 72 hours after birth.[89] Ebner et al prospectively evaluated 52 neonates born to opioid-maintained mothers and found that the mean duration from birth to requirement of NAS treatment was 33 hours for the morphine group, 34 hours for the buprenorphine group, and 58 hours for the methadone group.[90]

Buprenorphine, a partial μ-receptor agonist, is beginning to have a role in the treatment of opiate addiction and is an alternative to methadone-maintenance programs.[91] Though not FDA-approved in pregnancy, buprenorphine has been used in this regard and has been reported to have less incidence of NAS compared to methadone.[92-94] Despite this, several cases have described NAS in newborns born of buprenorphine-treated mothers.[92,95-97] Kayemba-Kay et al[95] describe 13 infants born to mothers on buprenorphine maintenance: 11 of the 13 infants experienced NAS, with 10 of the 11 requiring treatment. Compared to methadone, the onset of NAS varied among these patients, ranging from day 1 through day 5. The duration of NAS in these infants was quite prolonged, with a range of 14 to 30 days.[95] Further studies on buprenorphine and its effect on neonates are warranted. Until then, providers need to be familiar with buprenorphine use and its ability to induce NAS.

PHARMACOLOGIC CONSIDERATIONS FOR THE TREATMENT OF OPIOID-INDUCED NAS

Pharmacologic intervention must be individualized and based on the severity of NAS symptoms. Seizures represent a true emergency. Scoring tools are available and should be employed in the nursery to direct therapy. Well-recognized scoring tools include the Lipsitz tool[98] and the Finnegan method.[99] Nonpharmacologic strategies such as minimizing excessive noise and swaddling have been successfully employed.[100] Though managing these patients in the ED is extremely rare, it is worth a discussion on the available pharmacologic interventions. Very few studies compare the efficacy of different treatments for NAS. Management of opioid-induced NAS is predominantly treated with opioids. Tincture of opium is recommended over paregoric by the AAP.[101] Tincture of opium contains 10 mg/mL of morphine and 30% ethanol, and needs to be diluted prior to administration. A 25-fold dilution of tincture of opium (DTO) provides 0.4 mg/mL morphine. The dosing of DTO recommended by the AAP is 0.1 mL/kg or 2 drops/kg with feedings every 4 hours. Dosing can be increased by 2 drops/kg every 4 hours as needed to control withdrawal symptoms.[101] Paregoric has been used for many years for the treatment of NAS. Its primary active ingredient is anhydrous morphine (0.4 mg/mL) and it is dosed at 0.1 mL/kg (2 drops/kg) every 4 hours and can be titrated by 2 drops/kg every 4 hours as needed to control withdrawal symptoms.[101] In addition to containing anhydrous morphine, paregoric also contains antispasmodics, camphor, ethanol, and benzoic acid all of which are not without inherent toxicity. Because of these additives, the use of paregoric has declined in recent years. If oral morphine is employed, often supplied as 2 mg/mL and 4 mg/mL concentrations, it should be dosed to deliver a morphine equivalent as supplied by DTO or paregoric. Phenobarbital (PBT) has also been employed for opioid-induced NAS, although it is considered a second-line agent. In neonates withdrawing simultaneously from several drugs, however, PBT is considered the drug of choice. Despite identified therapeutic serum concentrations of PBT for the management of seizures, the serum concentration necessary for the control of withdrawal is unknown. Dose-dependent respiratory and mental status depression may accompany PBT administration and neonates should be monitored accordingly. Few studies demonstrate the efficacy of one particular treatment regimen over another. Ebner et al [90] and Jackson et al[90,102,103] prospectively compared morphine vs PBT for the treatment of NAS. The infants treated with morphine, in both studies, had a shorter duration of treatment and a reduced need for second-line agents.

▶ DRUGS UTILIZED IN CARDIOVASCULAR EMERGENCIES

PHARMACOLOGIC CONSIDERATIONS FOR THE MANAGEMENT OF PATENT DUCTUS ARTERIOSUS (PDA)

Congenital heart disease occurs in 0.01% of all live births.[104] (See Chapter 4 for a complete discussion on the pathophysiology and management of congenital heart disease.)

In a neonate presenting to the ED with cyanosis and respiratory distress and a ductal-dependent lesion is suspected, immediate treatment is required. In the preterm neonate, pharmacologic therapy for closure of patent ductus arteriosus (PDA) is achieved using indomethacin.[105] For the purpose of this chapter, we will focus on the emergent management of PDA in the neonate presenting to the ED.

Prostaglandin E_1 (Alprostadil) (PGE_1) is an essential therapeutic option in the management of PDA. It was first studied by Olley et al[106] and Coceani et al[107] and was shown to be involved in the patency of the ductus arteriosus. PGE_1 dilates the smooth muscle layer of the ductus arteriosus, thereby increasing the right-to-left or left-to-right blood flow and subsequently increasing pulmonary or systemic blood flow and decreasing pulmonary vascular resistance.

PGE_1 should be initiated in the ED as soon as the suspicion of a ductal-dependent lesion is entertained. PGE_1 infusion should be initiated at a rate of 0.05 µg/kg/min and can be increased to 0.1 µg/kg/min.[104,108]

The use of PGE_1 is not without risk and adverse events. Apnea can occur in up to 12%

of patients following initiation of PGE_1 infusion.[104] Talosi et al retrospectively reviewed 49 neonates that received PGE_1 infusions. The main adverse effect of the infusion was apnea in 15 of 49 cases; 5 of these 15 cases required mechanical ventilation. Fever was also fairly common in these patients and was managed by lowering the incubator temperature. One patient had a seizure during the infusion.[108]

Although aminophylline has been investigated and shown to be effective for the prevention of apnea during PGE_1 infusion via its bronchodilating effects,[109] this intervention may be associated with significant toxicity with small dosing errors and improper monitoring. Due to the risks, we do not recommend the administration of aminophylline in this setting.

Neonates given PGE_1 infusions in the ED should be monitored closely for apnea and mechanical ventilation should be performed if necessary. The administration of sedatives increases the incidence of apnea and should be used with caution. Frequent vital signs including blood pressure and temperature are imperative due to the risk of fever and hypotension secondary to the infusion.

After initial stabilization in the ED, the neonate should be monitored in a neonatal or pediatric intensive care unit.

▶ PHARMACOLOGIC CONSIDERATIONS IN THE MANAGEMENT OF SHOCK

There are several causes of shock. The mechanisms and causes of shock are discussed in detail in Chapters 4 and 5 of this text. This review will discuss the management of shock with the assumption that the underlying cause is being addressed.

Though hypovolemia is a rare cause of hypotension in neonates, volume expansion is often used as a first-line intervention.[110,111]

Crystalloid fluids should be the mainstay of volume expansion. The administration of colloids has been associated with increased morbidity and mortality and, when compared to normal saline, has shown no additional benefit.[112,113]

A single IV bolus over 10 min of 10-20 mL/kg of 0.9% sodium chloride should be administered for hypovolemia-induced shock.[114]

Vasopressors have been used for many years for the management of hypotension and shock of many different etiologies. There is little evidence suggesting that the use of vasopressors improves mortality in the neonatal population, although it makes reasonable sense that improving hypotension will improve overall outcomes as well as neurologic outcomes by increasing cerebral blood flow. Similarly, vasopressors have never been shown to improve mortality in the adult population, yet they are the standard of care.

DOPAMINE

Dopamine is the most commonly used agent in the treatment of hypotension in neonates.[111,115,116] Dopamine is an indirect vasopressor and is a precursor to norepinephrine. It exerts its pharmacologic action by a dose-dependent stimulation of dopaminergic receptors and alpha- and beta-adrenergic receptors. At low doses, dopaminergic receptor effects predominate and as the dose increases, beta-and alpha-receptor effects predominate. When the alpha- and beta-adrenergic receptors are stimulated, peripheral vasoconstriction, increased myocardial contractility, and increased cardiac output occur. Dopamine is administered by a continuous IV infusion and the dose is titratable from 2.5 µg/kg/min up to 20 µg/kg/min. Doses exceeding 20 µg/kg/min are not recommended due to profound alpha-receptor agonism and peripheral vasoconstriction.[111,115,116]

DOBUTAMINE

Dobutamine exerts its pharmacologic action by stimulating beta 1- and beta 2-adrenergic receptors, thereby increasing cardiac output by increasing stroke volume. It also causes a decrease in total peripheral vascular resistance by beta 2-adrenergic stimulation. Dopamine has been shown to be superior over dobutamine in the neonatal patient population.[112,117,118] Dobutamine should be used as adjunctive therapy in patients with known myocardial dysfunction.[119] Dobutamine is administered by a continuous IV infusion and the dose is titratable from 5-20 µg/kg/min.

EPINEPHRINE

Epinephrine is a direct-acting vasopressor and stimulates both alpha- and beta-adrenergic receptors. At lower doses, the beta-adrenergic receptor agonism predominates with a resultant increased myocardial contractility and peripheral vasodilatation. As the dose is increased, the alpha-adrenergic receptor agonism results in peripheral vasoconstriction and an increase in systemic vascular resistance. Epinephrine is widely used to treat neonatal resuscitation and refractory hypotension.[120,121] Epinephrine is administered by a continuous IV infusion and the dose is titratable from 0.05-2.5 µg/kg/min. Adverse effects of epinephrine result from excessive peripheral vasoconstriction and can include decreased cardiac output and impaired tissue perfusion. Norepinephrine is rarely used in neonates and therefore will not be discussed in detail.

CORTICOSTEROIDS

Adrenal insufficiency should also be a considered etiology of hypotension, particularly in the preterm infant.[122] When adrenal insufficiency is thought to be the cause of hypotension, corticosteroids should be administered. Corticosteroids increase the responsiveness to circulating catecholamines and subsequently can increase vascular tone.[111] Hydrocortisone is administered as an IV bolus of 2.5 µg/kg and repeated every 6 hours. Despite the known adverse events associated with long-term corticosteroid use, there are minimal risks associated with short-term use.[111]

REFERENCES

1. Painter M. Neonatal seizure disorders. In: Levene M, Chervenak F, Whittle MJ, Bennett MJ, Punt J, eds. *Fetal and Neonatal Neurology and Neurosurgery.* 3rd ed. New York: Churchill Livingstone; 2001:547-564.

2. Evans D, Levene M. Neonatal seizures.[erratum appears in arch dis child fetal neonatal ed 1998 jul;79(1):F80]. *Arch Dis Child Fetal Neonatal Ed.* 1998;78:F70-F75.

3. Volpe J. Neonatal seizures. In: Volpe J, ed. *Neurology of the Newborn.* 4th ed. Philadelphia, PA: WB Saunders; 2001:178-214.

4. Scher MS, Aso K, Beggarly ME, Hamid MY, Steppe DA, Painter MJ. Electrographic seizures in preterm and full-term neonates: clinical correlates, associated brain lesions, and risk for neurologic sequelae. *Pediatrics.* 1993;91:128-134.

5. Olney JW, Wozniak DF, Jevtovic-Todorovic V, Farber NB, Bittigau P, Ikonomidou C. Drug-induced apoptotic neurodegeneration in the developing brain. *Brain Pathol.* 2002;12:488-498.

6. Bittigau P, Sifringer M, Genz K, et al. Antiepileptic drugs and apoptotic neurodegeneration in the developing brain. *Proc Natl Acad Sci USA.* 2002;99:15089-15094.

7. Diaz J, Schain RJ, Bailey BG. Phenobarbital-induced brain growth retardation in artificially reared rat pups. *Biol Neonate.* 1977;32:77-82.

8. Bartha AI, Shen J, Katz KH, et al. Neonatal seizures: multicenter variability in current treatment practices. *Pediatr Neurol.* 2007;37:85-90.

9. Painter MJ, Scher MS, Stein AD, et al. Phenobarbital compared with phenytoin for the treatment of neonatal seizures. *N Engl J Med.* 1999;341:485-489.

10. Lockman LA, Kriel R, Zaske D, Thompson T, Virnig N. Phenobarbital dosage for control of neonatal seizures. *Neurology.* 1979;29:1445-1449.

11. Boylan GB, Rennie JM, Chorley G, et al. Second-line anticonvulsant treatment of neonatal seizures: a video-EEG monitoring study. *Neurology.* 2004;62:486-488.

12. Scher MS, Alvin J, Gaus L, Minnigh B, Painter MJ. Uncoupling of EEG-clinical neonatal seizures after antiepileptic drug use. *Pediatr Neurol.* 2003;28:277-280.

13. Boylan GB, Rennie JM, Pressler RM, Wilson G, Morton M, Binnie CD. Phenobarbitone, neonatal seizures, and video-EEG. *Arch Dis Child Fetal Neonatal Ed.* 2002;86:F165-F170.

14. Boylan GB, Rennie JM, Chorley G, et al. Second-line anticonvulsant treatment of neonatal seizures: a video-EEG monitoring study. *Neurology.* 2004;62:486-488.

15. McBride MC, Laroia N, Guillet R. Electrographic seizures in neonates correlate with poor neurodevelopmental outcome. *Neurology.* 2000; 55:506-513.

16. Ferriero DM. Neonatal brain injury.[see comment]. *N Engl J Med.* 2004;351:1985-1995.

17. Touw DJ, Graafland O, Cranendonk A, Vermeulen RJ, van Weissenbruch MM. Clinical pharmacokinetics of phenobarbital in neonates. *Eur J Pharm Sc.* 2000;12:111-116.

18. Gal P, Toback J, Boer HR, Erkan NV, Wells TJ. Efficacy of phenobarbital monotherapy in treatment of neonatal seizures—relationship to blood levels. *Neurology.* 1982;32:1401-1404.

19. Painter MJ, Pippenger C, MacDonald H, Pitlick W. Phenobarbital and diphenylhydantoin levels in neonates with seizures. *J Pediatr.* 1978;92:315-319.

20. Wilensky AJ, Friel PN, Levy RH, Comfort CP, Kaluzny SP. Kinetics of phenobarbital in normal subjects and epileptic patients. *Eur J Clin Pharmacol.* 1982;23:87-92.

21. Gilman JT, Gal P, Duchowny MS, Weaver RL, Ransom JL. Rapid sequential phenobarbital treatment of neonatal seizures. *Pediatrics.* 1989;83:674-678.

22. Kaindl AM, Asimiadou S, Manthey D, Hagen MV, Turski L, Ikonomidou C. Antiepileptic drugs and the developing brain. *Cell Mol Life Sc.* 2006;63:399-413.

23. Sicca F, Contaldo A, Rey E, Dulac O. Phenytoin administration in the newborn and infant. *Brain Dev.* 2000;22:35-40.

24. Riviello JJ. Drug therapy for neonatal seizures: Part 1. *NeoReviews.* 2004;5:e215.

25. Fischer JH, Patel TV, Fischer PA. Fosphenytoin: clinical pharmacokinetics and comparative advantages in the acute treatment of seizures. *Clin Pharmacokinet.* 2003;42:33-58.

26. Langslet A, Meberg A, Bredesen JE, Lunde PK. Plasma concentrations of diazepam and N-desmethyldiazepam in newborn infants after intravenous, intramuscular, rectal and oral administration. *Acta Paediatr Scand.* 1978;67:699-704.

27. Castro Conde JR, Hernandez Borges AA, Domenech Martinez E, Gonzalez Campo C, Perera Soler R. Midazolam in neonatal seizures with no response to phenobarbital. *Neurology.* 2005;64:876-879.

28. Shany E, Benzaqen O, Watemberg N. Comparison of continuous drip of midazolam or lidocaine in the treatment of intractable neonatal seizures. *J Child Neurol.* 2007;22:255-259.

29. Orr RA, Dimand RJ, Venkataraman ST, Karr VA, Kennedy KJ. Diazepam and intubation in emergency treatment of seizures in children. *Ann Emerg Med.* 1991;20:1009-1013.

30. Ng E, Klinger G, Shah V, Taddio A. Safety of benzodiazepines in newborns. *Ann Pharmacother.* 2002;36:1150-1155.

31. Sexson WR, Thigpen J, Stajich GV. Stereotypic movements after lorazepam administration in premature neonates: a series and review of the literature. *J Perinatol.* 1995;15:146-149.

32. Lee DS, Wong HA, Knoppert DC. Myoclonus associated with lorazepam therapy in very-low-birth-weight infants. *Biol Neonate.* 1994;66:311-315.

33. Chess PR, D'Angio CT. Clonic movements following lorazepam administration in full-term infants. *Arch Pediatr Adolesc Med.* 1998;152:98-99.

34. Flomenbaum NE, Goldfrank LR, Hoffman RS, Howland MA, Lewin NA, Nelson LS, eds. *Goldfrank's Toxicologic Emergencies.* 8th ed. New York: McGraw-Hill; 2006.

35. Gospe SM. Pyridoxine-dependent seizures: findings from recent studies pose new questions. *Pediatr Neurol.* 2002;26:181-185.

36. Gerdes JS. Diagnosis and management of bacterial infections in the neonate. *Pediatr Clin North Am.* 2004;51:939-959.

37. Sinha A, Yokoe D, Platt R. Intrapartum antibiotics and neonatal invasive infections caused by organisms other than group B streptococcus. *J Pediatr.* 2003;142:492-497.

38. Heath PT, Nik Yusoff NK, Baker CJ. Neonatal meningitis. *Arch Dis Child Fetal Neonatal Ed.* 2003;88:F173-F178.

39. Principles of appropriate use of vancomycin. In: Pickering L, Baker C, Long S, McMillan JA, eds. *Red Book: 2006 Report of the Committee on Infectious Diseases.* 27th ed. Elk Grove Village, IL: American Academy of Pediatrics; 2006:740-741.

40. McCollough M, Sharieff GQ. Common complaints in the first 30 days of life. *Emerg Med Clin North Am.* 2002;20:27-48.

41. Brunton LL, Lazo JS, Parker KL, eds. *Goodman & Gilman's: The Pharmacological Basis of Therapeutics.* 11th ed. New York: McGraw-Hill; 2006.

42. Group B streptococcal infections. In: Pickering L, Baker C, Long S, McMillan JA, eds. *Red Book: 2006 Report of the Committee on Infectious Diseases.* 27th ed. Elk Grove Village, IL: American Academy of Pediatrics; 2006:620-627.

43. Odio CM, Faingezicht I, Salas JL, Guevara J, Mohs E, McCracken GH, Jr. Cefotaxime vs. conventional therapy for the treatment of bacterial meningitis of infants and children. *Pediatr Infect Dis.* 1986;5:402-407.

44. Henry NK, Hoecker JL, Rhodes KH. Antimicrobial therapy for infants and children: guidelines for the inpatient and outpatient practice of pediatriac infectious diseases. *Mayo Clin Proc.* 2000;75:86-97.

45. *Rocephin (Ceftriaxone Sodium) Package Insert.* Nutley, New Jersey: Roche Laboratories; 2007; No. May.

46. Dawson PM. Vancomycin and gentamicin in neonates: hindsight, current controversies, and forethought. *J Perinat Neonatal Nurs.* 2002;16:54-72.

47. Nestaas E, Bangstad HJ, Sandvik L, Wathne KO. Aminoglycoside extended interval dosing in neonates is safe and effective: a meta-analysis. [see comment]. *Arch Dis Child Fetal Neonatal Ed.* 2005;90:F294-F300.

48. Tables of antibacterial drug dosages. In: Pickering L, Baker C, Long S, McMillan JA, eds. *Red Book: 2006 Report of the Committee on Infectious Diseases.* 27th ed. Elk Grove Village, IL: American Academy of Pediatrics; 2006:750-765.

49. de Hoog M, Mouton JW, van den Anker JN. New dosing strategies for antibacterial agents in the neonate. *Semin Fetal Neonatal Med.* 2005;10:185-194.

50. Winter M, ed. *Basic Clinical Pharmacokinetics.* 4th ed. Baltimore, MD: Lippincott Williams & Wilkins; 2004.

51. de Hoog M, Mouton JW, van den Anker JN. Vancomycin: pharmacokinetics and administration regimens in neonates. *Clin Pharmacokinet.* 2004;43:417-440.

52. Herpes simplex. In: Pickering L, Baker C, Long S, McMillan JA, eds. *Red Book: 2006 Report of the Committee on Infectious Diseases.* 27th ed. Elk Grove Village, IL: American Academy of Pediatrics; 2006:361-371.

53. Rudd C, Rivadeneira ED, Gutman LT. Dosing considerations for oral acyclovir following neonatal herpes disease. *Acta Paediatr.* 1994;83:1237-1243.

54. Baker KL, Baker SD, Morgan DL. Largest dose of acyclovir inadvertently administered to a neonate. *Pediatr Infect Dis J.* 2003;22:842.

55. McDonald LK, Tartaglione TA, Mendelman PM, Opheim KE, Corey L. Lack of toxicity in two cases of neonatal acyclovir overdose. *Pediatr Infect Dis J.* 1989;8:529-532.

56. Fitzgerald M, Beggs S. The neurobiology of pain: developmental aspects. *Neuroscientist.* 2001;7:246-257.

57. Maroney DI. Recognizing the potential effect of stress and trauma on premature infants in the NICU: How are outcomes affected? *J Perinatol.* 2003;23:679-683.

58. Anand KJ, Scalzo FM. Can adverse neonatal experiences alter brain development and subsequent behavior? *Biol Neonate.* 2000;77:69-82.

59. American Academy of Pediatrics Committee on Fetus and, Newborn, American Academy of Pediatrics Section on, Surgery, Canadian Paediatric Society Fetus and Newborn, Committee, Batton DG, Barrington KJ, Wallman C. Prevention and management of pain in the neonate: an update. *Pediatrics.* 2006;118:2231-2241.

60. Mace S, Brown L, Clark R, et al. Clinical policy: critical issues in sedation of pediatric patients in the emergency department. J Emerg Nurs. 2005;34:e33-e107.

61. Lefrak L, Burch K, Caravantes R, et al. Sucrose analgesia: identifying potentially better practices. *Pediatrics.* 2006;118:S197-S202.

62. Gradin M, Eriksson M, Holmqvist G, Holstein A, Schollin J. Pain reduction at venipuncture in newborns: oral glucose compared with local anesthetic cream. *Pediatrics.* 2002;110:1053-1057.

63. Fernandez M, Blass EM, Hernandez-Reif M, Field T, Diego M, Sanders C. Sucrose attenuates a negative electroencephalographic response to an aversive stimulus for newborns. *J Dev Behav Pediatr.* 2003;24:261-266.

64. Blass EM, Shah A. Pain-reducing properties of sucrose in human newborns. *Chem Senses.* 1995;20:29-35.

65. Blass EM, Shide DJ. Some comparisons among the calming and pain-relieving effects of sucrose, glucose, fructose and lactose in infant rats. *Chem Senses.* 1994;19:239-249.

66. Shah V, Taddio A, Ohlsson A. Randomised controlled trial of paracetamol for heel prick pain in neonates. *Arch Dis Child Fetal Neonatal Ed.* 1998;79:F209-F11.

67. van der Marel CD, Peters JW, Bouwmeester NJ, Jacqz-Aigrain E, van den Anker JN, Tibboel D. Rectal acetaminophen does not reduce morphine consumption after major surgery in young infants. *Br J Anaesth.* 2007;98:372-379.

68. Jacqz-Aigrain E, Anderson BJ. Pain control: non-steroidal anti-inflammatory agents. *Semin Fetal Neonatal Med.* 2006;11:251-259.

69. Walls L, Baker CF, Sarkar S. Acetaminophen-induced hepatic failure with encephalopathy in a newborn. *J Perinatol.* 2007;27:133-135.

70. Anand KJ, Hall RW. Pharmacological therapy for analgesia and sedation in the newborn. [erratum appears in arch dis child fetal neonatal ed. 2007 mar;92(2):F156 note: Dosage error in text]. *Arch Dis Child Fetal Neonatal Ed.* 2006;91:F448-F453.

71. Lehr VT, Taddio A. Topical anesthesia in neonates: clinical practices and practical considerations. *Semin Perinatol.* 2007;31:323-329.

72. Lemyre B, Hogan DL, Gaboury I, Sherlock R, Blanchard C, Moher D. How effective is tetracaine 4% gel, before a venipuncture, in

reducing procedural pain in infants: a randomized double-blind placebo controlled trial. *BMC Pediatrics.* 2007;7:7.

73. Saarenmaa E, Neuvonen PJ, Huttunen P, Fellman V. Ketamine for procedural pain relief in newborn infants. *Arch Dis Child Fetal Neonatal Ed.* 2001;85:F53-F56.

74. Osborn DA, Jeffery HE, Cole M. Opiate treatment for opiate withdrawal in newborn infants.[update of cochrane database syst rev. 2002;(3):CD002059; PMID: 12137642]. *Cochrane Database Syst Rev.* 2005:002059.

75. Richardson KA, Yohay AL, Gauda EB, McLemore GL. Neonatal animal models of opiate withdrawal. *ILAR J.* 2006;47:39-48.

76. Subhedar NV. Treatment of hypotension in newborns. *Semin Neonatol.* 2003;8:413-423.

77. Pichini S, Garcia-Algar O. In utero exposure to smoking and newborn neurobehavior: How to assess neonatal withdrawal syndrome?. *Ther Drug Monit.* 2006;28:288-290.

78. Reynolds EW, Riel-Romero RM, Bada HS. Neonatal abstinence syndrome and cerebral infarction following maternal codeine use during pregnancy. *Clin Pediatr (Phila).* 2007;46:639-645.

79. Schempf AH. Illicit drug use and neonatal outcomes: a critical review. *Obstet Gynecol Surv.* 2007;62:749-757.

80. Noori S, Seri I. Pathophysiology of newborn hypotension outside the transitional period. *Early Hum Dev.* 2005;81:399-404.

81. Pladys P, Wodey E, Beuchee A, Branger B, Betremieux P. Left ventricle output and mean arterial blood pressure in preterm infants during the 1st day of life. *Eur J Pediatr.* 1999;158:817-824.

82. Seri I, Somogyvari Z, Hovanyovszky S, Kiszel J, Tulassay T. Developmental regulation of the inhibitory effect of dopamine on prolactin release in the preterm neonate. *Biol Neonate.* 1998;73:137-144.

83. Weinstein LB. Mothers and methadone. *Am J Nurs.* 2000;100:13-14.

84. Watterberg KL. Adrenal insufficiency and cardiac dysfunction in the preterm infant. *Pediatr Res.* 2002;51:422-424.

85. Welsh CJ, Cargiulo TP. Response to "detoxification with buprenorphine of a pregnant heroin addict." *Am J Addict.* 2000;9:340-341.

86. Van Overmeire B, Chemtob S. The pharmacologic closure of the patent ductus arteriosus. *Semin Fetal Neonatal Med.* 2005;10:177-184.

87. McCollough M, Sharieff GQ. Common complaints in the first 30 days of life. *Emerg Med Clin North Am.* 2002;20:27-48.

88. Schneider DJ, Moore JW. Patent ductus arteriosus. *Circulation.* 2006;114:1873-1882.

89. Davids E, Gastpar M. Buprenorphine in the treatment of opioid dependence. *Eur Neuropsychopharmacol.* 2004;14:209-216.

90. Pacifico P, Nardelli E, Pantarotto MF. Neonatal heroin withdrawal syndrome; evaluation of different pharmacological treatments. *Pharmacol Res.* 1989;21:63-64.

91. Ebner N, Rohrmeister K, Winklbaur B, et al. Management of neonatal abstinence syndrome in neonates born to opioid maintained women. *Drug Alcohol Depend.* 2007;87:131-138.

92. Seri I, Noori S. Diagnosis and treatment of neonatal hypotension outside the transitional period. *Early Hum Dev.* 2005;81:405-411.

93. Ceger P, Kuhn CM. Opiate withdrawal in the neonatal rat: relationship to duration of treatment and naloxone dose. *Psychopharmacology (Berl).* 2000;150:253-259.

94. Dysart K, Hsieh HC, Kaltenbach K, Greenspan JS. Sequela of preterm versus term infants born to mothers on a methadone maintenance program: differential course of neonatal abstinence syndrome. *J Perinat Med.* 2007;35:344-346.

95. So KW, Fok TF, Ng PC, Wong WW, Cheung KL. Randomised controlled trial of colloid or crystalloid in hypotensive preterm infants. *Arch Dis Child Fetal Neonatal Ed.* 1997;76:F43-F46.

96. Smith GC. The pharmacology of the ductus arteriosus. *Pharmacol Rev.* 1998;50:35-58.

97. Osborn DA, Jeffery HE, Cole MJ. Sedatives for opiate withdrawal in newborn infants.[update of cochrane database syst rev. 2002;(3):CD002053; PMID: 12137641]. *Cochrane Database Syst Rev.* 2005:002053.

98. Dysart K, Hsieh HC, Kaltenbach K, Greenspan JS. Sequela of preterm versus term infants born to mothers on a methadone maintenance program: differential course of neonatal abstinence syndrome. *J Perinat Med.* 2007;35:344-346.

99. Ebbesen F, Joergensen A, Hoseth E, et al. Neonatal hypoglycaemia and withdrawal symptoms after exposure in utero to valproate. *Arch*

Dis Child Fetal Neonatal Ed. 2000;83:F124-F129.

100. Burns L, Mattick RP. Using population data to examine the prevalence and correlates of neonatal abstinence syndrome. *Drug Alcohol Rev.* 2007;26:487-492.

101. Coyle MG, Ferguson A, Lagasse L, Oh W, Lester B. Diluted tincture of opium (DTO) and phenobarbital versus DTO alone for neonatal opiate withdrawal in term infants. *J Pediatr.* 2002;140:561-564.

102. Sinha C, Ohadike P, Carrick P, Pairaudeau P, Armstrong D, Lindow SW. Neonatal outcome following maternal opiate use in late pregnancy. *Int J Gynaecol Obstet.* 2001;74:241-246.

103. Seri I, Noori S. Diagnosis and treatment of neonatal hypotension outside the transitional period. *Early Hum Dev.* 2005;81:405-411.

104. Greenough A, Cheeseman P, Kavvadia V, Dimitriou G, Morton M. Colloid infusion in the perinatal period and abnormal neurodevelopmental outcome in very low birth weight infants. *Eur J Pediatr.* 2002;161:319-323.

105. Zhu H, Barr GA. Naltrexone-precipitated morphine withdrawal in infant rat is attenuated by acute administration of NOS inhibitors but not NMDA receptor antagonists. *Psychopharmacology (Berl).* 2000;150:325-336.

106. Haddad PM, Pal BR, Clarke P, Wieck A, Sridhiran S. Neonatal symptoms following maternal paroxetine treatment: Serotonin toxicity or paroxetine discontinuation syndrome?. *J Psychopharmacol.* 2005;19:554-557.

107. Heckmann M, Trotter A, Pohlandt F, Lindner W. Epinephrine treatment of hypotension in very low birthweight infants. *Acta Paediatr.* 2002;91:566-570.

108. Neonatal drug withdrawal. American academy of pediatrics committee on drugs. *Pediatrics.* 1998;101:1079-1088.

109. Abrahams RR, Kelly SA, Payne S, Thiessen PN, Mackintosh J, Janssen PA. Rooming-in compared with standard care for newborns of mothers using methadone or heroin. *Can Fam Physician.* 2007;53:1722-1730.

110. Hermes-DeSantis ER, Clyman RI. Patent ductus arteriosus: Pathophysiology and management. [see comment]. *J Perinatol.* 2006;26:S14-S18.

111. Jackson L, Ting A, McKay S, Galea P, Skeoch C. A randomised controlled trial of morphine versus phenobarbitone for neonatal abstinence syndrome. *Arch Dis Child Fetal Neonatal Ed.* 2004;89:F300-F304.

112. Jansson LM, Dipietro JA, Elko A, Velez M. Maternal vagal tone change in response to methadone is associated with neonatal abstinence syndrome severity in exposed neonates. *J Matern Fetal Neonatal Med.* 2007;20:677-685.

113. Jazz Pharmaceuticals I, ed. *Antizol (R) (Fomepizole) Injection [Product Information].* Palo Alto, CA: Author; 2007.

114. Boluyt N, Bollen CW, Bos AP, Kok JH, Offringa M. Fluid resuscitation in neonatal and pediatric hypovolemic shock: a Dutch Pediatric evidence-based clinical practice guideline. *Intens Care Med.* 2006;32:995-1003.

115. Greenberg M. Ultrarapid opioid detoxification of two children with congenital heart disease. *J Addict Dis.* 2000;19:53-58.

116. Fischer G. Treatment of opioid dependence in pregnant women. *Addiction.* 2000;95:1141-1144.

117. Johnson K, Gerada C, Greenough A. Treatment of neonatal abstinence syndrome. *Arch Dis Child Fetal Neonatal Ed.* 2003;88:F2-F5.

118. Johnson RE, Jones HE, Jasinski DR, et al. Buprenorphine treatment of pregnant opioid—dependent women: maternal and neonatal outcomes. *Drug Alcohol Depend.* 2001;63:97-103.

119. Kahila H, Kivitie-Kallio S, Halmesmaki E, Valanne L, Autti T. Brain magnetic resonance imaging of infants exposed prenatally to buprenorphine. *Acta Radiol.* 2007;48:228-231.

120. Jones HE, Johnson RE, Jasinski DR, et al. Buprenorphine versus methadone in the treatment of pregnant opioid-dependent patients: effects on the neonatal abstinence syndrome. *Drug Alcohol Depend.* 2005;79:1-10.

121. Jones HE, Johnson RE, Jasinski DR, et al. Buprenorphine versus methadone in the treatment of pregnant opioid-dependent patients: effects on the neonatal abstinence syndrome. *Drug Alcohol Depend.* 2005;79:1-10.

122. Jones HE, Suess P, Jasinski DR, Johnson RE. Transferring methadone-stabilized pregnant patients to buprenorphine using an immediate release morphine transition: an open-label exploratory study. *Am J Addict.* 2006;15:61-70.

INDEX

Page numbers followed by *t* indicate tables; page numbers followed by *f* indicate figures.